Update on the Management of Non-Obstructive Azoospermia: Current Evidence and Unmet Needs

Update on the Management of Non-Obstructive Azoospermia: Current Evidence and Unmet Needs

Editors

Giovanni M. Colpi
Ettore Caroppo

MDPI • Basel • Beijing • Wuhan • Barcelona • Belgrade • Manchester • Tokyo • Cluj • Tianjin

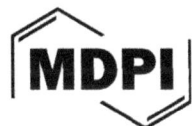

Editors
Giovanni M. Colpi
Scientific Director and Head of
Andrology Service, ProCrea
Swiss Fertility Center
Switzerland

Ettore Caroppo
Reproductive and IVF Unit,
Andrology Outpatients Clinic,
Asl Bari, PTA "F Jaia",
Conversano (Ba)
Italy

Editorial Office
MDPI
St. Alban-Anlage 66
4052 Basel, Switzerland

This is a reprint of articles from the Special Issue published online in the open access journal *Journal of Clinical Medicine* (ISSN 2077-0383) (available at: https://www.mdpi.com/journal/jcm/special_issues/NOA_Management).

For citation purposes, cite each article independently as indicated on the article page online and as indicated below:

LastName, A.A.; LastName, B.B.; LastName, C.C. Article Title. *Journal Name* **Year**, *Volume Number*, Page Range.

ISBN 978-3-0365-3433-6 (Hbk)
ISBN 978-3-0365-3434-3 (PDF)

© 2022 by the authors. Articles in this book are Open Access and distributed under the Creative Commons Attribution (CC BY) license, which allows users to download, copy and build upon published articles, as long as the author and publisher are properly credited, which ensures maximum dissemination and a wider impact of our publications.

The book as a whole is distributed by MDPI under the terms and conditions of the Creative Commons license CC BY-NC-ND.

Contents

About the Editors . . . . **vii**

Ettore Caroppo and Giovanni M. Colpi
Update on the Management of Non-Obstructive Azoospermia: Current Evidence and Unmet Needs
Reprinted from: *J. Clin. Med.* **2022**, *11*, 62, doi:10.3390/jcm11010062 . . . . **1**

Danilo L. Andrade, Marina C. Viana and Sandro C. Esteves
Differential Diagnosis of Azoospermia in Men with Infertility
Reprinted from: *J. Clin. Med.* **2021**, *10*, 3144, doi:10.3390/jcm10143144 . . . . **5**

Csilla Krausz and Francesca Cioppi
Genetic Factors of Non-Obstructive Azoospermia: Consequences on Patients' and Offspring Health
Reprinted from: *J. Clin. Med.* **2021**, *10*, 4009, doi:10.3390/jcm10174009 . . . . **25**

Ettore Caroppo and Giovanni Maria Colpi
Prediction Models for Successful Sperm Retrieval in Patients with Non-Obstructive Azoospermia Undergoing Microdissection Testicular Sperm Extraction: Is There Any Room for Further Studies?
Reprinted from: *J. Clin. Med.* **2021**, *10*, 5538, doi:10.3390/jcm10235538 . . . . **43**

Ettore Caroppo and Giovanni M. Colpi
Hormonal Treatment of Men with Nonobstructive Azoospermia: What Does the Evidence Suggest?
Reprinted from: *J. Clin. Med.* **2021**, *10*, 387, doi:10.3390/jcm10030387 . . . . **53**

Nahid Punjani, Caroline Kang and Peter N. Schlegel
Two Decades from the Introduction of Microdissection Testicular Sperm Extraction: How This Surgical Technique Has Improved the Management of NOA
Reprinted from: *J. Clin. Med.* **2021**, *10*, 1374, doi:10.3390/jcm10071374 . . . . **67**

Caroline Kang, Nahid Punjani and Peter N. Schlegel
Reproductive Chances of Men with Azoospermia Due to Spermatogenic Dysfunction
Reprinted from: *J. Clin. Med.* **2021**, *10*, 1400, doi:10.3390/jcm10071400 . . . . **77**

Giovanni M. Colpi and Ettore Caroppo
Performing Microdissection Testicular Sperm Extraction: Surgical Pearls from a High-Volume Infertility Center
Reprinted from: *J. Clin. Med.* **2021**, *10*, 4296, doi:10.3390/jcm10194296 . . . . **95**

Kaan Aydos and Oya Sena Aydos
Sperm Selection Procedures for Optimizing the Outcome of ICSI in Patients with NOA
Reprinted from: *J. Clin. Med.* **2021**, *10*, 2687, doi:10.3390/jcm10122687 . . . . **109**

Gary D. Smith, Clementina Cantatore and Dana A. Ohl
Microfluidic Systems for Isolation of Spermatozoa from Testicular Specimens of Non-Obstructive Azoospermic Men: Does/Can It Improve Sperm Yield?
Reprinted from: *J. Clin. Med.* **2021**, *10*, 3667, doi:10.3390/jcm10163667 . . . . **141**

Evangelia Billa, George A. Kanakis and Dimitrios G. Goulis
Endocrine Follow-Up of Men with Non-Obstructive Azoospermia Following Testicular Sperm Extraction
Reprinted from: *J. Clin. Med.* **2021**, *10*, 3323, doi:10.3390/jcm10153323 . . . . **151**

About the Editors

Giovanni M. Colpi is a specialist in Urology, Andrology and Endocrinology. He is the Scientific Director and Head of the Andrology Unit, Next Fertility ProCrea, Lugano, and Academician of the European Academy of Andrology. He was formerly the Head of AndroUrology and IVF Unit, San Paolo Hospital, University of Milan, Adjunct Professor in Andrology, Universities of Milan, Pavia, and L'Aquila. Member of the Committee for the Guidelines on OligoAsthenoTeratozoospermia of the European Academy of Andrology. He was also a former Member of the Health Care Office for Guidelines on Male Infertility of the European Association of Urology (2000–2008). He is a member of the Editorial Board of Andrologia and the International Journal of Fertility and Sterility. He is also the author of many articles in peer-reviewed international journals

Ettore Caroppo MD, is a specialist in Endocrinology and the course of Andrology. He has served as the Chief Clinical Andrologist at a Reproductive and IVF Unit since 1998. Since 2011 he has been a member of the Editorial Board of Fertility and Sterility, and since January 2022 he has been an Associate Editor of Human Reproduction. He has authored many articles in peer-reviewed international journals, in addition to book chapters of international manuals on male infertility.

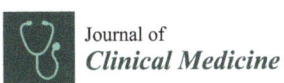

Editorial

Update on the Management of Non-Obstructive Azoospermia: Current Evidence and Unmet Needs

Ettore Caroppo [1,*] and Giovanni M. Colpi [2]

1. Andrology Outpatients Clinic, Asl Bari, PTA "F Jaia", Conversano, 70014 Bari, Italy
2. Andrology Unit, Procrea Institute, 6900 Lugano, Switzerland; gmcolpi@yahoo.com
* Correspondence: ecaroppo@teseo.it

Citation: Caroppo, E.; Colpi, G.M. Update on the Management of Non-Obstructive Azoospermia: Current Evidence and Unmet Needs. *J. Clin. Med.* **2022**, *11*, 62. https://doi.org/10.3390/jcm11010062

Received: 10 December 2021
Accepted: 21 December 2021
Published: 23 December 2021

Publisher's Note: MDPI stays neutral with regard to jurisdictional claims in published maps and institutional affiliations.

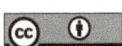

Copyright: © 2021 by the authors. Licensee MDPI, Basel, Switzerland. This article is an open access article distributed under the terms and conditions of the Creative Commons Attribution (CC BY) license (https://creativecommons.org/licenses/by/4.0/).

Azoospermia, defined as the absence of sperm in the ejaculate after examination of the centrifuged specimens, affects about 1% of the male population and 10–15% of infertile men. In about two-thirds of cases, this is caused by severe spermatogenic dysfunction [1], and it is commonly termed "nonobstructive azoospermia" (NOA) to differentiate it from the less severe form of azoospermia caused by the obstruction of the seminal tract (obstructive azoospermia—OA); the latter affects the remaining one-third of cases. Managing patients with NOA is challenging due to the severity of spermatogenic dysfunction and the lack of medical treatments, with surgical retrieval of testicular sperm being the only way of enabling some of these patients to father their own biological children. In-depth clinical knowledge is key for supporting clinical reasoning and decision making when counselling patients with NOA, and surgical skill is required to maximize the outcome of surgical procedures that aim to retrieve testicular sperm. Therefore, the present Special Issue was designed to provide young reproductive urologists and endocrinologists with an update of the scientific evidence in the field, together with surgical tips.

The differential diagnosis between OA and NOA is mandatory for the correct management of patients; men with OA have intact spermatogenesis, so that sperm may be surgically retrieved in the vast majority of cases by means of minimally invasive techniques [2]. Sperm retrieval is successful in no more than 58% of men with NOA, provided that the most effective surgical technique, namely, microdissection testicular sperm extraction (mTESE), is used [3]. In the first article of the present Special Issue, Danilo L. Andrade, Marina C. Viana and Sandro C. Esteves showed that the differential diagnosis between OA and NOA may be effectively accomplished in most patients by means of a standardized male infertility workup, which should include a detailed medical history, a careful physical examination with a focus on secondary sexual characteristics, a semen analysis obtained on at least two occasions and assessed according to the World Health Organization, hormonal evaluation (serum FSH, LH, prolactin and testosterone levels), genetic tests (karyotype and Y chromosome microdeletion analysis, screening for cystic fibrosis transmembrane conductance regulator gene mutations), and a scrotal and transrectal ultrasound, with testis biopsy being reserved only for the cases of doubt [4].

Genetic tests are useful for diagnostic and prognostic purposes in men with NOA. Csilla Krausz and Francesca Cioppi reviewed the most common genetic abnormalities found in men with NOA and illustrated their possible consequences on their general and reproductive health, as well as on their children's health. They also dedicated a chapter to the conflicting evidence regarding health issues in offspring conceived by ICSI with testicular sperm retrieved in patients with NOA, and highlighted the potential diagnostic utility of performing whole-exome sequencing in men with NOA due to meiotic arrest [5].

Management of men with NOA would undoubtedly benefit from the identification of clinical and laboratory markers of spermatogenesis able to individuate those patients really suited for mTESE. The evidence from the literature in this field, reviewed by our group for this Special Issue [6], clearly shows that, although few factors, including complete AZFc deletion or history of cryptorchidism, were associated with better chances of successful sperm retrieval (SSR), no clinical or laboratory marker is able to predict the outcome of mTESE, due to the anatomic singularity of the testes of men with NOA, which may hide few loci of spermatogenesis. Moreover, the great impact of the surgeon's skill and experience, together with the time and efforts dedicated to the search for sperm in the testicular specimens, may have an impact on mTESE outcome. Promising results arising from studies investigating the predictive ability of molecular markers expressed in the seminal plasma should be confirmed by further studies.

Azoospermia due to spermatogenic dysfunction is an untreatable condition, apart from the rare cases of patients with hypogonadotropic hypogonadism. Nonetheless, a role for the hormonal stimulation of spermatogenesis to improve sperm retrieval rates in these patients was proposed by some authors. As summarized in our review paper, while the optimization of serum testosterone level seems to be justifiable in men with hypogonadism, the available evidence is insufficient for recommending hormonal treatment before surgery in men with NOA [7].

The introduction of mTESE in 1999 greatly improved the chance of retrieving testicular sperm in patients with NOA, by enabling the identification of foci of spermatogenesis at high magnification even in patients with nearly atrophic testes. In the two review papers coauthored with Nahid Punjani and Caroline Kang, the pioneer of this surgical technique, Prof. Peter N. Schlegel, illustrates how to manage patients with NOA and optimize the success of mTESE [8], and sheds light on the reproductive chances of men with NOA according to the underlying etiologies (Klinefelter syndrome, Y chromosome microdeletions, chemotherapy-associated NOA, cryptorchidism) [9]. Both papers are a must read for reproductive urologists.

A learning curve is required to improve the outcome of mTESE. A detailed description of mTESE surgical procedures, accompanied by an extensive iconography, is provided by a review authored by our group, in view of the vast surgical experience in this field of our leading urologist [10].

The outcome of mTESE is greatly affected by the accuracy in testicular sperm processing techniques. Kaan Aydos and Oya Sena Aydos reviewed the available sperm selection procedures, as well as the different approaches to testicular sperm cryopreservation, providing valuable suggestions for embryologists and clinicians about how to effectively handle testicular specimens and testicular sperm to maximize the outcome of mTESE [11].

The laboratory techniques used for testicular sperm processing are highly labor-intensive and subject to inter-laboratory and intra-laboratory variability. In view of his pioneering studies in the field of microfluidic technology applied to gamete and embryo isolation and culture, Gary D. Smith, joined by Clementina Cantatore and Dana A. Ohl, analyzed the potential utility, benefits, and shortcomings of such a technology to the isolation of non-motile sperm from retrieved NOA testicular samples [12].

Testicular surgery is not devoid of complications. Testicular damage is often a complication of conventional testicular sperm extraction (cTESE), as well as of testicular aspiration, while mTESE may be a more conservative surgical strategy, since it enables the identification of subalbuginal vessels and possibly avoids residual bleeding inside the tunica albuginea, which often results in testicular tissue damage. Still, both cTESE and mTESE may result in transient or, less frequent, permanent hypogonadism due to Leydig cells dysfunction. Evangelia Billa, George A Kanakis and Dimitrios G Goulis reviewed this interesting topic, explaining how hypogonadism may depend upon the underlying histology, the number of previous testicular surgeries, the etiology of NOA, and the size of the testes; in some patients, e.g., those with Klinefelter syndrome, the decrease in testosterone levels may be more profound and of longer duration [13].

Author Contributions: E.C. drafted the manuscript; G.M.C. critically revised the manuscript. All authors have read and agreed to the published version of the manuscript.

Funding: This research received no external funding.

Conflicts of Interest: The authors declare no conflict of interest.

References

1. Esteves, S.C. Clinical management of infertile men with nonobstructive azoospermia. *Asian J. Androl.* **2015**, *17*, 459–470. [CrossRef] [PubMed]
2. Practice Committee of the American Society for Reproductive Medicine in Collaboration with the Society for Male Reproduction and Urology. The management of obstructive azoospermia: A committee opinion. *Fertil. Steril.* **2019**, *111*, 873–880. [CrossRef] [PubMed]
3. Bernie, A.M.; Mata, D.A.; Ramasamy, R.; Schlegel, P.N. Comparison of microdissection testicular sperm extraction, conventional testicular sperm extraction, and testicular sperm aspiration for nonobstructive azoospermia: A systematic review and meta-analysis. *Fertil. Steril.* **2015**, *104*, 1099–1103. [CrossRef] [PubMed]
4. Andrade, D.L.; Viana, M.C.; Esteves, S.C. Differential Diagnosis of Azoospermia in Men with Infertility. *J. Clin. Med.* **2021**, *10*, 3144. [CrossRef] [PubMed]
5. Krausz, C.; Cioppi, F. Genetic Factors of Non-Obstructive Azoospermia: Consequences on Patients' and Offspring Health. *J. Clin. Med.* **2021**, *10*, 4009. [CrossRef] [PubMed]
6. Caroppo, E.; Colpi, G.M. Prediction Models for Successful Sperm Retrieval in Patients with Non-Obstructive Azoospermia Undergoing Microdissection Testicular Sperm Extraction: Is There Any Room for Further Studies? *J. Clin. Med.* **2021**, *10*, 5538. [CrossRef] [PubMed]
7. Caroppo, E.; Colpi, G.M. Hormonal treatment of men with non-obstructive azoospermia: What does the evidence suggest? *J. Clin. Med.* **2021**, *10*, 387. [CrossRef] [PubMed]
8. Punjani, N.; Kang, C.; Schlegel, P.N. Two decades from the introduction of microdissection testicular sperm extraction: How this surgical technique has improved the management of NOA. *J. Clin. Med.* **2021**, *10*, 1374. [CrossRef] [PubMed]
9. Kang, C.; Punjani, N.; Schlegel, P.N. Reproductive chances of men with azoospermia due to spermatogenic dysfunction. *J. Clin. Med.* **2021**, *10*, 1400. [CrossRef] [PubMed]
10. Colpi, G.M.; Caroppo, E. Performing microdissection testicular sperm extraction: Surgical pearls from a high-volume infertility center. *J. Clin. Med.* **2021**, *10*, 4296. [CrossRef] [PubMed]
11. Aydos, K.; Aydos, O.S. Sperm selection procedures for optimizing the outcome of ICSI in patients with NOA. *J. Clin. Med.* **2021**, *10*, 2687. [CrossRef] [PubMed]
12. Smith, G.D.; Cantatore, C.; Ohl, D.A. Microfluidics systems for isolation of spermatozoa from testicular specimens of non-obstructive azoospermic men: Does/can it improve sperm yield? *J. Clin. Med.* **2021**, *10*, 3667. [CrossRef] [PubMed]
13. Billia, E.; Kanakis, G.A.; Goulis, D.G. Endocrine follow-up of men with non-obstructive azoospermia following testicular sperm extraction. *J. Clin. Med.* **2021**, *10*, 3323. [CrossRef] [PubMed]

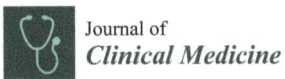

Review
Differential Diagnosis of Azoospermia in Men with Infertility

Danilo L. Andrade [1], Marina C. Viana [2] and Sandro C. Esteves [3,4,*]

[1] Department of Medical Physiopathology (Postgraduate Program), State University of Campinas (UNICAMP), Campinas 13083-887, SP, Brazil; danilo_landrade@hotmail.com
[2] Department of Surgery (Residency Program), Division of Urology, State University of Campinas (UNICAMP), Campinas 13083-887, SP, Brazil; marinacorreaviana@gmail.com
[3] ANDROFERT, Andrology & Human Reproduction Clinic, Campinas 13075-460, SP, Brazil
[4] Department of Surgery, Division of Urology, State University of Campinas (UNICAMP), Campinas 13083-887, SP, Brazil
* Correspondence: s.esteves@androfert.com.br

Abstract: The differential diagnosis between obstructive and nonobstructive azoospermia is the first step in the clinical management of azoospermic patients with infertility. It includes a detailed medical history and physical examination, semen analysis, hormonal assessment, genetic tests, and imaging studies. A testicular biopsy is reserved for the cases of doubt, mainly in patients whose history, physical examination, and endocrine analysis are inconclusive. The latter should be combined with sperm extraction for possible sperm cryopreservation. We present a detailed analysis on how to make the azoospermia differential diagnosis and discuss three clinical cases where the differential diagnosis was challenging. A coordinated effort involving reproductive urologists/andrologists, geneticists, pathologists, and embryologists will offer the best diagnostic path for men with azoospermia.

Keywords: azoospermia; diagnosis; male infertility; nonobstructive azoospermia; spermatogenic failure; testis biopsy; sperm retrieval; genetic testing; endocrine evaluation; review

1. Introduction

Azoospermia (a-, without + –zoo– » Greek zôion, animal + –spermia– » Greek sperma, sperm/seed) is defined by the absence of sperm in the ejaculate. Although the term does not imply an underlying etiology, azoospermia inevitably provokes infertility [1]. According to global estimates, 1 out of 100 men at reproductive age and up to 10% of men with infertility are azoospermic [2–4].

Azoospermia is broadly classified into obstructive and nonobstructive. This differentiation is clinically meaningful because it affects patient management and treatment outcomes [4]. Notably, nonobstructive azoospermia (NOA) relates to an intrinsic testicular defect caused by various conditions that ultimately affect sperm production profoundly.

The severe spermatogenic deficiency observed in NOA patients is often a consequence of primary testicular failure affecting mainly spermatogenic cells (spermatogenic failure (STF)) or related to a dysfunction of the hypothalamus-pituitary-gonadal axis (hypogonadotropic hypogonadism (HH)). From this point on, the acronyms STF and HH will distinguish these types of NOA, as appropriate [5]. The above-proposed terminology might be more intuitive for the clinician. It not only indicates the site of the problem (central or local) explicitly, but also makes it clear that the testicular disorder refers primarily to a spermatogenic defect, unlike the indistinct term 'testicular failure' that may relate to an isolated spermatogenic defect or such a defect combined with Leydig cell failure.

The differential diagnosis between STF and HH is also essential because the former is linked with severe and untreatable conditions, whereas the latter can be effectively treated with gonadotropin therapy [5,6]. By contrast, obstructive azoospermia (OA) originates from a mechanical block along the reproductive tract, namely, vas deferens, epididymis, or ejac-

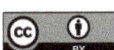

Citation: Andrade, D.L.; Viana, M.C.; Esteves, S.C. Differential Diagnosis of Azoospermia in Men with Infertility. *J. Clin. Med.* **2021**, *10*, 3144. https://doi.org/10.3390/jcm10143144

Academic Editors: Ettore Caroppo, Giovanni M. Colpi and Kent Doi

Received: 3 June 2021
Accepted: 13 July 2021
Published: 16 July 2021

Publisher's Note: MDPI stays neutral with regard to jurisdictional claims in published maps and institutional affiliations.

Copyright: © 2021 by the authors. Licensee MDPI, Basel, Switzerland. This article is an open access article distributed under the terms and conditions of the Creative Commons Attribution (CC BY) license (https://creativecommons.org/licenses/by/4.0/).

ulatory duct [7,8]. Unlike NOA, spermatogenesis is preserved, and both reconstructive procedures and sperm retrieval are typically highly successful in OA patients [7–10].

Nonobstructive azoospermia can be distinguished from OA using history, physical examination, semen analysis, hormonal assessment, and genetic testing in most patients [4,5,11]. However, in some instances, this distinction is not straightforward, and a testis biopsy is required. In this article, we first provide readers an overview of the azoospermia differential diagnosis. Secondly, we discuss the differential diagnosis in cases of doubt, including a workable clinical algorithm. Lastly, we present exemplary clinical cases to illustrate a difficult diagnosis and its outcomes.

2. Azoospermia Differential Diagnosis: An Overview

The primary goals of the differential diagnosis are the identification of:

- Potentially correctable forms of azoospermia (e.g., by surgery or medication).
- Irreversible types of azoospermia suitable for sperm retrieval and intracytoplasmic sperm injection (ICSI), using own sperm.
- Types of azoospermia in which donor insemination or adoption are the only possibilities.
- Health-threatening illness associated with azoospermia requiring medical attention.
- Genetic causes of azoospermia that may affect the patient or offspring's health, mainly if assisted reproductive technology is used.

It is critical to evaluate the azoospermic patient using a standardized workup to achieve these goals, as discussed in the next sections.

2.1. Medical History

A thorough medical history is pivotal to help determine the type of azoospermia. It must cover eight critical elements (Table 1), which are:

1. Infertility history
2. Sexual history
3. Childhood and development history
4. Personal medical history
5. Previous surgery/treatments
6. Gonadotoxic exposure
7. Family history
8. Current health status and lifestyle

The history may reveal the presence of congenital abnormalities, such as cryptorchidism, which could result in NOA-STF. Testicular infections (e.g., mumps orchitis), testicular trauma, testicular torsion, gonadotoxin exposure (e.g., radiotherapy/chemotherapy, anabolic steroid use, testosterone replacement therapy), or a history of brain surgery are informative to help establish a possible etiologic factor for NOA [5]. Hypogonadotropic hypogonadism is caused by congenital (e.g., Kallmann syndrome) or acquired conditions (e.g., prolactinomas, pituitary surgery, or testosterone replacement therapy) [6,12,13]. Notably, testosterone injections—commonly prescribed nowadays to men at reproductive age with signs of hypogonadism—suppress the hypothalamic-pituitary-gonadal axis. Consequently, intratesticular testosterone levels—critical for normal spermatogenesis—remain very low and, therefore, unable to sustain spermatogenesis [14].

On the other hand, a history of hernia repair, scrotal surgery, pelvic surgery, endoscopic urethral instrumentation, or genitourinary infection (e.g., epididymitis) may cause OA. Along these lines, a previous vasectomy is a typical OA etiology [8]. However, in many cases, the etiology cannot be determined, and additional tests are required, as explained in the following sections.

Table 1. Medical history outline. Adapted from Esteves et al. [11], Clinics 66, 691–700, 2011.

Elements	Components
(1) Infertility History	• Age of partners, length of time the couple has been attempting to conceive • Contraceptive methods/duration • Previous pregnancy/miscarriage (current partner/partner/another partner) • Previous treatments • Treatments/evaluations of female partner
(2) Sexual History	• Potency, libido, lubricant use • Ejaculation, timed intercourse, frequency of masturbation
(3) Childhood and Development	• Cryptorchidism, hernia, testicular trauma, testicular torsion, infection (e.g., mumps) • Sexual development, puberty onset
(4) Personal History	• Systemic diseases (e.g., diabetes, cirrhosis, hypertension) • Sexually transmitted diseases, tuberculosis, viral infections, genital and systemic bacterial infections, history of fever
(5) Previous Surgery/Treatment	• Orchidopexy, herniorrhaphy, orchiectomy (e.g., testicular cancer, torsion) • Retroperitoneal and pelvic surgery • Other inguinal, scrotal, or perineal surgery • Bariatric surgery, bladder neck surgery, transurethral resection of the prostate
(6) Gonadotoxin Exposure	• Pesticides, alcohol, cocaine, marijuana • Medication (e.g., chemotherapy agents, cimetidine, sulfasalazine, nitrofurantoin, allopurinol, colchicine, thiazide, α- and β-blockers, calcium blockers, finasteride) • Organic solvents, heavy metals • Anabolic steroids, tobacco use • High temperatures, electromagnetic energy • Radiation (e.g., therapeutic, nuclear power plant workers)
(7) Family History	• Cystic fibrosis, endocrine diseases • Infertility
(8) Current Health Status/Lifestyle	• Respiratory infection, anosmia • Galactorrhea, visual disturbances • Obesity, metabolic syndrome

2.2. Physical Examination

The physical exam is critical in the assessment of men presenting with azoospermia. It starts with the appraisal of the overall body characteristics, with a focus on secondary sexual characteristics. Abnormal body hair distribution and gynecomastia may be indicative of hypogonadism or hormonal disturbances [5,11]. Examination of inguinal and genital areas may unveil scars from previous surgeries that could have injured testicular blood supply and the vas deferens. Other physical defects, such as abnormalities of the penis (e.g., hypospadias, epispadias, short frenulum, phimosis, fibrotic nodules), should also be evaluated.

Testicular size, texture, and consistency should be assessed. In routine practice, testicular volume is estimated using the Prader's orchidometer. The mean testicular volume measured using the Prader's orchidometer in the general population is 20.0 ± 5.0 mL [15].

Testes of men with OA have a firm texture. About 85% of testicular parenchyma is implicated in spermatogenesis. By contrast, men with NOA usually have small testicles (<15 mL or ≤4.6 cm long axis) [16]. However, it should be noted that there is no threshold for testicular size to completely exclude the possibility of harvesting sperm on a retrieval attempt [17]. Moreover, both patients with OA and NOA-STF due to maturation arrest have normal-sized testicles [18]. Therefore, testicular size may not necessarily be informative for the differential diagnosis. Palpable abnormalities of the testis should be further evaluated with imaging studies because azoospermic men, particularly those with NOA-STF, have increased risks of developing testis malignancy [19].

The presence of the vas deferens and the epididymis' characteristics should always be determined. A normal and healthy epididymis is firm, whereas an obstructed epididymis is ingurgitated (soft) [11]. Patients with NOA typically have palpable vasa deferentia and flat epididymides [5].

The vas deferens is easily palpable inside the spermatic cord as a firm, round, "spaghetti-like" structure. The vas can be absent at both sides, indicating a congenital abnormality [5,11]. Congenital bilateral absence of vas deferens (CBAVD) is associated with OA, and approximately 10% of these men have concurrent unilateral renal agenesis and should undergo an ultrasound scan to uncover this potentially health-threatening condition. By contrast, most patients (~60%) with congenital unilateral absence of vas deferens (CUAVD) are non-azoospermic [20]. A gene mutation associated with cystic fibrosis causes bilateral vas agenesis; therefore, genetic screening is advisable for the affected couples planning assisted reproductive technology (ART) [11,12]. Mutations affecting the cystic fibrosis transmembrane conductance regulator (CFTR) gene have also been identified in about 10% of men with CUAVD and normal kidneys, and it has been suggested that these patients should undergo CFTR testing as recommended for CBAVD patients.

Assessment of the spermatic cord is mandatory as a varicocele may be found [5,11,21]. Varicocele is a prevalent congenital abnormality linked to infertility, impaired testicular growth, and hypogonadism [22–25]. Although varicocele is not uncommon in azoospermic men [24], it is debatable whether the vein dilation is coincident or contributory to spermatogenesis disruption in such patients [25]. Nonetheless, spermatogonia, spermatocytes, and spermatids are highly exposed to heat stress caused by varicocele. Furthermore, it was shown that varicocelectomy might ameliorate spermatogenesis and androgen production in azoospermic patients with spermatogenic failure [24–26].

The varicocele diagnosis is primarily made by a physical examination in a warm room with the patient standing. Palpable varicoceles are graded as (i) small (Grade 1): palpable during Valsalva maneuver, (ii) moderate size (Grade 2): palpable at rest, and (iii) large (Grade 3): visible and palpable at rest [22]. Scrotal Doppler ultrasound is indicated if a physical examination is inconclusive [11]. A maximum venous diameter of >3 mm in the upright position and during the Valsalva maneuver and venous reflux with a duration >2 s usually correlate with the presence of a palpable varicocele [27].

2.3. Semen Analysis

The term azoospermia essentially refers to a semen analysis result. The assessment of an azoospermic ejaculate with normal volume (i.e., >1.5 mL) should be followed by examining the pelleted semen after centrifugation to rule out cryptozoospermia, defined by the presence of rare sperm [5,28]. Centrifugation should be carried out at $3000\times g$ for 15 min or longer [29]. The finding of live sperm may allow ICSI to be carried out with ejaculated sperm, obviating surgical sperm harvesting. Azoospermia must be confirmed in at least two consecutive semen analyses because temporary azoospermia due to toxic, environmental, infectious, fever, or iatrogenic conditions can take place [30,31]. Assessment of azoospermic ejaculates on more than one occasion is also essential given the biological variability of the same individuals' specimens. However, a limit of semen analyses (e.g., 2–3) might be set from a practical standpoint, although the exact number is difficult to ascertain. An interval between analyses is also advisable (e.g., one month apart) [32], albeit the optimal interval between examinations has not been established.

The state-of-art on how human semen should be assessed in the laboratory is set out by the World Health Organization (WHO), which periodically issues manuals that include standard operating procedures and reference values [29,31]. The lower reference limits (5th centile) for semen characteristics according to the 2010 WHO manual are as follows: (i) Semen volume: 1.5 mL, (ii) Total sperm number: 39 million/mL, (iii) Sperm concentration: 15 million/mL, (iv) Total motility: 40%, (v) Progressive motility: 32%, (vi) Vitality: 58% alive, and (vii) Sperm morphology: 4% normal forms [29].

Ejaculates of men with NOA-STF usually exhibit normal volume and pH (>7.2), indicating functional seminal vesicles and patent ejaculatory ducts [5]. By contrast, hypospermia (ejaculate volume < 1.5 mL) is typical in patients with HH-NOA [5,6]. A combination of a low volume (<1.5 mL), acidic ejaculate (pH < 7.2), with low fructose (e.g., <13 µmol per ejaculate) indicates seminal vesicle hypoplasia or obstruction [11]. Both conditions are associated with OA; the former with CBAVD and the latter with ejaculatory duct obstruction [33,34]. Seminal neutral alpha-glucosidase levels can also be determined as they reflect the epididymal function [29]. It was reported that seminal α-glucosidase levels < 18 mU/ejaculate is a reliable indicator of congenital bilateral absence of the vas deferens [4].

2.4. Hormonal Evaluation

Assessment of reproductive hormones' serum levels may add relevant information to establish azoospermia type. Follicle-stimulating hormone (FSH) and testosterone are the essential hormones driving spermatogenesis [5,11]. Testosterone is produced by the Leydig cells under luteinizing hormone (LH) stimulation. Adequate levels of intratesticular testosterone are critical for sperm maturation [35]. By contrast, FSH is mainly responsible for increasing sperm production, and it collaborates with intratesticular testosterone to promote cell proliferation [36].

In general, there is an inverse relationship between FSH levels and spermatogonia quantity [37,38]. When spermatogonia number is absent or remarkably reduced, FSH levels increase; when spermatogonia number is normal, FSH levels are within normal ranges. FSH levels also relate to the proportion of seminiferous tubules exhibiting Sertoli cell-only on testicular biopsies [39]. Nevertheless, for patients subjected to sperm retrieval, FSH levels do not precisely predict whether spermatogenesis is present [40]. It is, therefore, possible to find focal sperm-producing areas in the testes of men with NOA-STF and elevated FSH levels during testicular sperm extraction [5,40–43].

Low FSH levels (e.g., <1.5 mIU/mL), combined with low LH (e.g., <1.5 mIU/mL), and low testosterone levels (e.g., <300 ng/dL) indicate primary or secondary HH [5,11]. In such cases, azoospermia is the result of an absence of testicular stimulation by pituitary gonadotropins. Pharmacotherapy using exogenous gonadotropins is highly effective in inducing sperm production in patients with congenital or acquired HH forms, with reported pregnancy rates of up to 65%, which are achieved naturally or with medically assisted reproduction [6,44].

Typically, patients with NOA-STF present with elevated FSH (>7.6 mIU/mL) and low testosterone (<300 ng/dL) levels, whereas those with OA show normal FSH and testosterone levels. Other hormones can also be assessed, including inhibin B, prolactin, estradiol, 17-hydroxyprogesterone, and sex hormone-binding globulin (SHBG) [11]. In particular, prolactin levels should be measured in patients with HH because prolactinoma may be the causative factor [11]. Inhibin-B levels reflect Sertoli cell integrity and spermatogenesis status [45]. However, its diagnostic value seems to be no better than that of FSH, and its use in clinical practice for azoospermia differentiation or sperm retrieval success prediction has not been broadly advocated [30,40].

2.5. Genetic Analysis

Azoospermia may have a genetic origin. The frequency of numerical autosomal and sex chromosome abnormalities, single-gene mutations, and partial or complete microdeletions of the Y-chromosome is increased in azoospermic patients [12,46]. Indeed, the incidence of genetic abnormalities increases as the sperm output decreases [47,48]. For instance, approximately 15% of men with NOA present with chromosomal anomalies, in contrast to ~5% of those with sperm concentration between 1 and 10 million/mL and <1% of men with >19 million/mL [49].

As a general rule, azoospermic men should undergo karyotype and Y chromosome microdeletion studies [5]. Exceptions apply to conditions in which azoospermia has an evident obstructive origin (e.g., vasectomy, ejaculatory duct obstruction) or a non-genetic-related etiology (e.g., post-chemotherapy/radiotherapy, post-orchitis). Karyotype and Y chromosome microdeletion tests are broadly available and are based on the screening of genomic deoxyribonucleic acid (DNA) taken mainly from peripheral blood samples.

The most common abnormal karyotypic finding in azoospermic men is Klinefelter syndrome (KS), detected in ~10% of cases [12]. Azoospermia in KS men is associated with reduced testicular growth, pre-pubertal degeneration of primordial germ cells, or spermatogenic maturation arrest. For this reason, all azoospermic KS men have NOA-STF. Two karyotypic patterns are typically noticed: non-mosaic (47,XXY; ~85% of cases) and mosaic (47,XXY/46,X; ~15% of cases) [12]. Residual foci of active spermatogenesis is found on microdissection testicular sperm extraction (micro-TESE) in about 30–50% of KS men [12,40,50]. The retrieved sperm may be used for ICSI and generate a healthy child [28,40]. However, KS patients seem to be at an increased risk of having aneuploid gametes, which might increase the chance of producing offspring with a chromosomal abnormality [48]. Although the finding of an extra X chromosome is confirmatory, KS is suspected during the initial workup stages. These patients classically present with extremely small (1–8 mL) testes, gynecomastia (~40% of cases), and hypogonadism (e.g., scanty facial and pubic hair, poor libido, and erectile dysfunction) [5,11,12]. Reduced testosterone levels are commonly noticed (~80% of cases) and are attributed to decreased Leydig cell population due to the small testicular size.

Microdeletions in the long arm of the Y chromosome are the second most common genetic cause of azoospermia [12]. This region aggregates 26 genes involved in spermatogenesis regulation, located in an interval named "AZF" (azoospermia factor); microdeletions at this interval are usually associated with azoospermia [38]. The AZF interval has three subregions, named AZFa, AZFb, and AZFc, each enclosing vital genes for spermatogenesis control. Approximately 10% of men with NOA-STF have microdeletions within the AZF interval that justify their condition [12,51].

The Y chromosome microdeletion study is based on a multiplex polymerase chain reaction (PCR), which amplifies Y chromosome sequences using specific sequence-tagged site primers [51]. Y-chromosome microdeletion testing allows detecting almost all clinically significant deletions. Hence, it helps identify the male infertility etiology, but it also provides information about treatment prognosis. Sperm retrieval success is determined by the type of Y microdeletion detected. Among men with AZFc deletions, sperm may be occasionally found in the ejaculate, or through testicular sperm extraction in at least 50% of individuals [5,51]. By contrast, patients with complete AZFa and/or AZFb microdeletions are not eligible for surgical sperm retrieval because large deletions involving these subregions are virtually incompatible with any residual spermatogenesis [5].

Notwithstanding the observations above, case reports showed sperm in the ejaculate of men with partial AZFb deletions [52,53]. While the AZFa region is relatively small and contains only two single-copy genes (*USP9Y* and *DDX3Y*), the AZFb and AZFc regions span over several megabase pairs and contain multiple relevant genes [51]. Notably, deletions usually remove more than one gene, but testing as currently performed only determines the presence or absence of a set of primers rather than gene-specific deletions.

Azoospermic patients with AZFc microdeletions in whom testicular sperm are successfully retrieved can father a child through ICSI [5,40,54]. The probability of biological parenthood by ICSI appears to be not affected by the microdeletion. However, the male offspring of such fathers will inherit the genetic defect and, consequently, be infertile [54]. Genetic counseling is, therefore, recommended before sperm retrieval. Preimplantation genetic testing may be proposed for embryo sex selection to couples undergoing ICSI with testicular sperm retrieved from patients with AZFc microdeletions to avoid transmitting this form of infertility to the offspring.

Cystic fibrosis transmembrane conductance regulator gene mutations usually result in CBAVD and, consequently, the affected patients have OA [12,55]. Over 2000 mutations have been discovered in the CFTR gene [56]. About eight out of ten patients with CBAVD harbor two CFTR mutations, usually in compound heterozygosity [57]. CFTR mutations were also implicated in bilateral epididymal obstruction in patients with palpable vasa. According to the 2020 European Association of Urology (EAU) guidelines on sexual and reproductive health, testing for CFTR gene mutations should be recommended for men with infertility and anatomical abnormalities of the vas deferens (unilateral or bilateral vas agenesis) when associated with normal kidneys [30]. In such cases, testing should be carried out in both partners of an infertile couple and has to include common point mutations (e.g., deltaF508, R117H, W1282X) and the 5T allele.

Screening for CFTR mutations is carried out in clinical molecular genetics laboratories. Methods for CFTR testing typically apply semiquantitative PCR analysis (e.g., multiplex ligation-dependent probe amplification) or quantitative fluorescent multiplex PCR [57]. The test report should be interpreted with prudence as not all mutations are implicated in disease. However, findings of mutations with clinical relevance confirm a genetic cause of OA [12]. In such patients, spermatogenesis is preserved, and therefore, sperm are easily retrieved from the testis or epididymis [8,33]. The retrieved sperm have to be used for ICSI, which results in adequate success rates [8,33]. The female partners should be screened for clinically relevant CFTR mutations. If the partner carries a CFTR mutation, the couple has up to a 50% risk of having a child with cystic fibrosis or CBAVD, depending on the parents' type of mutation [11,30]. Preimplantation genetic testing may be offered for embryo sex selection or to identify non-affected embryos.

Given the solid genetic background of NOA, additional genetic analysis beyond karyotyping and screening for Y-chromosome microdeletions has been investigated. Gene panels using whole-exome sequencing have been proposed as a way to detect genetic variants possibly explaining NOA [56,58]. At present, however, these advanced genetic assessments are not entirely validated and therefore not yet suitable for inclusion in the routine investigation.

2.6. Imaging Studies

Imaging studies may add information to help determine the type and cause of azoospermia.

Scrotal ultrasound (US) is useful to detect signs of testicular dysgenesis (e.g., microlithiasis, heterogeneous testis architecture) which are often related to NOA-STF [5]. As a general rule, men with suspected NOA-STF should undergo scrotal ultrasonography because these patients have an increased chance of testicular cancer [30]. A scrotal scan may also help to determine testis volume, epididymis characteristics, and presence of a varicocele if a physical examination is inconclusive (e.g., large hydrocele, inguinal testis, obesity) [11,21]. Additionally, indirect signs of obstruction might be seen during a scrotal US examination, including a dilated rete testis, enlarged epididymis, or absent/partially absent epididymis in patients with CBAVD [59]. Scrotal color Doppler US findings obtained from healthy fertile men provide reference ranges for clinicians [59,60]. For example, the lowest reference limit for testes volume (measured according to the ellipsoid formula) was about 12 mL, and thresholds for epididymis heal, tail, and vas deferens were 12, 6, and 4.5 mm [59].

Transrectal ultrasound (TRUS) is indicated in azoospermic patients with hypospermia (ejaculate volume < 1.5 mL) and seminal acidic pH if an obstruction is suspected [34]. Using TRUS, seminal vesicle abnormalities and prostatic cysts may be detected [34,59]. These lesions can obstruct the ejaculatory ducts and result in azoospermia [61]. Moreover, the presence of seminal vesical cysts should alert the clinician for possible concomitant genitourinary anomalies, including renal agenesis, dysgenesis, and autosomal dominant polycystic kidney disease [62,63]. Treatment to relieve the obstruction can be offered for these patients [8]. Besides, TRUS can help confirm CBAVD as the seminal vesicles of these patients are either absent or hypoplasic [11,28].

Magnetic resonance may also be used, and it is helpful to assess the distal parts of the seminal tract, the presence of prolactinomas, and an intra-abdominal location of an undescended testis [11]. Lastly, renal imaging studies should be performed in men with anatomical vas deferens abnormalities and no evidence of CFTR mutations. The unilateral absence of the vas deferens is usually associated with an ipsilateral absence of the kidney. Moreover, renal abnormalities (e.g., pelvic kidney) may be found in patients with bilateral absence of vas deferens without CFTR mutations [64].

3. Differential Diagnosis in Cases of Doubt: Testis Biopsy

Testis biopsy findings ultimately determine the type of azoospermia. However, from a practical standpoint, the differentiation is made in over 90% of cases using a detailed medical history, physical examination, semen analysis, hormonal assessment, and genetic and imaging studies [5,11,16]. Nevertheless, there are cases of doubt in which the differential diagnosis between OA and NOA remains undetermined unless a testis biopsy followed by histopathological analysis is carried out.

Congenital intratesticular obstruction and congenital epididymal obstruction—unrelated to anatomic vas deferens abnormalities—cause OA, and these conditions are not easily recognizable [65]. Equally challenging to recognize is the functional obstruction of the distal parts of ejaculatory ducts [34,66]. Additionally, patients with idiopathic NOA might have normal FSH levels and normal testicular size (e.g., maturation arrest) because FSH levels correlate primarily with the number of spermatogonia [18,37]. A prediction model for testis histology in men with NOA showed that FSH levels could not correctly identify patients with maturation arrest [67].

A diagnostic testicular biopsy is the gold-standard method to discriminate OA from NOA in men with normal FSH, normal testicular size, and no apparent obstruction signs found in history, physical examination, semen analysis, and imaging studies. The biopsy should be ideally made using an open approach [30]. However, our experience with percutaneous biopsies—using a large needle (18 G) and a Cameco syringe holder—has been reassuring in the clinical scenario described above, as confirmed by the adequate amount of tissue extracted and the number of seminiferous tubules' cross-sections examined. The extracted specimen is placed in a fixative solution, like Bouin's, Zenker's, or glutaraldehyde. Notably, formalin should not be used as a fixative because it disrupts tissue architecture.

Histopathology results will inform if spermatogenesis impairment exists. Histopathology findings include (i) absent germ cells in seminiferous tubules (Sertoli cell-only), (ii) spermatogenic maturation arrest (incomplete spermatogenesis), (iii) presence of all spermatogenic stages, including spermatozoa, but with an evident impairment in germ cell number (hypospermatogenesis), (iv) tubular hyalinization, and (v) normal spermatogenesis [68,69]. Sertoli cell-only, maturation arrest, hypospermatogenesis, and tubular hyalinization are indicative of NOA. These patterns come alone or in combination (mixed pattern). By contrast, normal spermatogenesis is indicative of OA.

Furthermore, intratubular germ cell neoplasia in situ (GCNIS) might be revealed in biopsy specimens taken from men with NOA-STF, mainly those with a history of cryptorchidism and/or multiple foci of testicular microlithiasis [30,70,71]. In general, GCNIS precedes the development of seminomas and non-seminoma tumors, and the risk of testicular cancer is increased in men with NOA [72].

Notably, diagnostic biopsies might harm the testis; therefore, they should be limited to very selected cases. Its routine use as a diagnostic tool to establish the azoospermia type is not recommended by relevant guidelines [30,32]. In our settings, one or more specimens are extracted and examined fresh in the in vitro fertilization (IVF) laboratory during a diagnostic biopsy [68,69,73]. In the presence of viable sperm, cryopreservation is offered [73–76]. Our approach is consistent with the EAU guidelines recommendations [30], stating that a biopsy should be combined with testicular sperm extraction (TESE) for possible sperm cryopreservation. Cryopreservation is carried out using isolated sperm suspensions or tissue fragments [74,75,77].

Along these lines, a formal scrotal exploration might be applied to identify an obstruction at the epididymis or proximal vas deferens level that could be ultimately treatable using microsurgery (e.g., vasoepididymostomy) at the same operative time [9]. In the above scenario, a testis biopsy should be taken and examined fresh to confirm the presence of active spermatogenesis. Moreover, even if signs of obstruction are evident and a reconstructive procedure is carried out, a testis specimen should be sent for formal histopathology examination as good clinical practice.

In cases of untreatable epididymal obstructions, microsurgical epididymal sperm aspiration may be applied to harvest sperm for cryopreservation [7,9,10,78,79]. By contrast, a testicular sperm retrieval technique (e.g., conventional TESE or microdissection TESE) should be carried out in the same operative time if no signs of obstruction are seen [10]. During the sperm extraction, a specimen should also be taken for histopathology examination to confirm the type of azoospermia.

A clinical algorithm to help distinguish OA from NOA related to HH or STF is provided in Figure 1.

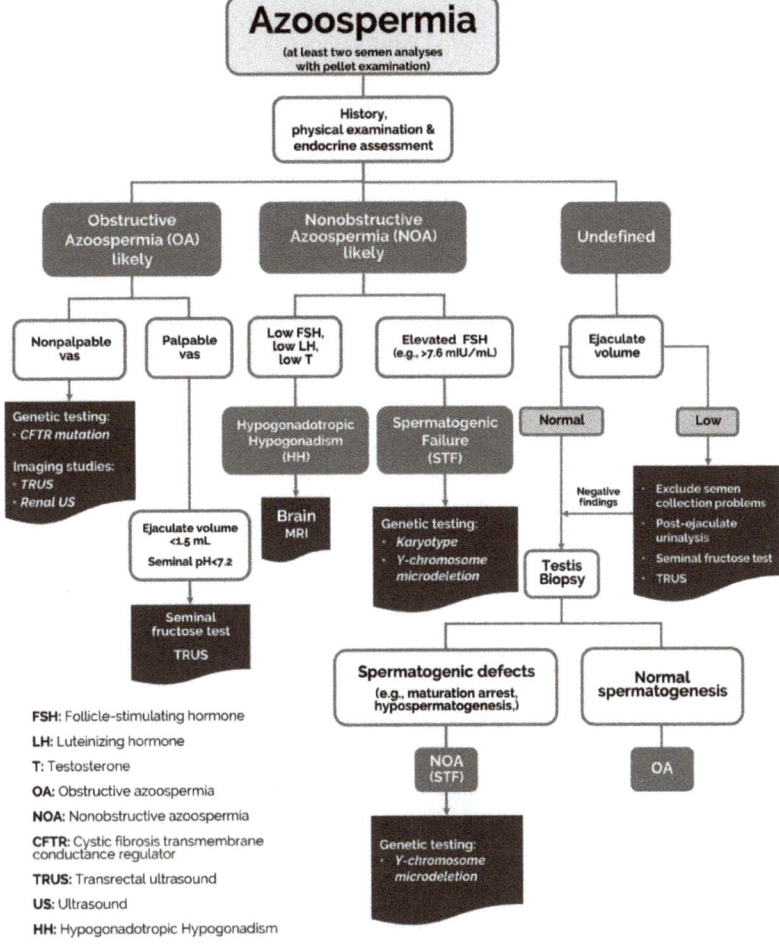

Figure 1. Algorithm for azoospermia differential diagnosis.

4. Clinical Cases: Difficult Differential Diagnosis

4.1. Case 1

A 36-year-old man presented for evaluation with a 7-year infertility history and azoospermia confirmed on multiple semen analyses. His wife was 27 years old and had no obvious female factor (e.g., eumenorrheic, patent tubes, normal-sized ovaries, normal ovarian reserve (Anti-Müllerian Hormone level of 2.5 ng/mL), no previous surgery, no medical comorbidities).

His childhood and adolescent history were unremarkable. In the sexual history, the patient complained of decreased libido and mild erectile dysfunction, which resulted in an irregular intercourse routine. He denied previous or current gonadotoxic exposure, medication use, or sexually transmitted diseases. However, he reported a history of a right-sided hernia repair at age 26 and noticed that the size of the right testis decreased after the operation.

Physical examination revealed a normal virilized man with no gynecomastia, a body mass index (BMI) of 30.1 kg/m^2, and a right inguinal scar from previous hernia repair. His right testis was atrophic (Prader orchidometry of 2 mL), whereas his left testis had a normal size (Prader orchidometry between 15 and 20 mL). The right epididymis was reduced in size, and the left epididymis was normal on palpation. Both vas deferens were palpable, and we did not detect varicocele on physical examination. Fasting blood tests taken in the morning (~10:00 a.m.) revealed a serum FSH level of 6.1 mIU/mL (reference: 1.4–8.1), LH level of 5.6 mIU/mL (reference: 1.5–9.3), estradiol level of 30.3 pg/mL (reference: <39.8 pg/mL), thyroid-stimulating hormone level (TSH) of 2.6 µIU/mL (reference range: 0.48–5.60 µIU/mL), thyroxin (T4) level of 0.99 ng/dL (reference: 0.85–1.50 ng/dL), prolactin level of 7.1 ng/mL (reference range: 2.1–17.7 ng/mL), total testosterone level of 266 ng/dL (reference range: 241–827 ng/dL), free testosterone level of 5 ng/dL (reference range: 3.03–14.8 ng/dL), and vitamin D of 52 ng/mL (reference: >20 ng/mL). Two additional semen analyses performed in the fertility clinic's andrology laboratory confirmed the presence of azoospermia after the examination of the centrifuged pellet, and these ejaculates had normal volume (4 and 3 mL) and pH (8.0 and 7.8). Genetic tests were ordered, which reported a normal (46,XY) karyotype and no Yq chromosome microdeletions.

Although the diagnosis of right testicular atrophy secondary to iatrogenic vascular damage during hernia repair was established, the type of azoospermia on the left testis was more equivocal. Therefore, a percutaneous testicular biopsy was undertaken on the left testis at the fertility center's operating theater and sent for both fresh and histopathology examinations (Figure 2). The fresh specimen contained abundant germ cells but no mature sperm or elongated spermatid (Figure 2B). The histopathology specimen revealed maturation arrest at the spermatocyte stage in all tubules examined (120 cross-sections) (Figure 2C).

With the diagnosis of NOA due to maturation arrest on the left testis, we recommended sperm retrieval. However, the patient was advised to undergo an off-label hormonal modulation, which seems justified in selected NOA cases, particularly those associated with hypogonadism [5,80,81]. He was started on human chorionic gonadotropin (recombinant hCG, 125 mcg twice weekly). After two months of treatment, his total testosterone levels improved to 476 ng/dL, his FSH levels dropped to <1.5 mIU/L, and his estradiol levels raised to 55 pg/mL. He was then started on FSH (recombinant FSH 150 IU twice weekly) and anastrozole 1 mg/day. Therapy lasted for six months, and during treatment, no sperm were found on the follow-up semen analysis.

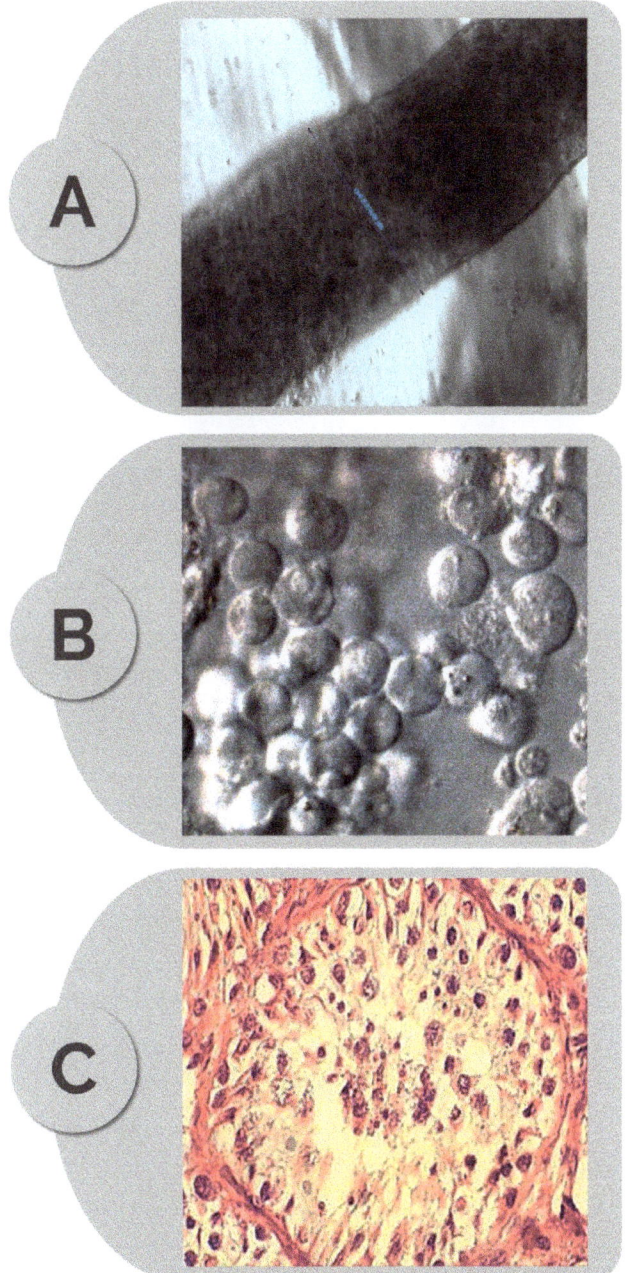

Figure 2. Photomicrographs illustrating: (**A**) intact seminiferous tubule (diameter 270 micrometers), (**B**) cell suspension obtained after mechanical tubule mincing, and (**C**) corresponding histopathology (hematoxylin/eosin) specimen revealing germ cell maturation arrest (MA). Images A and B obtained at 400× magnification using an inverted optical microscope (Nikon Eclipse Diaphot 300, Nikon, Japan, with phase contrast (Hoffman)).

He was then subjected to micro-TESE on the left side. At the time of surgery, his hormone levels were: FSH of 3.2 mIU/L, total testosterone of 578 ng/dL, and estradiol of 39 pg/mL. During the operation, we were able to harvest viable sperm with apparent adequate morphology from the seminiferous tubules, which were cryopreserved using conventional and vitrification methods [73,74]. A specimen taken for histopathology showed germ cell maturation arrest with focal areas of normal spermatogenesis. Subsequently, sperm injections were performed with frozen-thawed testicular sperm. At oocyte pick-up, seven metaphase-II oocytes were retrieved, five of which fertilized, and three developed until the blastocyst stage. A single embryo transfer was performed, which resulted in a term delivery of a baby boy at term. Two blastocysts remain cryopreserved.

4.2. Case 2

A 35-year-old man presented for evaluation with an 8-year infertility history and azoospermia confirmed on multiple semen analyses. His partner was 32 years old, eumenorrheic, with no evident female factor or medical co-morbidities, despite an ovarian reserve in the lower normal limits (Anti-Müllerian Hormone level of 1.2 ng/mL).

The couple's sexual history was unremarkable, as was the patient's childhood and adolescent medical history. He denied previous or current gonadotoxic exposure, medication use, or sexually transmitted diseases. The patient had a history of bilateral varicocele repair at age 27, with no apparent complications.

Physical examination revealed a normal virilized man with no gynecomastia, a BMI of 32.5 kg/m^2, and a bilateral inguinal scar from the previous varicocelectomy. His testes were found to have normal volume (Prader orchidometry of 15 cc). The epididymides were normal, and the vas deferens was palpable on both sides. Fasting blood tests taken in the morning (~10:00 a.m.) revealed a serum FSH level of 4.4 mIU/mL (reference range: 1.4–8.1), LH level of 3.8 mIU/mL (nl: 1.5–9.3), estradiol level of 28 pg/mL (reference: <39.8 pg/mL), TSH of 1.2 µIU/mL (reference range: 0.48–5.60 µIU/mL), T4 level of 1.1 ng/dL (reference: 0.85–1.50 ng/dL), prolactin level of 5.8 ng/mL (reference range: 2.1–17.7 ng/mL), total testosterone level of 360 ng/dL (reference range: 241–827 ng/dL), and free testosterone level of 8.8 ng/dL (reference range: 3.03–14.8 ng/dL).

Two semen analyses carried out in the fertility center's andrology laboratory confirmed the presence of azoospermia after the examination of the centrifuged specimens, and these ejaculates had normal volume (>1.5 mL) and pH (>7.2). The genetic analysis revealed a normal (46,XY) karyotype and absence of Yq chromosome microdeletions.

The differential diagnosis remained equivocal, and therefore the patient had a scrotal exploration, which revealed no signs of obstruction. A right micro-TESE was carried out in the same operative procedure. The examination of the seminiferous tubules showed a homogeneous pattern of healthy tubules. Random micro-biopsies were taken for fresh examination, which revealed abundant germ cells, typical of maturation arrest, and no mature sperm or elongated spermatid. We decided to terminate the operation without exploring the contralateral testis. A specimen was taken and sent for histopathology, which confirmed maturation arrest at the primary spermatocyte stage.

Four weeks postoperatively, the patient was started on human chorionic gonadotropin (recombinant hCG 125 mcg twice weekly) and FSH (recombinant FSH 150 IU twice weekly). His hormone levels were monitored monthly and medication adjusted whenever needed, with the goal to keep testosterone levels between 500 and 800 ng/dL and FSH levels within normal levels. Semen analyses were also performed from the third month of therapy onwards, and after five months of therapy, occasional motile sperm were found, all of which were morphologically abnormal (mainly globozoospermic sperm). Sperm cryopreservation was carried on several occasions, and the couple had an ICSI cycle performed with frozen-thawed ejaculated testicular sperm. Sperm injections were carried out in 7 metaphase II oocytes, two of which fertilized, and one day-3 embryo was replaced into the uterus, but implantation did not occur. The embryologists informed that the quality of sperm was unsuitable for ICSI.

We opted to continue with medication and proceed to micro-TESE on the left testis, which was carried out after 12 months of gonadotropin therapy. At the time of micro-TESE, his hormone levels were: FSH of 5.6 mIU/L, total testosterone of 738 ng/dL, and estradiol of 46 pg/mL. Mature sperm were found intraoperatively; however, all harvested sperm exhibited abnormal morphology, as seen in the cryptozoospermic semen analyses. ICSI was performed in five metaphase-II oocytes, two of which fertilized with fresh testicular sperm isolated from the micro-TESE procedure. These zygotes developed into embryos, which were replaced in the partner's uterus on the third day of development. Again, no pregnancy was obtained. The couple declined the offer to carry on with donor sperm insemination. To our knowledge, at the time of writing, the couple remained childless.

4.3. Case 3

A 40-year-old man presented to the fertility clinic with a 4-year infertility history and azoospermia confirmed on repeated semen analyses. His wife was 29 years old and had adequate ovarian reserve markers, patent tubes, and normal gynecological investigations.

The couple's sexual history was mostly unremarkable, although the patient complained of occasional perineal discomfort after ejaculation. His childhood and adolescent medical history were also not significant. He had previous chickenpox at age 12 but denied a history suggestive of mumps orchitis. The patient underwent typical pubertal changes and denied sexually transmitted diseases, previous/current medication use, or gonadotoxic exposure, except cigarette smoking since age 19. He also denied previous surgeries. The only possible relevant finding was his habit of equestrian sports, which he practiced at least twice a week since age 16.

Physical examination revealed a normal virilized man with no gynecomastia, BMI of 29.4 kg/m^2, no inguinal/scrotal scars, and normal-sized testicles (Prader orchidometry of 20 cc). The epididymides had normal characteristics, the vasa deferentia were palpable, and the spermatic cords had no signs of varicocele; however, a small hydrocele was noted on both hemiscrotum. Fasting blood tests taken in the morning revealed a serum FSH level of 6.2 mIU/mL (reference range: 1.4–8.1), LH level of 3.6 mIU/mL (nl: 1.5–9.3), estradiol level of 23 pg/mL (reference: <39.8 pg/mL), TSH level of 2.1 µIU/mL (reference range: 0.48–5.60 µIU/mL), T4 level of 1.2 ng/dL (reference: 0.85–1.50 ng/dL), prolactin level of 13.5 ng/mL (reference range: 2.1–17.7 ng/mL), total testosterone level of 418 ng/dL (reference range: 241–827 ng/dL), and free testosterone level of 11.5 ng/dL (reference range: 3.03–14.8 ng/dL).

Semen analysis was carried out in the fertility center's andrology laboratory, which confirmed azoospermia after examining the centrifuged specimen. The ejaculate had a normal pH (8.0), but its volume was at the lower normal limits (1.5 mL). A TRUS was ordered to evaluate the complaint of perineal discomfort and borderline semen volume further, but its results were not suggestive of any signs of obstruction. A post-ejaculation urinalysis was also performed to check for retrograde ejaculation, yet no sperm were found. Additionally, a scrotum ultrasound confirmed the physical exam findings, but it did not add any relevant information to ascertain whether the azoospermia was obstructive or nonobstructive. The genetic analysis revealed a normal (46,XY) karyotype and no Yq chromosome microdeletions.

The patient had a scrotal exploration that revealed bilateral epididymal obstruction signs, possibly idiopathic or post-traumatic (equestrian sports). The testicles and the vasa deferentia were normal, and small-volume hydroceles were indeed present. A healthy epididymal tubule was isolated and incised using a microsurgical technique. Subsequently, the fluid was collected and sent to the laboratory for examination, revealing abundant motile sperm. The harvested epididymal sperm were cryopreserved. A microsurgical vasoepididymostomy was carried out using the intussusception technique applying three double-arm sutures in a triangular fashion [9]. The procedure was repeated on the contralateral side. Testicular specimens taken for histopathology showed normal spermatogenesis.

Follow-up semen analyses at 6 and 9 months postoperatively revealed a sperm concentration of 7 and 12 million/mL, 29% and 38% progressive motility, 4% and 7% strict morphology, and 4.7 and 9.2 million total motile sperm count, respectively. The couple achieved natural pregnancy one year postoperatively, which resulted in the delivery of a healthy baby girl at 38 gestational weeks.

5. Discussion

The clinical assessment and management of infertile men with azoospermia should consider the (i) differential diagnosis of azoospermia, (ii) identification of patients eligible for reconstructive procedures (e.g., OA), gonadotropin therapy (e.g., NOA-HH), or sperm retrieval, (iii) identification of patients with NOA-STF that might benefit from interventions (e.g., varicocele repair, hormonal modulation) before a sperm retrieval attempt, (iv) use of an optimal surgical method to harvest sperm, and (v) utilization of state-of-the-art IVF techniques when applicable. A detailed discussion of these aspects is outside the scope of this article and can be found elsewhere [5,9,10].

Nevertheless, the most challenging azoospermic patient to manage clinically is probably that with NOA-STF. Table 2 outlines the essential aspects to be considered under this scenario. Among several critical factors, a sensitive matter relates to hormonal modulation for men with NOA, as briefly described in clinical cases 1 and 2. The reason stems from the fact that it is generally believed that empirical medical treatment for men with NOA-STF is ineffective because gonadotropins' plasma levels are usually high. Yet, many patients with NOA-STF present with hypogonadism and might thus lack adequate levels of intratesticular testosterone, which are essential for spermatogenesis in combination with adequate Sertoli cell stimulation by FSH [80–82]. Furthermore, gonadotropin action is determined by the frequency, amplitude, and duration of its secretory pulses. Due to the high baseline levels of endogenous gonadotropins commonly seen in patient with NOA-STF, the relative amplitudes of FSH and LH are low, leading to a paradoxically weak stimulation of Leydig and Sertoli cells [35,83]. Therefore, there may be a potential role for pharmacotherapy in men with NOA [84,85].

Table 2. Interventions and recommended actions in the clinical management of azoospermic men with nonobstructive azoospermia seeking fertility.

Clinical Management Step	Intervention	Action	Interpretation
Differential diagnosis	Medical history, physical examination, endocrine profile (FSH and testosterone levels at a minimum; LH, prolactin, thyroid hormones, 17-hydroxiprogesterone and estradiol are added as needed), and examination of pelleted semen on multiple occasions. Testicular biopsy could be considered in selected cases in which the differential diagnosis could not be determined.	Confirm that azoospermia is due to spermatogenic failure, and identify men with severely impaired spermatogenesis having few sperm in the ejaculate (cryptozoospermia).	A differential diagnosis between obstructive azoospermia, hypogonadotropic hypogonadism, and spermatogenic failure should be established as management varies according to the type of azoospermia.
Determination of proper candidates for sperm retrieval	Y chromosome microdeletion screening using multiplex PCR blood test. The basic set of PCR primers recommended by the EAA/EMQN for the diagnosis of Yq microdeletion includes: sY14 (SRY), ZFX/ZFY, sY84 and sY86 (AZFa), sY127 and sY134 (AZFb), sY254, and sY255 (AZFc).	Deselect men with microdeletions involving subregions AZFa, AZFb, and AZFb+c.	Approximately 10% of men with NOA-STF harbor microdeletions within the AZF region. SR success in men with YCMD involving the subregions AZFa, AZFb, and AZFb+c are virtually nil, and such patients should be counseled accordingly. SR success in men with AZFc deletions range from 50% to 70%. Genetic counseling should be offered to men with AZFc deletions because testicular spermatozoa used for ICSI will invariably transmit the deletion from father to son.

Table 2. Cont.

Clinical Management Step	Intervention	Action	Interpretation
Identification of patients who could benefit from medical therapy or varicocele repair before sperm retrieval	Serum levels of FSH, total testosterone and estradiol.	Consider medical treatment with gonadotropins, aromatase inhibitors, or selective estrogen receptor modulators for NOA-STF patients with hypogonadism (TT < 300 ng/dL) or T/E ratio < 10. FSH therapy might be needed if FSH drop to below 1.5 mIU/mL during hCG treatment.	Patients should be informed that the evidence of a positive effect of medical treatment remains equivocal.
	Physical examination to identify the presence of clinical varicocele and analysis of testicular biopsy results (if available)	Consider microsurgical repair of clinical varicocele.	Microsurgical varicocele repair is associated with better outcomes concerning recurrence and postoperative complications. Patients with testicular histopathology indicating Sertoli cell-only are unlikely to benefit from varicocele repair. Evidence of a positive effect of varicocele repair is limited, and patients should be counseled accordingly.
Selection of the most effective surgical method for testicular sperm acquisition	Analysis of testicular biopsy results (if available) and of whether sperm have been obtained in previous treatment and by which method.	Microdissection testicular sperm extraction. Conventional testicular sperm extraction may be considered in cases of previous success with TESE, particularly when testicular histopathology indicates hypospermatogenesis.	Micro-TESE in NOA-STF is associated with higher SR success than conventional TESE. The lower tissue removal facilitates sperm processing and lessens testicular damage.
State-of-the-art laboratory techniques to handle surgically extracted testicular spermatozoa	Extraction of a minimum volume of tissue by micro-TESE facilitates tissue processing and search for sperm. Testicular tissue preparation techniques include mechanical and enzymatic mincing and erythrocyte lysis.	Sterile techniques, stable pH and temperature, and high laboratory air quality conditions are helpful to optimize micromanipulation efficiency and safety assurance. Excess sperm not used for ICSI should be cryopreserved for future attempts.	Spermatozoa collected from NOA-STF men are often compromised in quality and are more fragile than ejaculated counterparts. The reproductive potential of such gametes used for ICSI is differentially affected by NOA-STF.

EAA: European Association of Andrology; EMQN: European Molecular Genetics Quality Network; AZF: azoospermia factor; FSH: Follicle-stimulating hormone; ICSI: intracytoplasmic sperm injection; LH: luteinizing hormone; micro-TESE: microdissection testicular sperm extraction; NOA-STF: nonobstructive azoospermia due to spermatogenic failure; PCR: polymerase chain reaction; SR: sperm retrieval; T/E: testosterone to estradiol ratio; TESE: testicular sperm extraction; TT: total testosterone; YCMD: Y-chromosome microdeletions. Adapted from Esteves [5], Asian J. Androl. 17, 459–470, 2015, an Open Access article distributed under the terms of the Creative Commons Attribution Non-Commercial License.

Selective estrogen receptor modulators, aromatase inhibitors, human chorionic gonadotropin (hCG), and FSH have been used off-label to manipulate male reproductive hormones and optimize intratesticular testosterone production [5,84,86–88]. The goals are to induce recovery of sperm to the ejaculate or improve surgical sperm retrieval rates. Case series and a few cohort studies suggested that these treatments might increase sperm retrieval rates, and in some cases, treatment was associated with the return of minimal numbers of sperm to the ejaculate [5,84–88]. Despite that, no randomized controlled trial exists, making it difficult to make clear recommendations on this matter.

Notwithstanding these observations, limited data indicate that treatment with hCG and recombinant FSH could lead to 10–15% higher sperm retrieval rates than sperm retrieval with no previous treatment [35]. Furthermore, hCG treatment was shown to improve intratesticular testosterone production remarkably in men with NOA [89]. Based on these concepts and with the goals of inducing return of sperm to the ejaculate or improving surgical sperm retrieval rates, we have used hCG alone or in combination with recombinant FSH off-label to optimize intratesticular testosterone production and FSH action, as previously described [5]. Our treatment protocol, utilized in clinical cases 1 and 2, relies primarily on hCG to boost intratesticular production. Additionally, hCG treatment was shown to decrease FSH levels, which are typically elevated in most of these patients [51]. Based on limited data from animal and human studies, it has been speculated that FSH reset to normal levels might reduce Sertoli cell desensitization caused by excessive circulating endogenous gonadotropins [90–95]. Consequently, an increased Sertoli cell function and expression of FSH receptors could be obtained. Our patients are followed with a monthly hormonal assessment, and we add an aromatase inhibitor in the course of treatment when the testosterone (ng/dL) to estradiol (pg/mL) ratio becomes less than 10. We also prescribe recombinant FSH when, after hCG treatment, the FSH levels drop below 1.5 IU/L [4,51]. The ultimate goal is to increase intratesticular testosterone to optimal levels through hCG stimulation while securing adequate FSH levels within normal ranges. Although we need more data in this area, hormone stimulation for men with NOA may be worth considering in selected cases.

6. Conclusions

The differential diagnosis between OA and the two forms of NOA, namely NOA-STF and NOA-HH, can be effectively established in most patients based on a standardized male infertility workup. This is the first and critical step in the clinical decision-making process, and it will guide the physician on how to optimally manage these patients, thus providing the couples with an optimal path for parenthood.

A testicular biopsy should be reserved for the cases of doubt, mainly in patients whose history, physical examination, semen analysis, hormonal evaluation, genetic tests, and imaging studies are inconclusive. Histopathology findings will indicate if spermatogenesis is preserved or disrupted, confirming whether azoospermia is obstructive or nonobstructive. Besides providing specimens for a formal histopathology examination, a diagnostic testis biopsy allows for a concomitant fresh examination of one or more extracted specimens; in the presence of viable sperm, cryopreservation should be offered. Alternatively, a formal surgical scrotal exploration may be utilized in cases of doubt, provided the surgeon is prepared to fix an obstruction at the level of epididymis or vas deferens or perform epididymal or testicular sperm retrieval as appropriate. Therefore, these procedures should be carried out at properly equipped facilities.

A coordinated multidisciplinary effort involving reproductive urologists/andrologists, reproductive gynecologists, geneticists, and embryologists is vital to offer infertility patients with azoospermia the best chance of achieving biological parenthood.

Author Contributions: Conceptualization, S.C.E.; writing—original draft preparation, D.L.A. and M.C.V.; writing—review and editing, S.C.E.; supervision, S.C.E. All authors have read and agreed to the published version of the manuscript.

Funding: Author processing charges were funded by Next Fertility Procrea Lugano, Switzerland.

Institutional Review Board Statement: Not applicable.

Informed Consent Statement: The case studies were presented in accordance with the CARE (CAse Reports) guidelines https://www.care-statement.org/ (accessed on 15 May 2021).

Data Availability Statement: All data related to this manuscript are provided in the text.

Acknowledgments: We thank our patients who consented to sharing their cases.

Conflicts of Interest: The authors declare no conflict of interest.

References

1. Aziz, N. The importance of semen analysis in the context of azoospermia. *Clinics* **2013**, *6* (Suppl. 1), 35–38. [CrossRef]
2. Cocuzza, M.; Alvarenga, C.; Pagani, R. The epidemiology and etiology of azoospermia. *Clinics* **2013**, *68* (Suppl. 1), 15–26. [CrossRef]
3. Tüttelmann, F.; Werny, F.; Cooper, T.G.; Kliesch, S.; Simoni, M.; Nieschlag, E. Clinical experience with azoospermia: Aetiology and chances for spermatozoa detection upon biopsy. *Int. J. Androl.* **2011**, *34*, 291–298. [CrossRef]
4. Olesen, I.A.; Andersson, A.M.; Aksglaede, L.; Skakkebaek, N.E.; Rajpert-de Meyts, E.; Joergensen, N.; Juul, A. Clinical, genetic, biochemical, and testicular biopsy findings among 1213 men evaluated for infertility. *Fertil. Steril.* **2017**, *107*, 74–82.e7. [CrossRef]

5. Esteves, S.C. Clinical management of infertile men with nonobstructive azoospermia. *Asian J. Androl.* **2015**, *17*, 459–470. [CrossRef]
6. Fraietta, R.; Zylberstejn, D.S.; Esteves, S.C. Hypogonadotropic hypogonadism revisited. *Clinics* **2013**, *68* (Suppl. 1), 81–88. [CrossRef]
7. Miyaoka, R.; Esteves, S.C. Predictive factors for sperm retrieval and sperm injection outcomes in obstructive azoospermia: Do etiology, retrieval techniques and gamete source play a role? *Clinics* **2013**, *68* (Suppl. 1), 111–119. [CrossRef]
8. Esteves, S.C.; Lee, W.; Benjamin, D.J.; Seol, B.; Verza, S., Jr.; Agarwal, A. Reproductive potential of men with obstructive azoospermia undergoing percutaneous sperm retrieval and intracytoplasmic sperm injection according to the cause of obstruction. *J. Urol.* **2013**, *189*, 232–237. [CrossRef] [PubMed]
9. Esteves, S.C.; Miyaoka, R.; Agarwal, A. Surgical treatment of male infertility in the era of intracytoplasmic sperm injection—New insights. *Clinics* **2011**, *66*, 1463–1478. [CrossRef] [PubMed]
10. Miyaoka, R.; Orosz, J.E.; Achermann, A.P.; Esteves, S.C. Methods of surgical sperm extraction and implications for assisted reproductive technology success. *Panminerva Med.* **2019**, *61*, 164–177. [CrossRef]
11. Esteves, S.C.; Miyaoka, R.; Agarwal, A. An update on the clinical assessment of the infertile male. *Clinics* **2011**, *66*, 691–700, Erratum in *Clinics* **2012**, *67*, 203. [CrossRef] [PubMed]
12. Hamada, A.J.; Esteves, S.C.; Agarwal, A. A comprehensive review of genetics and genetic testing in azoospermia. *Clinics* **2013**, *68* (Suppl. 1), 39–60. [CrossRef]
13. Thakker, S.; Persily, J.; Najari, B.B. Kallman syndrome and central non-obstructive azoospermia. *Best Pract. Res. Clin. Endocrinol. Metab.* **2020**, *34*, 101475. [CrossRef]
14. Patel, A.S.; Leong, J.Y.; Ramos, L.; Ramasamy, R. Testosterone Is a Contraceptive and Should Not Be Used in Men Who Desire Fertility. *World J. Men's Health* **2019**, *37*, 45–54. [CrossRef]
15. Boeri, L.; Capogrosso, P.; Ventimiglia, E.; Cazzaniga, W.; Pozzi, E.; Belladelli, F.; Pederzoli, F.; Alfano, M.; Abbate, C.; Montanari, E.; et al. Testicular volume in infertile versus fertile white-European men: A case-control investigation in the real-life setting. *Asian J. Androl.* **2021**. [CrossRef]
16. Schoor, R.A.; Elhanbly, S.; Niederberger, C.S.; Ross, L.S. The role of testicular biopsy in the modern management of male infertility. *J Urol.* **2002**, *167*, 197–200. [CrossRef]
17. Majzoub, A.; Arafa, M.; Khalafalla, K.; AlSaid, S.; Burjaq, H.; Albader, M.; Al-Marzooqi, T.; Esteves, S.C.; Elbardisi, H. Predictive model to estimate the chances of successful sperm retrieval by testicular sperm aspiration in patients with nonobstructive azoospermia. *Fertil. Steril.* **2021**, *115*, 373–381. [CrossRef] [PubMed]
18. Hung, A.J.; King, P.; Schlegel, P.N. Uniform testicular maturation arrest: A unique subset of men with nonobstructive azoospermia. *J. Urol.* **2007**, *178*, 608–612, discussion 612. [CrossRef] [PubMed]
19. Jungwirth, A.; Giwercman, A.; Tournaye, H.; Diemer, T.; Kopa, Z.; Dohle, G.; Krausz, C. European Association of Urology Working Group on Male Infertility. European Association of Urology guidelines on Male Infertility: The 2012 update. *Eur. Urol.* **2012**, *62*, 324–332. [CrossRef]
20. Mieusset, R.; Bieth, E.; Daudin, M.; Isus, F.; Delaunay, B.; Bujan, L.; Monteil, L.; Fauquet, I.; Huyghe, E.; Hamdi, S.M. Male partners of infertile couples with congenital unilateral absence of the vas deferens are mainly non-azoospermic. *Andrology* **2020**, *8*, 645–653. [CrossRef] [PubMed]
21. Cocuzza, M.S.; Tiseo, B.C.; Srougi, V.; Wood, G.J.A.; Cardoso, J.P.G.F.; Esteves, S.C.; Srougi, M. Diagnostic accuracy of physical examination compared with color Doppler ultrasound in the determination of varicocele diagnosis and grading: Impact of urologists' experience. *Andrology* **2020**, *8*, 1160–1166. [CrossRef]
22. Miyaoka, R.; Esteves, S.C. A critical appraisal on the role of varicocele in male infertility. *Adv. Urol.* **2012**, *2012*, 597495. [CrossRef] [PubMed]
23. Lira Neto, F.T.; Roque, M.; Esteves, S.C. Effect of varicocelectomy on sperm deoxyribonucleic acid fragmentation rates in infertile men with clinical varicocele: A systematic review and meta-analysis. *Fertil. Steril.* **2021**. [CrossRef]
24. Esteves, S.C.; Miyaoka, R.; Roque, M.; Agarwal, A. Outcome of varicocele repair in men with nonobstructive azoospermia: Systematic review and meta-analysis. *Asian J. Androl.* **2016**, *18*, 246–253. [CrossRef]
25. Esteves, S.C. Pro: Should Varicocele Be Repaired in Azoospermic Infertile Men? In *Varicocele and Male Infertility*, 1st ed.; Esteves, S., Cho, C.L., Majzoub, A., Agarwal, A., Eds.; Springer: Cham, Switzerland, 2019. [CrossRef]
26. Dabaja, A.A.; Goldstein, M. When is a varicocele repair indicated: The dilemma of hypogonadism and erectile dysfunction? *Asian J. Androl.* **2016**, *18*, 213–216. [CrossRef]
27. Hamada, A.; Esteves, S.C.; Agarwal, A. Varicocele Classification. In *Varicocele and Male Infertility: Current Concepts, Controversies and Consensus*; Hamada, A., Esteves, S.C., Agarwal, A., Eds.; SpringerBriefs in Reproductive Biology, Springer International Publishing: Cham, Switzerland; Heidelberg, Germany; New York, NY, USA; London, UK, 2016; pp. 37–43.
28. Esteves, S.C.; Roque, M.; Bedoschi, G.; Haahr, T.; Humaidan, P. Intracytoplasmic sperm injection for male infertility and consequences for offspring. *Nat. Rev. Urol.* **2018**, *15*, 535–562. [CrossRef] [PubMed]
29. World Health Organization. *WHO Laboratory Manual for the Examination and Processing of Human Semen*, 5th ed.; WHO Press: Geneva, Switzerland, 2010.

30. Salonia, A.; Bettocchi, C.; Carvalho, J.; Corona, G.; Jones, T.H.; Kadioğlu, A.; Martinez-Salamanca, J.I.; Minhas, S.; Serefoğlu, E.C.; Verze, P. *European Association of Urology Guidelines on Sexual and Reproductive Health*; European Association of Urology, 2020. Available online: https://uroweb.org/wp-content/uploads/EAU-Guidelines-on-Sexual-and-Reproductive-Health-2020.pdf (accessed on 15 May 2021).
31. Esteves, S.C. Clinical relevance of routine semen analysis and controversies surrounding the 2010 World Health Organization criteria for semen examination. *Int. Braz. J. Urol.* **2014**, *40*, 443–453. [CrossRef] [PubMed]
32. Schlegel, P.N.; Sigman, M.; Collura, B.; De Jonge, C.J.; Eisenberg, M.L.; Lamb, D.J.; Mulhall, J.P.; Niederberger, C.; Sandlow, J.I.; Sokol, R.Z.; et al. Diagnosis and treatment of infertility in men: AUA/ASRM guideline part I. *Fertil. Steril.* **2021**, *115*, 54–61. [CrossRef] [PubMed]
33. Esteves, S.C. Percutaneous epididymal sperm aspiration as a method for sperm retrieval in men with obstructive azoospermia seeking fertility: Operative and laboratory aspects. *Int. Braz. J. Urol.* **2015**, *41*, 817–818. [CrossRef]
34. Achermann, A.P.P.; Esteves, S.C. Diagnosis and management of infertility due to ejaculatory duct obstruction: Summary evidence. *Int. Braz. J. Urol.* **2021**, *47*, 868–881. [CrossRef]
35. Shiraishi, K.; Ohmi, C.; Shimabukuro, T.; Matsuyama, H. Human chorionic gonadotrophin treatment prior to microdissection testicular sperm extraction in non-obstructive azoospermia. *Hum. Reprod.* **2012**, *27*, 331–339. [CrossRef]
36. Oduwole, O.O.; Peltoketo, H.; Huhtaniemi, I.T. Role of Follicle-Stimulating Hormone in Spermatogenesis. *Front. Endocrinol.* **2018**, *9*, 763. [CrossRef]
37. Ishikawa, T.; Fujioka, H.; Fujisawa, M. Clinical and hormonal findings in testicular maturation arrest. *BJU Int.* **2004**, *94*, 1314–1316. [CrossRef]
38. Martin-du-Pan, R.C.; Bischof, P. Increased follicle stimulating hormone in infertile men. Is increased plasma FSH always due to damaged germinal epithelium? *Hum. Reprod.* **1995**, *10*, 1940–1945. [CrossRef]
39. Bergmann, M.; Behre, H.M.; Nieschlag, E. Serum FSH and testicular morphology in male infertility. *Clin. Endocrinol.* **1994**, *40*, 133–136. [CrossRef] [PubMed]
40. Arshad, M.A.; Majzoub, A.; Esteves, S.C. Predictors of surgical sperm retrieval in non-obstructive azoospermia: Summary of current literature. *Int. Urol. Nephrol.* **2020**, *52*, 2015–2038. [CrossRef] [PubMed]
41. Esteves, S.C. Microdissection testicular sperm extraction (micro-TESE) as a sperm acquisition method for men with nonobstructive azoospermia seeking fertility: Operative and laboratory aspects. *Int. Braz. J. Urol.* **2013**, *39*, 440–441. [CrossRef]
42. Esteves, S.C.; Agarwal, A. Reproductive outcomes, including neonatal data, following sperm injection in men with obstructive and nonobstructive azoospermia: Case series and systematic review. *Clinics* **2013**, *68* (Suppl. 1), 141–150. [CrossRef]
43. Esteves, S.C.; Ramasamy, R.; Colpi, G.M.; Carvalho, J.F.; Schlegel, P.N. Sperm retrieval rates by micro-TESE versus conventional TESE in men with non-obstructive azoospermia-the assumption of independence in effect sizes might lead to misleading conclusions. *Hum. Reprod. Update* **2020**, *26*, 603–605. [CrossRef] [PubMed]
44. Behre, H.M. Clinical Use of FSH in Male Infertility. *Front. Endocrinol.* **2019**, *10*, 322. [CrossRef]
45. Adamopoulos, D.A.; Koukkou, E.G. 'Value of FSH and inhibin-B measurements in the diagnosis of azoospermia'—A clinician's overview. *Int. J. Androl.* **2010**, *33*, e109–e113. [CrossRef] [PubMed]
46. Krausz, C.; Riera-Escamilla, A. Genetics of male infertility. *Nat. Rev. Urol.* **2018**, *15*, 369–384. [CrossRef] [PubMed]
47. Kohn, T.P.; Kohn, J.R.; Owen, R.C.; Coward, R.M. The Prevalence of Y-chromosome Microdeletions in Oligozoospermic Men: A Systematic Review and Meta-analysis of European and North American Studies. *Eur. Urol.* **2019**, *76*, 626–636. [CrossRef] [PubMed]
48. Peña, V.N.; Kohn, T.P.; Herati, A.S. Genetic mutations contributing to non-obstructive azoospermia. *Best Pract. Res. Clin. Endocrinol. Metab.* **2020**, *34*, 101479. [CrossRef] [PubMed]
49. Liu, J.L.; Peña, V.; Fletcher, S.A.; Kohn, T.P. Genetic testing in male infertility—Reassessing screening thresholds. *Curr. Opin. Urol.* **2020**, *30*, 317–323. [CrossRef] [PubMed]
50. Corona, G.; Minhas, S.; Giwercman, A.; Bettocchi, C.; Dinkelman-Smit, M.; Dohle, G.; Fusco, F.; Kadioglou, A.; Kliesch, S.; Kopa, Z.; et al. Sperm recovery and ICSI outcomes in men with non-obstructive azoospermia: A systematic review and meta-analysis. *Hum. Reprod. Update* **2019**, *25*, 733–757. [CrossRef] [PubMed]
51. Krausz, C.; Hoefsloot, L.; Simoni, M.; Tüttelmann, F. European Academy of Andrology; European Molecular Genetics Quality Network. EAA/EMQN best practice guidelines for molecular diagnosis of Y-chromosomal microdeletions: State-of-the-art 2013. *Andrology* **2014**, *2*, 5–19. [CrossRef]
52. Kleiman, S.E.; Yogev, L.; Lehavi, O.; Hauser, R.; Botchan, A.; Paz, G.; Yavetz, H.; Gamzu, R. The likelihood of finding mature sperm cells in men with AZFb or AZFb-c deletions: Six new cases and a review of the literature (1994–2010). *Fertil. Steril.* **2011**, *95*, 2005–2012.e4. [CrossRef]
53. Stouffs, K.; Vloeberghs, V.; Gheldof, A.; Tournaye, H.; Seneca, S. Are AZFb deletions always incompatible with sperm production? *Andrology* **2017**, *5*, 691–694. [CrossRef]
54. Simoni, M.; Tuüttelmann, F.; Gromoll, J.; Nieschlag, E. Clinical consequences of microdeletions of the Y chromosome: The extended Muünster experience. *Reprod. Biomed. Online* **2008**, *16*, 289–303. [CrossRef]
55. Bieniek, J.M.; Lapin, C.D.; Jarvi, K.A. Genetics of CFTR and male infertility. *Transl. Androl. Urol.* **2021**, *10*, 1391–1400. [CrossRef]
56. Cioppi, F.; Rosta, V.; Krausz, C. Genetics of Azoospermia. *Int. J. Mol. Sci.* **2021**, *22*, 3264. [CrossRef] [PubMed]

57. Dequeker, E.; Stuhrmann, M.; Morris, M.A.; Casals, T.; Castellani, C.; Claustres, M.; Cuppens, H.; des Georges, M.; Ferec, C.; Macek, M.; et al. Best practice guidelines for molecular genetic diagnosis of cystic fibrosis and CFTR-related disorders–updated European recommendations. *Eur. J. Hum. Genet.* **2009**, *17*, 51–65. [CrossRef]
58. Fakhro, K.A.; Elbardisi, H.; Arafa, M.; Robay, A.; Rodriguez-Flores, J.L.; Al-Shakaki, A.; Syed, N.; Mezey, J.G.; Abi Khalil, C.; Malek, J.A.; et al. Point-of-care whole-exome sequencing of idiopathic male infertility. *Genet. Med.* **2018**, *20*, 1365–1373. [CrossRef] [PubMed]
59. Lotti, F.; Frizza, F.; Balercia, G.; Barbonetti, A.; Behre, H.M.; Calogero, A.E.; Cremers, J.F.; Francavilla, F.; Isidori, A.M.; Kliesch, S.; et al. The European Academy of Andrology (EAA) ultrasound study on healthy, fertile men: Scrotal ultrasound reference ranges and associations with clinical, seminal, and biochemical characteristics. *Andrology* **2021**, *9*, 559–576. [CrossRef] [PubMed]
60. Lotti, F.; Maggi, M. Ultrasound of the male genital tract in relation to male reproductive health. *Hum. Reprod. Update* **2015**, *21*, 56–83. [CrossRef]
61. Netto, N.R., Jr.; Esteves, S.C.; Neves, P.A. Transurethral resection of partially obstructed ejaculatory ducts: Seminal parameters and pregnancy outcomes according to the etiology of obstruction. *J. Urol.* **1998**, *159*, 2048–2053. [CrossRef]
62. Kim, B.; Kawashima, A.; Ryu, J.A.; Takahashi, N.; Hartman, R.P.; King, B.F., Jr. Imaging of the seminal vesicle and vas deferens. *Radiographics* **2009**, *29*, 1105–1121. [CrossRef]
63. Danaci, M.; Akpolat, T.; Baştemir, M.; Sarikaya, S.; Akan, H.; Selçuk, M.B.; Cengiz, K. The prevalence of seminal vesicle cysts in autosomal dominant polycystic kidney disease. *Nephrol. Dial. Transplant.* **1998**, *13*, 2825–2828. [CrossRef]
64. Kolettis, P.N.; Sandlow, J.I. Clinical and genetic features of patients with congenital unilateral absence of the vas deferens. *Urology* **2002**, *60*, 1073–1076. [CrossRef]
65. Peng, J.; Yuan, Y.; Cui, W.; Zhang, Z.; Gao, B.; Song, W.; Xin, Z. Causes of suspected epididymal obstruction in Chinese men. *Urology* **2012**, *80*, 1258–1261. [CrossRef] [PubMed]
66. Font, M.D.; Pastuszak, A.W.; Case, J.R.; Lipshultz, L.I. An infertile male with dilated seminal vesicles due to functional obstruction. *Asian J. Androl.* **2017**, *19*, 256–257.
67. Caroppo, E.; Colpi, E.M.; D'Amato, G.; Gazzano, G.; Colpi, G.M. Prediction model for testis histology in men with non-obstructive azoospermia: Evidence for a limited predictive role of serum follicle-stimulating hormone. *J. Assist. Reprod. Genet.* **2019**, *36*, 2575–2582. [CrossRef]
68. Esteves, S.C.; Prudencio, C.; Seol, B.; Verza, S.; Knoedler, C.; Agarwal, A. Comparison of sperm retrieval and reproductive outcome in azoospermic men with testicular failure and obstructive azoospermia treated for infertility. *Asian J. Androl.* **2014**, *16*, 602–606. [CrossRef]
69. Esteves, S.C.; Agarwal, A. Re: Sperm retrieval rates and intracytoplasmic sperm injection outcomes for men with non-obstructive azoospermia and the health of resulting offspring. *Asian J. Androl.* **2014**, *16*, 642. [CrossRef]
70. Barbonetti, A.; Martorella, A.; Minaldi, E.; D'Andrea, S.; Bardhi, D.; Castellini, C.; Francavilla, F.; Francavilla, S. Testicular Cancer in Infertile Men With and Without Testicular Microlithiasis: A Systematic Review and Meta-Analysis of Case-Control Studies. *Front. Endocrinol.* **2019**, *10*, 164. [CrossRef]
71. van Casteren, N.J.; Looijenga, L.H.; Dohle, G.R. Testicular microlithiasis and carcinoma in situ overview and proposed clinical guideline. *Int. J. Androl.* **2009**, *32*, 279–287. [CrossRef]
72. Montironi, R. Intratubular germ cell neoplasia of the testis: Testicular intraepithelial neoplasia. *Eur. Urol.* **2002**, *41*, 651–654. [CrossRef]
73. Esteves, S.C.; Varghese, A.C. Laboratory handling of epididymal and testicular spermatozoa: What can be done to improve sperm injections outcome. *J. Hum. Reprod. Sci.* **2012**, *5*, 233–243. [CrossRef] [PubMed]
74. Esteves, S.C. Novel concepts in male factor infertility: Clinical and laboratory perspectives. *J. Assist. Reprod. Genet.* **2016**, *33*, 1319–1335. [CrossRef] [PubMed]
75. Yovich, J.L.; Esteves, S.C. Storage of sperm samples from males with azoospermia. *Reprod. Biomed. Online* **2018**, *37*, 509–510. [CrossRef] [PubMed]
76. Esteves, S.C.; Lombardo, F.; Garrido, N.; Alvarez, J.; Zini, A.; Colpi, G.M.; Kirkman-Brown, J.; Lewis, S.E.M.; Björndahl, L.; Majzoub, A.; et al. SARS-CoV-2 pandemic and repercussions for male infertility patients: A proposal for the individualized provision of andrological services. *Andrology* **2021**, *9*, 10–18. [CrossRef]
77. Salzbrunn, A.; Benson, D.M.; Holstein, A.F.; Schulze, W. A new concept for the extraction of testicular spermatozoa as a tool for assisted fertilization (ICSI). *Hum. Reprod.* **1996**, *11*, 752–755. [CrossRef] [PubMed]
78. McBride, J.A.; Kohn, T.P.; Mazur, D.J.; Lipshultz, L.I.; Coward, R.M. Sperm retrieval and intracytoplasmic sperm injection outcomes in men with cystic fibrosis disease versus congenital bilateral absence of the vas deferens. *Asian J. Androl.* **2021**, *23*, 140–145. [CrossRef] [PubMed]
79. Hayon, S.; Moustafa, S.; Boylan, C.; Kohn, T.P.; Peavey, M.; Coward, R.M. Surgically Extracted Epididymal Sperm from Men with Obstructive Azoospermia Results in Similar In Vitro Fertilization/Intracytoplasmic Sperm Injection Outcomes Compared with Normal Ejaculated Sperm. *J. Urol.* **2021**, *205*, 561–567. [CrossRef]
80. Sussman, E.M.; Chudnovsky, A.; Niederberger, C.S. Hormonal evaluation of the infertile male: Has it evolved? *Urol. Clin. N. Am.* **2008**, *35*, 147–155. [CrossRef] [PubMed]
81. Bobjer, J.; Naumovska, M.; Giwercman, Y.L.; Giwercman, A. High prevalence of androgen deficiency and abnormal lipid profile in infertile men with non-obstructive azoospermia. *Int. J. Androl.* **2012**, *35*, 688–694. [CrossRef]

82. Ramaswamy, S.; Weinbauer, G.F. Endocrine control of spermatogenesis: Role of FSH and LH/testosterone. *Spermatogenesis* **2015**, *4*, e996105. [CrossRef]
83. Shiraishi, K.; Matsuyama, H. Gonadotoropin actions on spermatogenesis and hormonal therapies for spermatogenic disorders. *Endocr. J.* **2017**, *64*, 123–131. [CrossRef]
84. Laursen, R.J.; Elbaek, H.O.; Povlsen, B.B.; Lykkegaard, J.; Jensen, K.B.S.; Esteves, S.C.; Humaidan, P. Hormonal stimulation of spermatogenesis: A new way to treat the infertile male with non-obstructive azoospermia? *Int. Urol. Nephrol.* **2019**, *51*, 453–456. [CrossRef]
85. Caroppo, E.; Colpi, G.M. Hormonal Treatment of Men with Nonobstructive Azoospermia: What Does the Evidence Suggest? *J. Clin. Med.* **2021**, *10*, 387. [CrossRef] [PubMed]
86. Reifsnyder, J.E.; Ramasamy, R.; Husseini, J.; Schlegel, P.N. Role of optimizing testosterone before microdissection testicular sperm extraction in men with nonobstructive azoospermia. *J. Urol.* **2012**, *188*, 532–536. [CrossRef] [PubMed]
87. Ramasamy, R.; Ricci, J.A.; Palermo, G.D.; Gosden, L.V.; Rosenwaks, Z.; Schlegel, P.N. Successful fertility treatment for Klinefelter's syndrome. *J. Urol.* **2009**, *182*, 1108–1113. [CrossRef] [PubMed]
88. Hussein, A.; Ozgok, Y.; Ross, L.; Rao, P.; Niederberger, C. Optimization of spermatogenesis-regulating hormones in patients with non-obstructive azoospermia and its impact on sperm retrieval: A multicentre study. *BJU Int.* **2013**, *111*, E110–E114. [CrossRef] [PubMed]
89. Shinjo, E.; Shiraishi, K.; Matsuyama, H. The effect of human chorionic gonadotropin-based hormonal therapy on intratesticular testosterone levels and spermatogonial DNA synthesis in men with non-obstructive azoospermia. *Andrology* **2013**, *1*, 929–935. [CrossRef]
90. Foresta, C.; Bettella, A.; Spolaore, D.; Merico, M.; Rossato, M.; Ferlin, A. Suppression of the high endogenous levels of plasma FSH in infertile men are associated with improved Sertoli cell function as reflected by elevated levels of plasma inhibin B. *Hum. Reprod.* **2004**, *19*, 1431–1437. [CrossRef]
91. Themmen, A.P.; Blok, L.J.; Post, M.; Baarends, W.M.; Hoogerbrugge, J.W.; Parmentier, M.; Vassart, G.; Grootegoed, J.A. Follitropin receptor down-regulation involves a cAMP-dependent post-transcriptional decrease of receptor mRNA expression. *Mol. Cell Endocrinol.* **1991**, *78*, R7–R13. [CrossRef]
92. Gnanaprakasam, M.S.; Chen, C.J.; Sutherland, J.G.; Bhalla, V.K. Receptor depletion and replenishment processes: In vivo regulation of gonadotropin receptors by luteinizing hormone, follicle stimulating hormone and ethanol in rat testis. *Biol. Reprod.* **1979**, *20*, 991–1000. [CrossRef]
93. Namiki, M.; Nakamura, M.; Okuyama, A.; Sonoda, T.; Itatani, H.; Sugao, H.; Sakurai, T.; Nishimune, Y.; Matsumoto, K. Reduction of human and rat testicular follicle stimulating hormone receptors by human menopausal gonadotrophin in vivo and in vitro. *Clin. Endocrinol.* **1987**, *26*, 675–684. [CrossRef] [PubMed]
94. Namiki, M.; Okuyama, A.; Sonoda, T.; Miyake, A.; Aono, T.; Matsumoto, K. Down-regulation of testicular follicle-stimulating hormone receptors by human menopausal gonadotropin in infertile men. *Fertil. Steril.* **1985**, *44*, 710–712. [CrossRef]
95. Zhang, S.; Li, W.; Zhu, C.; Wang, X.; Li, Z.; Zhang, J.; Zhao, J.; Hu, J.; Li, T.; Zhang, Y. Sertoli cell-specific expression of metastasis-associated protein 2 (MTA2) is required for transcriptional regulation of the follicle-stimulating hormone receptor (FSHR) gene during spermatogenesis. *J. Biol. Chem.* **2012**, *287*, 40471–40483. [CrossRef] [PubMed]

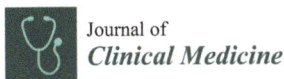

Review

Genetic Factors of Non-Obstructive Azoospermia: Consequences on Patients' and Offspring Health

Csilla Krausz * and Francesca Cioppi

Department of Experimental and Clinical Sciences "Mario Serio", University of Florence, 50139 Florence, Italy; francesca.cioppi@unifi.it
* Correspondence: csilla.krausz@unifi.it

Abstract: Non-Obstructive Azoospermia (NOA) affects about 1% of men in the general population and is characterized by clinical heterogeneity implying the involvement of several different acquired and genetic factors. NOA men are at higher risk to be carriers of known genetic anomalies such as karyotype abnormalities and Y-chromosome microdeletions in respect to oligo-normozoospermic men. In recent years, a growing number of novel monogenic causes have been identified through Whole Exome Sequencing (WES). Genetic testing is useful for diagnostic and pre-TESE prognostic purposes as well as for its potential relevance for general health. Several epidemiological observations show a link between azoospermia and higher morbidity and mortality rate, suggesting a common etiology for NOA and some chronic diseases, including cancer. Since on average 50% of NOA patients has a positive TESE outcome, the identification of genetic factors in NOA patients has relevance also to the offspring's health. Although still debated, the observed increased risk of certain neurodevelopmental disorders, as well as impaired cardiometabolic and reproductive health profile in children conceived with ICSI from NOA fathers may indicate the involvement of transmissible genetic factors. This review provides an update on the reproductive and general health consequences of known genetic factors causing NOA, including offspring's health.

Keywords: azoospermia; infertility; genetics; exome; WES; Y chromosome; cancer; NOA; genes; general health; ICSI; offspring health

Citation: Krausz, C.; Cioppi, F. Genetic Factors of Non-Obstructive Azoospermia: Consequences on Patients' and Offspring Health. *J. Clin. Med.* **2021**, *10*, 4009. https://doi.org/10.3390/jcm10174009

Academic Editor: Giovanni M. Colpi

Received: 30 July 2021
Accepted: 31 August 2021
Published: 5 September 2021

Publisher's Note: MDPI stays neutral with regard to jurisdictional claims in published maps and institutional affiliations.

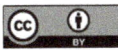

Copyright: © 2021 by the authors. Licensee MDPI, Basel, Switzerland. This article is an open access article distributed under the terms and conditions of the Creative Commons Attribution (CC BY) license (https://creativecommons.org/licenses/by/4.0/).

1. Introduction

Azoospermia (absence of spermatozoa in the ejaculate) is a relatively frequent cause of infertility occurring in about 1–2% of men in the general population. Its origin can be congenital or acquired and can be divided into: (i) hypothalamic–pituitary axis dysfunction, (ii) primary quantitative spermatogenic disturbances, and (iii) urogenital duct obstruction causing obstructive azoospermia (OA), including anatomic and genetic (e.g., *CFTR* mutation causes) [1]. While central hypogonadism is a rare etiology of Non-Obstructive Azoospermia (NOA), accounting for approximately 5% of cases, primary testicular failure is responsible for the large majority of azoospermia (>75%) [2].

NOA is a symptom which can be the consequence of different types of testicular failure such as: (i) Sertoli-Cell-Only Syndrome (SCOS), (ii) Maturation Arrest (MA) at different stages of germ cell maturation (such as Spermatogonial and Spermatocyte Arrest (SGA, SCA)), (iii) hypospermatogenesis; (iv) mixed forms. Similar to histology, follicle-stimulating hormone (FSH) and luteinizing hormone (LH) levels, testis volume, and degree of androgenization can vary among NOA men. This intrinsic clinical heterogeneity implies the involvement of several different acquired and congenital genetic factors. The known genetic factors underlying the NOA phenotype account for almost 30% of cases and include primarily chromosomal abnormalities (such as 47, XXY Klinefelter syndrome and 46, XX male), followed by Y-chromosome microdeletions and monogenic defects. Three comprehensive reviews on this topic were recently published providing a complete list of NOA-related genetic factors [3–5]. NOA is receiving a growing attention, not only because it is the most severe infertility phenotype but also because epidemiological observations show a link between azoospermia and a higher incidence of morbidity and lower life expectancy [6–14] (Table 1).

Table 1. List of studies reporting increased mortality and/or morbidity in azoospermic men.

Increased Mortality Rate (HR)	Increased Morbidity Rate (Yes/No)	Reference
n.a.	Yes *	[8]
2.29, 95% CI: 1.12–4.65	n.a.	[9]
n.a.	Yes **	[11]
3.66, 95% CI: 2.18–6.16	n.a.	[13]
2.01, 95% CI: 1.60–2.53	n.a.	[14]

HR: Hazard Ratio; n.a.: not available; * Cancer risk (HR = 2.9, 95% CI:1.4–5.4); ** The top three related-conditions are: (i) renal disease (HR = 2.26, 95% CI:1.20–4.27), (ii) alcohol abuse (HR = 1.94, 95% CI:1.11–3.39), (iii) depression (HR = 1.45, 95% CI:1.13–1.85).

It is worth noting that a 10-fold increased risk of hypogonadism among azoospermic men has been reported [15], which by itself can be linked to adverse health outcomes, i.e., higher risks of metabolic syndrome [16], cardiovascular disease [17], rheumatic autoimmune diseases [18] and overall mortality [16]. In addition, a significantly increased risk of developing testis cancer in infertile men has been well-documented [19,20]. In particular, men with azoospermia present a 2.9 times higher risk to develop cancer in respect to the general population [8].

Following the above observations, semen phenotype has been proposed as a biomarker of general health [12,13,19,21]. Since on average 50% of NOA patients will have a positive Testicular Sperm Extraction (TESE) outcome, the routine testing for known genetic anomalies has relevance not only for the carrier but also for his future child. Elucidating the genetic causes underlying azoospermia would allow improving the management of patients, identifying those azoospermic men who are unlikely to have testicular spermatozoa, those who are at higher risk for general health problems and would also have an impact on the health of their descendants (Figure 1).

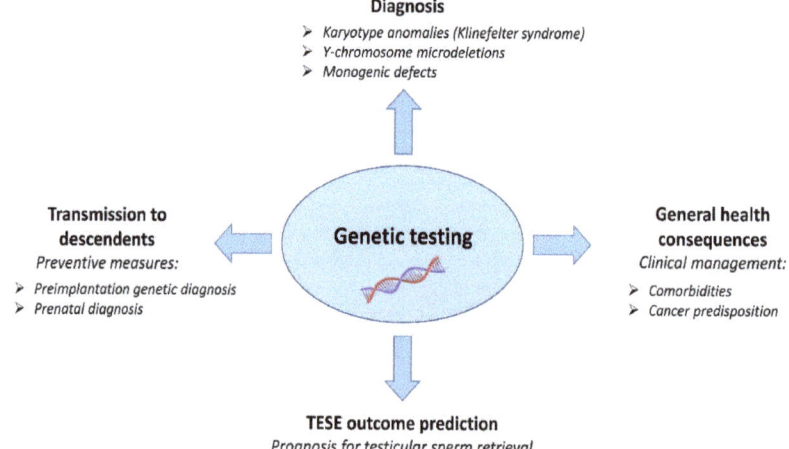

Figure 1. Clinical relevance of genetic testing in azoospermic men.

This review focuses on the reproductive and general health consequences of known genetic factors causing NOA including offspring's health.

2. Consequences of Chromosomal Anomalies

2.1. Klinefelter Syndrome (47,XXY)

Is the most common genetic disorder causing NOA, which is characterized by the presence of an extra X chromosome. Its prevalence is 0.1–0.2% in newborn male infants, and it increases in relation to the age of diagnosis. Its frequency has been estimated as 3–4% among infertile males and 10–12% in azoospermic subjects [22,23]. The severity of the clinical phenotype of KS males may vary, and testosterone level, number of CAG repeats in the androgen receptor and/or supernumerary X chromosome could be involved in the clinical signs/symptoms of KS [24].

Reproductive consequences: the sex chromosome aneuploidy leads to a progressive deterioration of the testicular tissue and both the germinal epithelium and testosterone-producing Leydig cells are affected. There is a progressive deposition of ialine, which is responsible for the typical hard consistency of the testes. Azoospermia is present in about 95% of KS patients [25]. However, very rarely, non-mosaic KS patients can have spermatozoa in their ejaculate, leading to spontaneous pregnancy. The success rate for the recovery of spermatozoa through microsurgical TESE (m-TESE) in KS men is 34–44% [26]. As for other NOA patients, also in this case, the fertility status of the female partner is essential for achieving pregnancy through Intracytoplasmic Sperm Injection (ICSI). A growing number of KS patients are diagnosed during their fetal life, through pre-natal genetic diagnosis. This novel trend raises the issue about the correct management of these patients during their transition period from childhood to adulthood [23]. There are still debated questions such as the right timing for testosterone replacement therapy (for its potential interference with residual spermatogenesis) and m-TESE in young post-pubertal KS boys [27,28].

General health consequences: besides azoospermia, a wide spectrum of clinical manifestations including several comorbidities are present, i.e., metabolic syndrome, type 2 diabetes mellitus, anaemia, cardiovascular diseases (ischemic heart disease, deep vein thrombosis, lung embolism), osteopenia/osteoporosis, breast cancer, extra-gonadal germ cell tumours, non-Hodgkin lymphoma, haematological cancers and some autoimmune diseases and psychiatric disorders [23,25,29,30]. Part of the above pathological conditions are the consequence of impaired testosterone production (e.g., metabolic syndrome, osteopenia/osteoporosis), others may be due to X-linked gene dosage effect or epigenetic factors [3]. Given the complexity of this disease, patients care in dedicated multidisciplinary centres is advocated [23,31].

Consequences on offspring's health: it is expected that spermatozoa from KS subjects are likely to be originated from euploid spermatogonia, i.e., the testis shows a mosaic condition where the majority of tubules contains 46,XXY spermatogonia while in a few of them spermatogonia carry a normal chromosomal asset (46,XY) [32]. Accordingly, data in the literature do not show an increased risk of having a KS child compared to infertile men with normal karyotype [32]. In fact, more than 200 healthy offspring were born worldwide from KS fathers and only a few cases of 47,XXY fetus/newborns were reported [33–35]. Despite the encouraging data that KS offspring seem not to be affected by the genetic disease of the father, it remains still an open question whether Preimplantation Genetic Diagnosis (PGD) or pre-natal genetic analyses should be recommended [23].

2.2. 46,XX Testicular/ovo-Testicular Disorder of Sex Development (DSD)

Also known as 46,XX male, referring to a rare, heterogeneous clinical condition with an incidence of about 1:20,000–25,000 male newborns [36,37]. The phenotype is largely dependent on the presence or absence of the master gene of male sex determination (SRY), mapping to the short arm of Y chromosome.

Reproductive consequences: due to the lack of Y chromosome linked AZF regions, which are essential for physiological spermatogenesis, all patients with this genetic anomaly are azoospermic. In addition, the gonadal development may be affected.

General health: apart from NOA, additional features characterize these patients. Testosterone levels may range from normal to low with increased FSH and LH levels leading to the progressive development of hypogonadism [37,38]. Short stature, due to the absence of growth-regulation genes on the Y chromosome, is also a relatively common finding.

Consequences on offspring's health: the chance to find spermatozoa in the testes of a 46,XX male with sperm harvesting methods is zero. If the couple desires to have children, sperm donation is the only viable option, or adoption.

3. Consequences of Y-Chromosome Microdeletions

The loss of specific chromosomal sequences on the long arm of the Y (Yq) is a the most frequent molecular genetic cause of NOA [39]. The so called AZoospermia Factor (AZF) regions [40,41] contain genes involved in spermatogenesis and their removal causes different reproductive phenotypes. Many AZF genes are multicopy genes and most of them are involved in post-transcriptional and post-translational control in germ cells [42]. The AZF regions are surrounded by highly homologous repeated sequences with the same direction, representing an optimal substrate for Non-Allelic Homologous Recombination (NAHR) leading to deletions. The frequency of AZF deletions in the general population is 1:4000 but in NOA patients it can be as high as 7–10% [39,43]. The most frequently affected region is the AZFc region accounting for >60% of deletions. Due to the peculiar structure of this region, with many potential NAHR substrates, partial deletions with different breakpoints may occur at a relatively high frequency [44]. Among them, the gr/gr deletion, removing half of the AZFc gene content, is considered a proven genetic risk factor for oligozoospermia [45].

Reproductive consequences: depending on which type of AZF regions is removed, the semen phenotype can be azoospermia or severe oligozoospermia [39]. The complete removal of the AZFa region (approximately 792 kb) causes SCOS, whereas the complete removal of the AZFb deletion (with the extension marker sY1192 absent) leads to meiotic arrest [46]. In both conditions the probability of finding testicular spermatozoa through TESE is virtually zero. The complete removal of the AZFc is associated with a highly variable phenotype, ranging from the complete absence of germ cells in the testis (SCOS) to severe oligozoospermia. The TESE success rate in these patients is around 50%, but it is highly variable in different reports.

General health: haploinsufficiency of the *SHOX* gene, located in the pseudoautosomal region PAR1 of the Y chromosome, has been reported by Jorgez and colleagues in men with AZF microdeletion and normal karyotype [47]. The authors proposed that AZF deletion carriers are at higher risk for incurring SHOX-haploinsufficiency, which is responsible for short stature and skeletal anomalies. This alarming finding was not confirmed in a subsequent large, multicentre study [48]. In accordance with this latter study, Castro and colleagues reported PAR abnormalities only in those AZF deletion carriers who presented concomitant karyotype anomalies (isochromosome Yp and/ or Y nullisomy) [49]. In addition to PAR abnormalities, 5/7 patients with terminal AZFbc deletion and abnormal karyotype presented neuropsychiatric disorders. The authors hypothesize that CNVs in the pseudoautosomal regions (PARs) and/or the removal of MSY genes (some of them are expressed also in the brain) may play a role in the observed neuropsychiatric disorders [49]. However, the association between neuropsychiatric disorders and terminal AZFbc deletions needs further confirmation especially in view of the lack of such neurodevelopmental disorders in 46,XX males [37].

Consequences on offspring's health: complete AZFc and partial AZFa or AZFb deletions are compatible with the presence of spermatozoa in the ejaculate or in the testis, therefore these patients will obligatorily transmit the deletion to their male descendants. Recent meta-analysis reported a reduced fertilization rate, but a similar clinical pregnancy rate, miscarriage rate, live birth rate and baby boy rate to those couple where the male partner did not carry AZF deletions [50]. It is expected that the semen phenotype of the son will be either azoospermia or oligozoospermia, however the exact semen phenotype is not predictable, since the genetic background and exposure to environmental factors may modulate the phenotypic expression of AZFc deletions. Some studies reported an association between Yq microdeletions and an overall Y-chromosomal instability, which might result in the formation of 45,X0 bearing spermatozoa [51,52]. This finding is in accordance with the relatively high incidence of AZF deletion in patients bearing a mosaic 46,XY/45,X0 karyotype with sexual ambiguity and/or Turner stigmata [53–56]. The PGD has been performed by two groups with conflicting data about the risk of monosomy X in embryos [57,58]. The limited data on children born from AZF deletion carriers show that they are apparently healthy [59].

4. Consequences of Monogenic Defects

Known monogenic anomalies with definitive clinical evidence are relatively rare in NOA [3]. Among them two *X-linked* genes reached diagnostic relevance: the *AR* and the *TEX11* genes.

4.1. AR Gene

The androgen receptor (AR) is a DNA-binding transcription factor, which is critical for several biological functions including male sex development. Upon binding of testosterone to the cytoplasmic AR, the complex translocates into the nucleus and binds to the regulatory regions of specific chromosomal DNA sequences to activate androgen dependent genes. Mutations in *AR* gene are responsible for the androgen insensitivity syndrome (AIS), with an estimated prevalence of 1:20,000 to 1:64,000 live male births [60]. This condition is associated with a high variety of phenotypes, ranging from complete androgen insensitivity (CAIS) with a female phenotype (Morris syndrome) to milder degrees of undervirilization (partial form or PAIS; Refenstein syndrome) or men with only infertility (mild form or MAIS) [61]. Beside pathogenic mutations in the coding exons of the *AR* causing AIS, a polymorphic CAG repeat in exon 1 has a functional effect on the receptor's activity. The number of the CAG repeats is inversely associated with the ligand-induced transactivational activity of the receptor and, in physiological conditions, (CAG)n directly correlates with serum testosterone levels [62]. This polymorphism has been associated with various androgen-dependent conditions including impaired sperm production (for review see [63]).

Reproductive consequences: in the PAIS/MAIS form of disease, patients may present with quantitative spermatogenic disturbances, i.e., azoospermia or oligozoospermia. The negative effect of longer (CAG)n on spermatogenesis is a debated issue. Although the majority of studies report a higher than average (CAG)n in infertile patients, it is not possible to define a cut-off value above which infertility risk is increased and to estimate the effect size of such a risk [63].

General health: a positive correlation between CAG repeat number and depressed mood, anxiety, and low bone mineral density with accelerated age-dependent bone loss have been reported [64,65]. Smaller CAG repeat number is associated with benign prostatic hypertrophy [66] and faster prostate growth during testosterone treatment [67]. The polymorphic range in the general population is up to 39 CAG repeats, the expansion over 39 CAG is a pathological condition leading to the Kennedy disease [68]. Kennedy disease is a rare form of X-linked spinal and bulbar muscular atrophy (SBMA), characterized by progressive neuromuscular atrophy and ataxia [69] and a progressive set up of mild androgen insensitivity associated to varying traits of hypogonadism, including gynecomastia, testicular atrophy, disorders of spermatogenesis, elevated serum gonadotropins, and diabetes mellitus [70].

Consequences on offspring's health: *AR* mutations compatible with sperm production will be obligatory transmitted to the female offspring with potential health consequences on her future male children. Concerning the (CAG)n repeats, it is worth noting that repeat expansions are inherently dynamic, often changing size when transmitted to the next generation [71]. This phenomenon, known as clinical anticipation, explains the tendency for disease severity to increase in successive generations of a family. Patients affected by Kennedy's disease may conceive their own biological children and, similarly to *AR* mutations, the expanded CAG repeats will be transmitted to the female child, who can generate a male offspring affected by Kennedy disease. As far as the polymorphic range of CAG repeats (up to 39 CAG) is concerned, the proposed relationship between longer CAG tract and male infertility indicates a theoretical higher risk for oligozoospermic men to conceive a female child presenting a pathological expansion of CAG repeats leading to a future son with Kennedy disease [60,71].

4.2. TEX11 Gene

This gene belongs to the family of Testis Expressed genes, and it is crucial for chromosome synapsis and formation of crossovers during meiosis. By using high-resolution array-Comparative Genomic Hybridization (a-CGH) to screen men with NOA, a recurring deletion of three exons of *TEX11* in two patients has been identified [72]. Furthermore, by sequencing *TEX11* in larger groups of azoospermic men, more disease-causing mutations were detected [72–75]. Overall, mutations in *TEX11* were identified in more than 1% of azoospermic men and in as many as 15% of patients with meiotic arrest.

Reproductive consequences: recessive mutations in this gene lead to NOA due to MA [72–74]. Very recently, Krausz and colleagues demonstrated that defects in the human gene showed a complete metaphase arrest, suggested by a residual spermatocytic development together with the dramatic increase in the number of apoptotic metaphases [75].

General health: apart from NOA, no additional features have been reported in mutated men.

Consequences on offspring's health: the chance to find mature spermatozoa in the testes of a man carrying loss of function *TEX11* mutations is virtually zero. If the couple desires to have children, sperm donation is the only viable option, or adoption.

4.3. Shared Genes between Spermatogenesis and Tumorigenesis

As stated in the introduction, an increased risk of various cancers has been documented in NOA patients which in part may be due to defects in biological pathways regulating genomic integrity [8,21,76–80]. It is plausible that spermatogenesis and tumorigenesis may share common genetic factors, especially those involved in stem cell renewal/differentiation, mismatch repair mechanisms and apoptosis. Particularly, germline alterations in DNA repair genes, which are fundamental for maintaining the genomic integrity and stability in the early stages of the male germline, may confer hereditable predisposition to impaired spermatogenesis and cancer.

Recent studies integrating omics and literature search revealed a significant genetic overlap between male infertility and particular types of cancer, including urologic neoplasms/carcinomas and B cell lymphoma [81,82]. By using mouse model data such as Mouse Genome Informatics (MGI) database, the integration of human orthologues to mouse male factor infertility with a curated list of known cancer genes (COSMIC genes) has identified 25 candidate genes that may confer risk of experiencing both conditions in humans [21]. In particular, there is a five-fold enrichment of COSMIC genes in the MGI male infertility list compared with genes that are not on the MGI list, suggesting that this overlap is highly non-random [21].

Apart from the bioinformatics models and epidemiological observations, there is a growing number of genes predisposing to cancer, which have been found mutated in men affected by NOA.

4.3.1. Rare Pathogenic Mutations

A recent example is related to *FANCA* mutations, which may cause both the classic early onset and the rarely observed late-onset Fanconi Anaemia (FA). Both manifestations are characterized by genomic instability leading to progressive bone marrow failure, congenital malformations and predisposition to typical cancers such as head and neck squamous cell carcinoma and leukaemia [83]. By performing exome analysis in NOA patients, Krausz and colleagues (2019), identified three subjects affected by SCOS with biallelic *FANCA* mutations [79]. All three subjects were unaware about having Fanconi anaemia, although two of them showed slightly abnormal blood cell count at the time of the genetic diagnosis. This study was the first in the literature reporting the accidental finding of Late onset FA (occult FA) in the absence of severe comorbidities of FA. In fact, occult FA is usually diagnosed in subjects following the diagnosis of typical malignancies. The three patients are now under surveillance by oncohematologists. This paper showed the importance of checking blood count, especially in patients presenting idiopathic SCOS, since the combined phenotype of SCOS with borderline low blood cell count indicates a higher risk for occult FA. Given that the carrier frequency of *FANCA* defects is relatively rare in the general population, pre-ICSI screening in the female partners of male carriers is not recommended. However, in case of consanguinity in the couple PGD should be offered given the severity of FA.

Fanconi anaemia and related malignancies can also be caused by recessive mutations in the *XRCC2* gene [84]. Interestingly, a homozygous *XRCC2* mutation has been reported in a consanguineous family causing isolated meiotic arrest without cancer predisposition [85]. This observation leads the authors to conclude that meiosis-specific mutations may exist when the linker region of XRCC2, essential for protein–protein interactions, is affected [85,86]. In support of this, knock-in mice carrying the same *XRCC2* mutation exhibited only meiotic arrest, leading to azoospermia in males and premature ovarian failure in females [85].

Another member of the FA pathway, *FANCM*, involved in DNA double-strand breaks (DSB) repair, was reported as the cause of NOA [78,80]. The *FANCM* gene is significantly associated with hereditary breast and ovarian cancers [87], in line with published data on female homozygous knock-out (KO) mice [88,89]. Recessive mutations in this gene seem to cause a wide spectrum of seminal phenotypes, ranging from oligoasthenozoospermia to azoospermia due to SCOS [78,80].

Biallelic mutations in two other DNA DBS repair genes, *MCM8* and *TEX15* were reported in azoospermia and oligo/crypto/azoospermia, respectively [90–93]. Very recently, germline mutations in the *MCM8* gene following a recessive pattern of inheritance, were detected in cancer patients [94]. One male patient affected by Lynch syndrome with fertility problems and two patients affected by breast cancer were found to be carriers of biallelic *MCM8* mutations, suggesting a role of this gene in the germline predisposition to breast cancer and hereditary colorectal cancer (CRC) [94]. Concerning *TEX15*, a rare heterozygous mutation predicted as deleterious by four bioinformatics tools was found to be significantly associated with prostate cancer risk [95].

Also the *X-linked WNK3* gene, involved in cell signalling, survival and proliferation has been linked both to NOA and cancer [96]. A *WNK3* mutation has been found to co-segregate with NOA due to SCOS in a family from Oman [97]. Concerning the role of this gene in oncology, several *WNK3* mutations in patient-derived xenografts of colorectal cancer liver metastasis were predicted to be deleterious, which might contribute to the initiation and progression of distant metastasis [98].

4.3.2. Genetic Polymorphisms

Besides rare mutations, common polymorphisms have been reported in a total of 8 mismatch repair genes, which could account for a shared aetiology between tumorigenesis and quantitative spermatogenic failure [21].

Homozygous or compound heterozygous mutations in the *MLH1* gene have been reported in the early-onset hereditary cancer disorder Lynch syndrome, as well as in haematological malignancies and brain tumours [99], often associated with features of neurofibromatosis type 1 (NF1) syndrome [100]. Besides its known carcinogenic role, an intronic SNP in *MLH1* seem to be a risk factor for the development of azoospermia or oligozoospermia [101].

Germline *MLH3* variants have been reported in hereditary Lynch syndrome-associated brain tumours patients [102], and a common polymorphism (C2531T) in the 3′UTR of the gene has been associated with clinical outcomes of colorectal cancer, in terms of increased risks of relapse or metastasis in patients with heterozygous genotype [103]. Interestingly, Xu and colleagues have observed an increased risk of azoospermia or severe oligozoospermia associated with the above-mentioned polymorphism in 3′UTR of the *MLH3* gene [104].

MSH5 has been reported as a pleiotropic susceptibility locus for lung, prostate, colorectal and serous ovarian cancers [105,106], and several polymorphisms in this gene have been associated with quantitative spermatogenic defects [101,104]. Further, one low-frequency *MSH5* variant associated with an increased risk of NOA has been reported in Han Chinese men [107].

Biallelic germline mutations of the *PMS2* gene cause the constitutional mismatch repair deficiency, characterized by early-onset malignancies [108]. In addition, a founder heterozygous frameshift mutation in the same gene is responsible for the Lynch syndrome [109]. Concerning the role of *PMS2* gene in spermatogenesis, the presence of a common polymorphism in the gene leads to a reduced interaction of MLH1 and PMS2 proteins, which may result in impaired sperm production [101].

Carriers of mutations in the *ATM* gene have been reported to have a higher mortality rate and an earlier age at death from cancer and ischemic heart disease than non-carriers [110]. Besides this finding, germline loss-of-function *ATM* mutations seem to be enriched in men with prostate cancer and multiple primary malignancies [111]. Concerning the role of this gene in spermatogenesis, both the homozygous and heterozygous genotypes for a common variant in the *ATM* gene promoter were associated with an increased risk for idiopathic NOA [112].

Two SNPs in the *XRCC1* gene were associated with increased bladder cancer risk among Asians [113], whilst another one, the R339Q, has been implicated in susceptibility for both idiopathic azoospermia and different types of cancer, such as hepatocellular cancer in Asians and breast cancer in Indians [114–118].

An identical SNP (C8092A) in 3′UTR of the *ERCC1* gene has independently been linked to both idiopathic azoospermia and various types of cancer, including breast carcinoma, head and neck carcinoma, adult glioma [119–122].

In this context, the identification of shared genetic aetiologies between azoospermia and cancer may have a significant clinical impact, for improving patient care and genetic counselling.

5. Health Issues in ICSI Offspring from NOA Fathers

The introduction of ICSI among Assisted Reproductive Techniques (ART) has opened an unforeseen perspective for fatherhood in NOA patients. NOA men may father their own biological child by using non-ejaculated spermatozoa, retrieved by conventional or micro-TESE with an average success rate of 50%. As stated above, it is well known that NOA patients are at higher risk for genetic anomalies than he general population; therefore, concerns were raised regarding offspring's health.

Various parameters have been evaluated in ICSI children (from birth to young adulthood) born to fathers affected by spermatogenic disturbances.

Many reports describe a high frequency of chromosomal abnormalities in ICSI babies, especially of the sex chromosomes, even when peripheral chromosome studies in the parents are normal [123–125]. A possible explanation for this phenomenon could depend on the testicular tubular alteration, which may determine abnormalities in the meiotic process leading to chromosomal anomalies in the spermatozoa [126]. Therefore, other forms of chromosome diploidy beyond sex chromosomes should be expected as well [127,128]. Overall, the risk of having chromosomal abnormalities, particularly sexual chromosome aneuploidy, is approximately 1% in children conceived through ICSI, which is higher than that of naturally conceived children (~0.2%) and of those conceived with conventional in vitro fertilization (IVF) (~0.7%) (see reference in [129]). In addition, children conceived by IVF and/or ICSI are at significantly increased risk for birth defects, although no risk difference between children conceived with the two ARTs has been observed [130]. A systematic review and meta-analysis showed that congenital malformations in ICSI-conceived children when compared to naturally conceived children translates into an increased risk of 7.1% of having a malformation for individuals born after ICSI versus 4.0% for naturally conceived children [131]. The most commonly observed congenital malformation involves the genitourinary tract which is significantly more frequent in ICSI children compared to both naturally conceived children and IVF children [132,133].

Besides chromosomal and birth defects, cognitive and neurodevelopmental disorders in offspring from an ICSI father have also been evaluated [134,135]. In one study a modestly increased risk of mental retardation and autism was reported in ICSI derived children [136], but this finding was not replicated in independent studies [137–139]. The largest of these studies, involving 10,718 children conceived with ICSI, 19,445 children conceived with IVF and 2,510,166 spontaneously conceived children, observed the greatest risk of mental retardation in children conceived through ICSI (RR 2.35, 95%; CI = 1.03–2.09) [136]. Importantly, treatment factors, i.e., ICSI and embryo cryopreservation, also appear to influence this risk [136]. In addition, an increased risk of autism in children conceived with ICSI using surgically extracted sperm (RR 4.60, 95%; CI = 2.14–9.88) was also observed [136]. This finding was not confirmed by Kissin and colleagues in the group of children conceived with ICSI for male factor infertility (HR 1.23, 95%; CI = 0.92–1.64) [139]. On the other hand, the severity of male factor does not seem to influence the cognitive development in early childhood [140–142].

In addition to neurodevelopmental aspects, other long-term outcomes of children conceived via ICSI due to severe male factor have been evaluated, but findings are conflicting and it is difficult to evaluate the impact of NOA on these disorders [135]. Among the large population registry studies that have examined growth and cardiometabolic factors, there is evidence that ICSI adolescents may be at risk of increased adiposity, especially girls [143–147]. Very recently, in male ICSI adolescents significant higher estradiol and lower testosterone/estradiol ratio, as well as a tendency towards lower inhibin B levels, was found [148]. Concerning reproductive outcomes in men conceived with ICSI, there is some evidence for impaired spermatogenesis [149–151]. In fact, a Belgian study, evaluating young men in the age interval 18–22 years, found reduced semen parameters among men conceived with ICSI, reporting a median sperm count and total motile sperm count being half that of their spontaneously conceived peers [151]. In addition, ICSI men showed a tendency to have lower inhibin B levels and higher FSH levels compared with spontaneously conceived peers [151].

Despite the growing number of studies, several uncertainties remain about whether any increases in risk are due to NOA or to the ICSI procedure itself [135]. To date, the global number of babies born as a result of ART techniques, such as ICSI, is more than 8 million (ESHRE: https://www.eshre.eu/ 31 August 2021), therefore it should be of paramount importance to reach to a final conclusion on safety issues. It is expected that with the extensive use of ICSI for non-male factor, a comparison of short and long-term outcomes between ICSI children derived from male factor versus non-male factor will elucidate the impact of azoospermia on the descendant's health.

6. Conclusions

Azoospermia, the most severe form of infertility, may represent a biomarker of overall health, serving as a harbinger for higher morbidity and mortality. As reported above, certain chromosomal anomalies and gene defects underlying azoospermia can be responsible for a wide spectrum of health issues beside azoospermia, including metabolic/cardiovascular disorders, autoimmune diseases, hypogonadism, syndromic conditions and cancers. After the exclusion of all known acquired causes and after performing routine genetic testing, the etiology remains unknown in a substantial proportion of patients and it could be related to yet unidentified genetic/epigenetic factors [3]). The clinical impact of discovering such "hidden" genetic factors is important to predict not only the fertility status but also the general health of these men. For instance, by performing a-CGH analyses, a "CNV burden" (especially deletions) in idiopathic infertile patients have been reported by three research groups [152–154], suggesting a higher genomic instability potentially relevant also for general health. CNV burden together with the above listed shared monogenic factors could be one of the many possible explanations for the higher morbidity and lower life expectancy observed in infertile men in respect to fertile men [6,7,19,152]. Similarly to monogenic disorders, the inheritance of an unstable genome may also have clinical consequences on the offspring's health.

Thanks to the diffusion of Whole Exome Sequencing (WES) in the frame of fruitful international collaborations, the number of genes involved in NOA is rapidly increasing [3,5,155]. Exome analysis has proven to be very efficient in diagnosing the cause of meiotic arrest [75], with potential implications for TESE prognosis. WES allowed the identification of many novel genes, potentially relevant also for tumorigenesis. It can be hypothesized that inherited genetic/epigenetic factors are responsible for the increased risk of certain neurodevelopmental disorders, as well as impaired cardiometabolic and reproductive health profile in children conceived with ICSI from NOA fathers. In this context, the discovery of genetic cause underlying azoospermia would allow not only to improve the management of NOA patients, but also to predict the clinical consequences on the offspring inheriting the certain gene defect(s) (Figure 1).

While the list of genetic defects with potential impact on general health increases, it is important to note that apart from a few exceptions, we are still missing a direct evidence for a clear-cut genetic link between NOA and higher morbidity, especially in terms of cancer predisposition. Multicentre efforts are needed in order to collect long-term follow-up data on large groups of genetically well-characterized NOA patients. Apart from the routine karyotype and Y chromosome deletion analysis, we hope that WES analysis will become soon part of the genetic diagnostic work-up of NOA patients allowing diagnosis, TESE prognosis and prevention for general health.

Author Contributions: C.K. conceived the manuscript. C.K. and F.C. designed and wrote the manuscript. Both authors have read and agreed to the published version of the manuscript.

Funding: The publication of this review article was supported by Next Fertility Procrea, Lugano, Switzerland.

Institutional Review Board Statement: Not applicable.

Informed Consent Statement: Not applicable.

Data Availability Statement: Not applicable.

Conflicts of Interest: The authors declare no conflict of interest.

References

1. Tournaye, H.; Krausz, C.; Oates, R.D. Novel concepts in the aetiology of male reproductive impairment. *Lancet Diabetes Endocrinol.* **2017**, *5*, 544–553. [CrossRef]
2. Krausz, C.; Riera-Escamilla, A. Genetics of male infertility. *Nat. Rev. Urol.* **2018**, *15*, 369–384. [CrossRef] [PubMed]
3. Cioppi, F.; Rosta, V.; Krausz, C. Genetics of Azoospermia. *Int. J. Mol. Sci.* **2021**, *22*, 3264. [CrossRef]
4. Kasak, L.; Laan, M. Monogenic causes of non-obstructive azoospermia: Challenges, established knowledge, limitations and perspectives. *Hum. Genet.* **2021**, *140*, 135–154. [CrossRef]

5. Capalbo, A.; Poli, M.; Riera-Escamilla, A.; Shukla, V.; Høffding, M.K.; Krausz, C.; Hoffmann, E.R.; Simon, C. Preconception genome medicine: Current state and future perspectives to improve infertility diagnosis and reproductive and health outcomes based on individual genomic data. *Hum. Reprod. Update* 2021, 27, 254–279. [CrossRef] [PubMed]
6. Jensen, T.K.; Jacobsen, R.; Christensen, K.; Nielsen, N.C.; Bostofte, E. Good Semen Quality and Life Expectancy: A Cohort Study of 43,277 Men. *Am. J. Epidemiol.* 2009, 170, 559–565. [CrossRef] [PubMed]
7. Salonia, A.; Matloob, R.; Gallina, A.; Abdollah, F.; Saccà, A.; Briganti, A.; Suardi, N.; Colombo, R.; Rocchini, L.; Guazzoni, G.; et al. Are Infertile Men Less Healthy than Fertile Men? Results of a Prospective Case-Control Survey. *Eur. Urol.* 2009, 56, 1025–1032. [CrossRef]
8. Eisenberg, M.L.; Betts, P.; Herder, D.; Lamb, D.J.; Lipshultz, L.I. Increased risk of cancer among azoospermic men. *Fertil. Steril.* 2013, 100, 681–685.e1. [CrossRef]
9. Eisenberg, M.L.; Li, S.; Behr, B.; Cullen, M.R.; Galusha, D.; Lamb, D.J.; Lipshultz, L.I. Semen quality, infertility and mortality in the USA. *Hum. Reprod.* 2014, 29, 1567–1574. [CrossRef]
10. Ventimiglia, E.; Capogrosso, P.; Boeri, L.; Serino, A.; Colicchia, M.; Ippolito, S.; Scano, R.; Papaleo, E.; Damiano, R.; Montorsi, F.; et al. Infertility as a proxy of general male health: Results of a cross-sectional survey. *Fertil. Steril.* 2015, 104, 48–55. [CrossRef]
11. Eisenberg, M.L.; Shufeng, L.; Cullen, M.R.; Baker, L.C. Increased risk of incident chronic medical conditions in infertile men: Analysis of United States claims data. *Fertil. Steril.* 2016, 105, 629–636. [CrossRef] [PubMed]
12. Choy, J.T.; Eisenberg, M.L. Male infertility as a window to health. *Fertil. Steril.* 2018, 110, 810–814. [CrossRef] [PubMed]
13. Glazer, C.H.; Eisenberg, M.L.; Tøttenborg, S.S.; Giwercman, A.; Flachs, E.M.; Bräuner, E.V.; Vassard, D.; Pinborg, A.; Schmidt, L.; Bonde, J.P. Male factor infertility and risk of death: A nationwide record-linkage study. *Hum. Reprod.* 2019, 34, 2266–2273. [CrossRef] [PubMed]
14. Del Giudice, F.; Kasman, A.M.; Li, S.; Belladelli, F.; Ferro, M.; de Cobelli, O.; De Bernardinis, E.; Busetto, G.M.; Eisenberg, M.L. Increased Mortality among Men Diagnosed with Impaired Fertility: Analysis of US Claims Data. *Urology* 2021, 147, 143–149. [CrossRef]
15. Bobjer, J.; Naumovska, M.; Giwercman, Y.L.; Giwercman, A. High prevalence of androgen deficiency and abnormal lipid profile in infertile men with non-obstructive azoospermia. *Int. J. Androl.* 2012, 35, 688–694. [CrossRef] [PubMed]
16. Ferlin, A.; Garolla, A.; Ghezzi, M.; Selice, R.; Pelago, P.; Caretta, N.; Di Mambro, A.; Valente, U.; De Rocco Ponce, M.; Dipresa, S.; et al. Sperm Count and Hypogonadism as Markers of General Male Health. *Eur. Urol. Focus* 2021, 7, 205–213. [CrossRef] [PubMed]
17. Corona, G.; Rastrelli, G.; Vignozzi, L.; Mannucci, E.; Maggi, M. Testosterone, cardiovascular disease and the metabolic syndrome. *Best Pract. Res. Clin. Endocrinol. Metab.* 2011, 25, 337–353. [CrossRef]
18. Baillargeon, J.; Al Snih, S.; Raji, M.A.; Urban, R.J.; Sharma, G.; Sheffield-Moore, M.; Lopez, D.S.; Baillargeon, G.; Kuo, Y.F. Hypogonadism and the risk of rheumatic autoimmune disease. *Clin. Rheumatol.* 2016, 35, 2983–2987. [CrossRef]
19. Eisenberg, M.L.; Li, S.; Brooks, J.D.; Cullen, M.R.; Baker, L.C. Increased Risk of Cancer in Infertile Men: Analysis of U.S. Claims Data. *J. Urol.* 2015, 193, 1596–1601. [CrossRef]
20. Del Giudice, F.; Kasman, A.M.; Ferro, M.; Sciarra, A.; De Bernardinis, E.; Belladelli, F.; Salonia, A.; Eisenberg, M.L. Clinical correlation among male infertility and overall male health: A systematic review of the literature. *Investig. Clin. Urol.* 2020, 61, 355–371. [CrossRef]
21. Nagirnaja, L.; Aston, K.I.; Conrad, D.F. Genetic intersection of male infertility and cancer. *Fertil. Steril.* 2018, 109, 20–26. [CrossRef] [PubMed]
22. Vloeberghs, V.; Verheyen, G.; Santos-Ribeiro, S.; Staessen, C.; Verpoest, W.; Gies, I.; Tournaye, H. Is genetic fatherhood within reach for all azoospermic Klinefelter men? *PLoS ONE* 2018, 13, e0200300. [CrossRef]
23. Zitzmann, M.; Aksglaede, L.; Corona, G.; Isidori, A.M.; Juul, A.; T'Sjoen, G.; Kliesch, S.; D'Hauwers, K.; Toppari, J.; Słowikowska-Hilczer, J.; et al. European academy of andrology guidelines on Klinefelter Syndrome Endorsing Organization: European Society of Endocrinology. *Andrology* 2021, 9, 145–167. [CrossRef]
24. Visootsak, J.; Graham, J.M. Klinefelter syndrome and other sex chromosomal aneuploidies. *Orphanet J. Rare Dis.* 2006, 1, 42. [CrossRef] [PubMed]
25. Gravholt, C.H.; Chang, S.; Wallentin, M.; Fedder, J.; Moore, P.; Skakkebæk, A. Klinefelter syndrome: Integrating genetics, neuropsychology, and endocrinology. *Endocr. Rev.* 2018, 39, 389–423. [CrossRef]
26. Corona, G.; Pizzocaro, A.; Lanfranco, F.; Garolla, A.; Pelliccione, F.; Vignozzi, L.; Ferlin, A.; Foresta, C.; Jannini, E.A.; Maggi, M.; et al. Sperm recovery and ICSI outcomes in Klinefelter syndrome: A systematic review and meta-analysis. *Hum. Reprod. Update* 2017, 23, 265–275. [CrossRef] [PubMed]
27. Rohayem, J.; Nieschlag, E.; Zitzmann, M.; Kliesch, S. Testicular function during puberty and young adulthood in patients with Klinefelter's syndrome with and without spermatozoa in seminal fluid. *Andrology* 2016, 4, 1178–1186. [CrossRef] [PubMed]
28. Franik, S.; Hoeijmakers, Y.; D'Hauwers, K.; Braat, D.D.; Nelen, W.L.; Smeets, D.; Claahsen-van der Grinten, H.L.; Ramos, L.; Fleischer, K. Klinefelter syndrome and fertility: Sperm preservation should not be offered to children with Klinefelter syndrome. *Hum. Reprod.* 2016, 31, 1952–1959. [CrossRef]
29. Seminog, O.O.; Seminog, A.B.; Yeates, D.; Goldacre, M.J. Associations between Klinefelter's syndrome and autoimmune diseases: English national record linkage studies. *Autoimmunity* 2015, 48, 125–128. [CrossRef]

30. Panimolle, F.; Tiberti, C.; Granato, S.; Semeraro, A.; Gianfrilli, D.; Anzuini, A.; Lenzi, A.; Radicioni, A. Screening of endocrine organ-specific humoral autoimmunity in 47,XXY Klinefelter's syndrome reveals a significant increase in diabetes-specific immunoreactivity in comparison with healthy control men. *Endocrine* **2016**, *52*, 157–164. [CrossRef]
31. Nieschlag, E.; Ferlin, A.; Gravholt, C.H.; Gromoll, J.; Köhler, B.; Lejeune, H.; Rogol, A.D.; Wistuba, J. The Klinefelter syndrome: Current management and research challenges. *Andrology* **2016**, *4*, 545–549. [CrossRef]
32. Greco, E.; Scarselli, F.; Minasi, M.G.; Casciani, V.; Zavaglia, D.; Dente, D.; Tesarik, J.; Franco, G. Birth of 16 healthy children after ICSI in cases of nonmosaic Klinefelter syndrome. *Hum. Reprod.* **2013**, *28*, 1155–1160. [CrossRef]
33. Denschlag, D.; Tempfer, C.; Kunze, M.; Wolff, G.; Keck, C. Assisted reproductive techniques in patients with Klinefelter syndrome: A critical review. *Fertil. Steril.* **2004**, *82*, 775–779. [CrossRef]
34. Fullerton, G.; Hamilton, M.; Maheshwari, A. Should non-mosaic Klinefelter syndrome men be labelled as infertile in 2009? *Hum. Reprod.* **2010**, *25*, 588–597. [CrossRef] [PubMed]
35. Brilli, S.; Forti, G. Managing infertility in patients with Klinefelter syndrome. *Expert Rev. Endocrinol. Metab.* **2014**, *9*, 239–250. [CrossRef]
36. McElreavey, K.; Vilain, E.; Abbas, N.; Herskowitz, I.; Fellous, M. A regulatory cascade hypothesis for mammalian sex determination: SRY represses a negative regulator of male development. *Proc. Natl. Acad. Sci. USA* **1993**, *90*, 3368–3372. [CrossRef]
37. Vorona, E.; Zitzmann, M.; Gromoll, J.; Schüring, A.N.; Nieschlag, E. Clinical, endocrinological, and epigenetic features of the 46,XX male syndrome, compared with 47,XXY Klinefelter patients. *J. Clin. Endocrinol. Metab.* **2007**, *92*, 3458–3465. [CrossRef]
38. Kousta, E.; Papathanasiou, A.; Skordis, N. Sex determination and disorders of sex development according to the revised nomenclature and classification in 46,XX individuals. *Hormones* **2010**, *9*, 218–231. [CrossRef] [PubMed]
39. Krausz, C.; Hoefsloot, L.; Simoni, M.; Tüttelmann, F.; European Academy of Andrology. European Molecular Genetics Quality Network EAA/EMQN best practice guidelines for molecular diagnosis of Y-chromosomal microdeletions: State-of-the-art 2013. *Andrology* **2014**, *2*, 5–19. [CrossRef]
40. Tiepolo, L.; Zuffardi, O. Localization of factors controlling spermatogenesis in the nonfluorescent portion of the human Y chromosome long arm. *Hum. Genet.* **1976**, *34*, 119–124. [CrossRef] [PubMed]
41. Vogt, P.H.; Edelmann, A.; Kirsch, S.; Henegariu, O.; Hirschmann, P.; Kiesewetter, F.; Köhn, F.M.; Schill, W.B.; Farah, S.; Ramos, C.; et al. Human Y chromosome azoospermia factors (AZF) mapped to different subregions in Yq11. *Hum. Mol. Genet.* **1996**, *5*, 933–943. [CrossRef]
42. Skaletsky, H.; Kuroda-Kawaguchi, T.; Minx, P.J.; Cordum, H.S.; Hillier, L.; Brown, L.G.; Repping, S.; Pyntikova, T.; Ali, J.; Bieri, T.; et al. The male-specific region of the human Y chromosome is a mosaic of discrete sequence classes. *Nature* **2003**, *423*, 825–837. [CrossRef]
43. Lo Giacco, D.; Chianese, C.; Sánchez-Curbelo, J.; Bassas, L.; Ruiz, P.; Rajmil, O.; Sarquella, J.; Vives, A.; Ruiz-Castañé, E.; Oliva, R.; et al. Clinical relevance of Y-linked CNV screening in male infertility: New insights based on the 8-year experience of a diagnostic genetic laboratory. *Eur. J. Hum. Genet.* **2014**, *22*, 754–761. [CrossRef] [PubMed]
44. Rozen, S.G.; Marszalek, J.D.; Irenze, K.; Skaletsky, H.; Brown, L.G.; Oates, R.D.; Silber, S.J.; Ardlie, K.; Page, D.C. AZFc Deletions and Spermatogenic Failure: A Population-Based Survey of 20,000 Y Chromosomes. *Am. J. Hum. Genet.* **2012**, *91*, 890–896. [CrossRef] [PubMed]
45. Krausz, C.; Casamonti, E. Spermatogenic failure and the Y chromosome. *Hum. Genet.* **2017**, *136*, 637–655. [CrossRef] [PubMed]
46. Stouffs, K.; Vloeberghs, V.; Gheldof, A.; Tournaye, H.; Seneca, S. Are AZFb deletions always incompatible with sperm production? *Andrology* **2017**, *5*, 691–694. [CrossRef] [PubMed]
47. Jorgez, C.J.; Weedin, J.W.; Sahin, A.; Tannour-Louet, M.; Han, S.; Bournat, J.C.; Mielnik, A.; Cheung, S.W.; Nangia, A.K.; Schlegel, P.N.; et al. Aberrations in pseudoautosomal regions (PARs) found in infertile men with Y-chromosome microdeletions. *J. Clin. Endocrinol. Metab.* **2011**, *96*, E674–E679. [CrossRef] [PubMed]
48. Chianese, C.; Lo Giacco, D.; Tüttelmann, F.; Ferlin, A.; Ntostis, P.; Vinci, S.; Balercia, G.; Ars, E.; Ruiz-Castañé, E.; Giglio, S.; et al. Y-chromosome microdeletions are not associated with SHOX haploinsufficiency. *Hum. Reprod.* **2013**, *28*, 3155–3160. [CrossRef]
49. Castro, A.; Rodríguez, F.; Flórez, M.; López, P.; Curotto, B.; Martínez, D.; Maturana, A.; Lardone, M.C.; Palma, C.; Mericq, V.; et al. Pseudoautosomal abnormalities in terminal AZFb+c deletions are associated with isochromosomes Yp and may lead to abnormal growth and neuropsychiatric function. *Hum. Reprod.* **2017**, *32*, 465–475. [CrossRef]
50. Li, X.; Li, X.; Sun, Y.; Han, J.; Ma, H.; Sun, Y. Effect of Y Chromosome Microdeletions on the Pregnancy Outcome of Assisted Reproduction Technology: A Meta-analysis. *Reprod. Sci.* **2021**, *28*, 2413–2421. [CrossRef]
51. Siffroi, J.P.; Le Bourhis, C.; Krausz, C.; Barbaux, S.; Quintana-Murci, L.; Kanafani, S.; Rouba, H.; Bujan, L.; Bourrouillou, G.; Seifer, I.; et al. Sex chromosome mosaicism in males carrying Y chromosome long arm deletions. *Hum. Reprod.* **2000**, *15*, 2559–2562. [CrossRef]
52. Jaruzelska, J.; Korcz, A.; Wojda, A.; Jedrzejczak, P.; Bierla, J.; Surmacz, T.; Pawelczyk, L.; Page, D.C.; Kotecki, M. Mosaicism for 45,X cell line may accentuate the severity of spermatogenic defects in men with AZFc deletion. *J. Med. Genet.* **2001**, *38*, 798–802. [CrossRef]
53. Papadimas, J.; Goulis, D.G.; Giannouli, C.; Papanicolaou, A.; Tarlatzis, B.; Bontis, J.N. Ambiguous genitalia, 45,X/46,XY mosaic karyotype, and Y chromosome microdeletions in a 17-year-old man. *Fertil. Steril.* **2001**, *76*, 1261–1263. [CrossRef]

54. Papanikolaou, A.D.; Goulis, D.G.; Giannouli, C.; Gounioti, C.; Bontis, J.N.; Papadimas, J. Intratubular germ cell neoplasia in a man with ambiguous genitalia, 45,X/46,XY mosaic karyotype, and Y chromosome microdeletions. *Endocr. Pathol.* **2003**, *14*, 177–182. [CrossRef] [PubMed]
55. Patsalis, P.C.; Sismani, C.; Quintana-Murci, L.; Taleb-Bekkouche, F.; Krausz, C.; McElreavey, K. Effects of transmission of Y chromosome AZFc deletions. *Lancet* **2002**, *360*, 1222–1224. [CrossRef]
56. Patsalis, P.C.; Skordis, N.; Sismani, C.; Kousoulidou, L.; Koumbaris, G.; Eftychi, C.; Stavrides, G.; Ioulianos, A.; Kitsiou-Tzeli, S.; Galla-Voumvouraki, A.; et al. Identification of high frequency of Y chromosome deletions in patients with sex chromosome mosaicism and correlation with the clinical phenotype and Y-chromosome instability. *Am. J. Med. Genet.* **2005**, *135*, 145–149. [CrossRef] [PubMed]
57. Mateu, E.; Rodrigo, L.; Martínez, M.C.; Peinado, V.; Milán, M.; Gil-Salom, M.; Martínez-Jabaloyas, J.M.; Remohí, J.; Pellicer, A.; Rubio, C. Aneuploidies in embryos and spermatozoa from patients with Y chromosome microdeletions. *Fertil. Steril.* **2010**, *94*, 2874–2877. [CrossRef] [PubMed]
58. Stouffs, K.; Lissens, W.; Tournaye, H.; Van Steirteghem, A.; Liebaers, I. The choice and outcome of the fertility treatment of 38 couples in whom the male partner has a Yq microdeletion. *Hum. Reprod.* **2005**, *20*, 1887–1896. [CrossRef]
59. Golin, A.P.; Yuen, W.; Flannigan, R. The effects of Y chromosome microdeletions on in vitro fertilization outcomes, health abnormalities in offspring and recurrent pregnancy loss. *Transl. Androl. Urol.* **2021**, *10*, 1457–1466. [CrossRef] [PubMed]
60. Francomano, D.; Greco, E.A.; Lenzi, A.; Aversa, A. CAG repeat testing of androgen receptor polymorphism: Is this necessary for the best clinical management of hypogonadism? *J. Sex. Med.* **2013**, *10*, 2373–2381. [CrossRef]
61. Krausz, C.; Cioppi, F.; Riera-Escamilla, A. Testing for genetic contributions to infertility: Potential clinical impact. *Expert Rev. Mol. Diagn.* **2018**, *18*, 331–346. [CrossRef] [PubMed]
62. Crabbe, P.; Bogaert, V.; De Bacquer, D.; Goemaere, S.; Zmierczak, H.; Kaufman, J.M. Part of the interindividual variation in serum testosterone levels in healthy men reflects differences in androgen sensitivity and feedback set point: Contribution of the androgen receptor polyglutamine tract polymorphism. *J. Clin. Endocrinol. Metab.* **2007**, *92*, 3604–3610. [CrossRef] [PubMed]
63. Davis-Dao, C.A.; Tuazon, E.D.; Sokol, R.Z.; Cortessis, V.K. Male Infertility and Variation in CAG Repeat Length in the Androgen Receptor Gene: A Meta-analysis. *J. Clin. Endocrinol. Metab.* **2007**, *92*, 4319–4326. [CrossRef]
64. Zitzmann, M.; Brune, M.; Kornmann, B.; Gromoll, J.; von Eckardstein, S.; von Eckardstein, A.; Nieschlag, E. The CAG repeat polymorphism in the AR gene affects high density lipoprotein cholesterol and arterial vasoreactivity. *J. Clin. Endocrinol. Metab.* **2001**, *86*, 4867–4873. [CrossRef]
65. Schneider, G.; Nienhaus, K.; Gromoll, J.; Heuft, G.; Nieschlag, E.; Zitzmann, M. Sex hormone levels, genetic androgen receptor polymorphism, and anxiety in ≥50-year-old males. *J. Sex. Med.* **2011**, *8*, 3452–3464. [CrossRef]
66. Mitsumori, K.; Terai, A.; Oka, H.; Segawa, T.; Ogura, K.; Yoshida, O.; Ogawa, O. Androgen Receptor CAG Repeat Length Polymorphism in Benign Prostatic Hyperplasia (BPH): Correlation with Adenoma Growth. *Prostate* **1999**, *41*, 253–257. [CrossRef]
67. Zitzmann, M.; Depenbusch, M.; Gromoll, J.; Nieschlag, E. Prostate volume and growth in testosterone-substituted hypogonadal men are dependent on the CAG repeat polymorphism of the androgen receptor gene: A longitudinal pharmacogenetic study. *J. Clin. Endocrinol. Metab.* **2003**, *88*, 2049–2054. [CrossRef]
68. La Spada, A.R.; Wilson, E.M.; Lubahn, D.B.; Harding, A.E.; Fischbeck, K.H. Androgen receptor gene mutations in X-linked spinal and bulbar muscular atrophy. *Nature* **1991**, *352*, 77–79. [CrossRef] [PubMed]
69. Gelmann, E.P. Molecular biology of the androgen receptor. *J. Clin. Oncol.* **2002**, *20*, 3001–3015. [CrossRef]
70. Sobue, G.; Doyu, M.; Morishima, T.; Mukai, E.; Yasuda, T.; Kachi, T.; Mitsuma, T. Aberrant androgen action and increased size of tandem CAG repeat in androgen receptor gene in X-linked recessive bulbospinal neuronopathy. *J. Neurol. Sci.* **1994**, *121*, 167–171. [CrossRef]
71. Paulson, H. Repeat expansion diseases. *Handb. Clin. Neurol.* **2018**, *147*, 105. [CrossRef] [PubMed]
72. Yatsenko, A.N.; Georgiadis, A.P.; Röpke, A.; Berman, A.J.; Jaffe, T.; Olszewska, M.; Westernströer, B.; Sanfilippo, J.; Kurpisz, M.; Rajkovic, A.; et al. X-linked TEX11 mutations, meiotic arrest, and azoospermia in infertile men. *N. Engl. J. Med.* **2015**, *372*, 2097–2107. [CrossRef] [PubMed]
73. Yang, F.; Silber, S.; Leu, N.A.; Oates, R.D.; Marszalek, J.D.; Skaletsky, H.; Brown, L.G.; Rozen, S.; Page, D.C.; Wang, P.J. TEX11 is mutated in infertile men with azoospermia and regulates genome-wide recombination rates in mouse. *EMBO Mol. Med.* **2015**, *7*, 1198–1210. [CrossRef] [PubMed]
74. Sha, Y.; Zheng, L.; Ji, Z.; Mei, L.; Ding, L.; Lin, S.; Wang, X.; Yang, X.; Li, P. A novel TEX11 mutation induces azoospermia: A case report of infertile brothers and literature review. *BMC Med. Genet.* **2018**, *19*, 63. [CrossRef] [PubMed]
75. Krausz, C.; Riera-Escamilla, A.; Moreno-Mendoza, D.; Holleman, K.; Cioppi, F.; Algaba, F.; Pybus, M.; Friedrich, C.; Wyrwoll, M.J.; Casamonti, E.; et al. Genetic dissection of spermatogenic arrest through exome analysis: Clinical implications for the management of azoospermic men. *Genet. Med.* **2020**, *22*, 1956–1966. [CrossRef]
76. Chalmel, F.; Lardenois, A.; Primig, M. Toward understanding the core meiotic transcriptome in mammals and its implications for somatic cancer. *Ann. N. Y. Acad. Sci.* **2007**, *1120*, 1–15. [CrossRef]
77. Hanson, H.A.; Anderson, R.E.; Aston, K.I.; Carrell, D.T.; Smith, K.R.; Hotaling, J.M. Subfertility increases risk of testicular cancer: Evidence from population-based semen samples. *Fertil. Steril.* **2016**, *105*, 322–328. [CrossRef]

78. Kasak, L.; Punab, M.; Nagirnaja, L.; Grigorova, M.; Minajeva, A.; Lopes, A.M.; Punab, A.M.; Aston, K.I.; Carvalho, F.; Laasik, E.; et al. Bi-allelic Recessive Loss-of-Function Variants in FANCM Cause Non-obstructive Azoospermia. *Am. J. Hum. Genet.* **2018**, *103*, 200–212. [CrossRef]
79. Krausz, C.; Riera-Escamilla, A.; Chianese, C.; Moreno-Mendoza, D.; Ars, E.; Rajmil, O.; Pujol, R.; Bogliolo, M.; Blanco, I.; Rodríguez, I.; et al. From exome analysis in idiopathic azoospermia to the identification of a high-risk subgroup for occult Fanconi anemia. *Genet. Med.* **2019**, *21*, 189–194. [CrossRef]
80. Yin, H.; Ma, H.; Hussain, S.; Zhang, H.; Xie, X.; Jiang, L.; Jiang, X.; Iqbal, F.; Bukhari, I.; Jiang, H.; et al. A homozygous FANCM frameshift pathogenic variant causes male infertility. *Genet. Med.* **2019**, *21*, 62–70. [CrossRef]
81. Liu, C.C.; Tseng, Y.T.; Li, W.; Wu, C.Y.; Mayzus, I.; Rzhetsky, A.; Sun, F.; Waterman, M.; Chen, J.J.; Chaudhary, P.M.; et al. DiseaseConnect: A comprehensive web server for mechanism-based disease-disease connections. *Nucleic Acids Res.* **2014**, *42*, W137–W146. [CrossRef]
82. Tarín, J.J.; García-Pérez, M.A.; Hamatani, T.; Cano, A. Infertility etiologies are genetically and clinically linked with other diseases in single meta-diseases. *Reprod. Biol. Endocrinol.* **2015**, *13*, 31. [CrossRef] [PubMed]
83. Ceccaldi, R.; Sarangi, P.; D'Andrea, A.D. The Fanconi anaemia pathway: New players and new functions. *Nat. Rev. Mol. Cell Biol.* **2016**, *17*, 337–349. [CrossRef] [PubMed]
84. Nepal, M.; Che, R.; Zhang, J.; Ma, C.; Fei, P. Fanconi Anemia Signaling and Cancer. *Trends Cancer* **2017**, *3*, 840–856. [CrossRef] [PubMed]
85. Yang, Y.; Guo, J.; Dai, L.; Zhu, Y.; Hu, H.; Tan, L.; Chen, W.; Liang, D.; He, J.; Tu, M.; et al. XRCC2 mutation causes meiotic arrest, azoospermia and infertility. *J. Med. Genet.* **2018**, *55*, 628–636. [CrossRef]
86. Kuznetsov, S.; Pellegrini, M.; Shuda, K.; Fernandez-Capetillo, O.; Liu, Y.; Martin, B.K.; Burkett, S.; Southon, E.; Pati, D.; Tessarollo, L.; et al. RAD51C deficiency in mice results in early prophase I arrest in males and sister chromatid separation at metaphase II in females. *J. Cell Biol.* **2007**, *176*, 581–592. [CrossRef]
87. Cavaillé, M.; Uhrhammer, N.; Privat, M.; Ponelle-Chachuat, F.; Gay-Bellile, M.; Lepage, M.; Molnar, I.; Viala, S.; Bidet, Y.; Bignon, Y.J. Analysis of 11 candidate genes in 849 adult patients with suspected hereditary cancer predisposition. *Genes. Chromosomes Cancer* **2021**, *60*, 73–78. [CrossRef]
88. Bakker, S.T.; van de Vrugt, H.J.; Rooimans, M.A.; Oostra, A.B.; Steltenpool, J.; Delzenne-Goette, E.; van der Wal, A.; van der Valk, M.; Joenje, H.; te Riele, H.; et al. Fancm-deficient mice reveal unique features of Fanconi anemia complementation group M. *Hum. Mol. Genet.* **2009**, *18*, 3484–3495. [CrossRef]
89. Luo, Y.; Hartford, S.A.; Zeng, R.; Southard, T.L.; Shima, N.; Schimenti, J.C. Hypersensitivity of Primordial Germ Cells to Compromised Replication-Associated DNA Repair Involves ATM-p53-p21 Signaling. *PLoS Genet.* **2014**, *10*, e1004730. [CrossRef]
90. Tenenbaum-Rakover, Y.; Weinberg-Shukron, A.; Renbaum, P.; Lobel, O.; Eideh, H.; Gulsuner, S.; Dahary, D.; Abu-Rayyan, A.; Kanaan, M.; Levy-Lahad, E.; et al. Minichromosome maintenance complex component 8 (MCM8) gene mutations result in primary gonadal failure. *J. Med. Genet.* **2015**, *52*, 391–399. [CrossRef] [PubMed]
91. Ruan, J.; He, X.J.; Du, W.D.; Chen, G.; Zhou, Y.; Xu, S.; Zuo, X.B.; Fang, L.B.; Cao, Y.X.; Zhang, X.J. Genetic variants in TEX15 gene conferred susceptibility to spermatogenic failure in the Chinese Han population. *Reprod. Sci.* **2012**, *19*, 1190–1196. [CrossRef]
92. Okutman, O.; Muller, J.; Baert, Y.; Serdarogullari, M.; Gultomruk, M.; Piton, A.; Rombaut, C.; Benkhalifa, M.; Teletin, M.; Skory, V.; et al. Exome sequencing reveals a nonsense mutation in TEX15 causing spermatogenic failure in a Turkish family. *Hum. Mol. Genet.* **2015**, *24*, 5581–5588. [CrossRef]
93. Colombo, R.; Pontoglio, A.; Bini, M. Two novel TEX15 mutations in a family with nonobstructive azoospermia. *Gynecol. Obstet. Investig.* **2017**, *82*, 283–286. [CrossRef] [PubMed]
94. Golubicki, M.; Bonjoch, L.; Acuña-Ochoa, J.G.; Díaz-Gay, M.; Muñoz, J.; Cuatrecasas, M.; Ocaña, T.; Iseas, S.; Mendez, G.; Cisterna, D.; et al. Germline biallelic Mcm8 variants are associated with early-onset Lynch-like syndrome. *JCI Insight* **2020**, *5*, e140698. [CrossRef] [PubMed]
95. Lin, X.; Chen, Z.; Gao, P.; Gao, Z.; Chen, H.; Qi, J.; Liu, F.; Ye, D.; Jiang, H.; Na, R.; et al. TEX15: A DNA repair gene associated with prostate cancer risk in Han Chinese. *Prostate* **2017**, *77*, 1271–1278. [CrossRef] [PubMed]
96. Moniz, S.; Jordan, P. Emerging roles for WNK kinases in cancer. *Cell. Mol. Life Sci.* **2010**, *67*, 1265–1276. [CrossRef]
97. Fakhro, K.A.; Elbardisi, H.; Arafa, M.; Robay, A.; Rodriguez-Flores, J.L.; Al-Shakaki, A.; Syed, N.; Mezey, J.G.; Abi Khalil, C.; Malek, J.A.; et al. Point-of-care whole-exome sequencing of idiopathic male infertility. *Genet. Med.* **2018**, *20*, 1365–1373. [CrossRef] [PubMed]
98. Wang, J.; Xing, B.; Liu, W.; Li, J.; Wang, X.; Li, J.; Yang, J.; Ji, C.; Li, Z.; Dong, B.; et al. Molecularly annotation of mouse avatar models derived from patients with colorectal cancer liver metastasis. *Theranostics* **2019**, *9*, 3485–3500. [CrossRef] [PubMed]
99. Gallinger, S.; Aronson, M.; Shayan, K.; Ratcliffe, E.M.; Gerstle, J.T.; Parkin, P.C.; Rothenmund, H.; Croitoru, M.; Baumann, E.; Durie, P.R.; et al. Gastrointestinal cancers and neurofibromatosis type 1 features in children with a germline homozygous MLH1 mutation. *Gastroenterology* **2004**, *126*, 576–585. [CrossRef]
100. Alotaibi, H.; Ricciardone, M.D.; Ozturk, M. Homozygosity at variant MLH1 can lead to secondary mutation in NF1, neurofibromatosis type I and early onset leukemia. *Mutat. Res.* **2008**, *637*, 209–214. [CrossRef]
101. Ji, G.; Long, Y.; Zhou, Y.; Huang, C.; Gu, A.; Wang, X. Common variants in mismatch repair genes associated with increased risk of sperm DNA damage and male infertility. *BMC Med.* **2012**, *10*, 49. [CrossRef]

102. Duraturo, F.; Liccardo, R.; Izzo, P. Coexistence of MLH3 germline variants in colon cancer patients belonging to families with Lynch syndrome-associated brain tumors. *J. Neurooncol.* **2016**, *129*, 577–578. [CrossRef]
103. Vymetalkova, V.; Pardini, B.; Rosa, F.; Di Gaetano, C.; Novotny, J.; Levy, M.; Buchler, T.; Slyskova, J.; Vodickova, L.; Naccarati, A.; et al. Variations in mismatch repair genes and colorectal cancer risk and clinical outcome. *Mutagenesis* **2014**, *29*, 259–265. [CrossRef]
104. Xu, K.; Lu, T.; Zhou, H.; Bai, L.; Xiang, Y. The role of MSH5 C85T and MLH3 C2531T polymorphisms in the risk of male infertility with azoospermia or severe oligozoospermia. *Clin. Chim. Acta.* **2010**, *411*, 49–52. [CrossRef]
105. Saunders, E.J.; Dadaev, T.; Leongamornlert, D.A.; Al Olama, A.A.; Benlloch, S.; Giles, G.G.; Wiklund, F.; Gronberg, H.; Haiman, C.A.; Schleutker, J.; et al. Gene and pathway level analyses of germline DNA-repair gene variants and prostate cancer susceptibility using the iCOGS-genotyping array. *Br. J. Cancer* **2016**, *114*, 945–952. [CrossRef]
106. Scarbrough, P.M.; Weber, R.P.; Iversen, E.S.; Brhane, Y.; Amos, C.I.; Kraft, P.; Hung, R.J.; Sellers, T.A.; Witte, J.S.; Pharoah, P.; et al. A Cross-Cancer Genetic Association Analysis of the DNA Repair and DNA Damage Signaling Pathways for Lung, Ovary, Prostate, Breast, and Colorectal Cancer. *Cancer Epidemiol. Biomarkers Prev.* **2016**, *25*, 193–200. [CrossRef]
107. Ni, B.; Lin, Y.; Sun, L.; Zhu, M.; Li, Z.; Wang, H.; Yu, J.; Guo, X.; Zuo, X.; Dong, J.; et al. Low-frequency germline variants across 6p22.2-6p21.33 are associated with non-obstructive azoospermia in Han Chinese men. *Hum. Mol. Genet.* **2015**, *24*, 5628–5636. [CrossRef] [PubMed]
108. Ramchander, N.C.; Ryan, N.A.; Crosbie, E.J.; Evans, D.J. Homozygous germ-line mutation of the PMS2 mismatch repair gene: A unique case report of constitutional mismatch repair deficiency (CMMRD). *BMC Med. Genet.* **2017**, *18*, 40. [CrossRef] [PubMed]
109. Clendenning, M.; Senter, L.; Hampel, H.; Lagerstedt Robinson, K.; Sun, S.; Buchanan, D.; Walsh, M.D.; Nilbert, M.; Green, J.; Potter, J.; et al. A frame-shift mutation of PMS2 is a widespread cause of Lynch syndrome. *J. Med. Genet.* **2008**, *45*, 340–345. [CrossRef] [PubMed]
110. Su, Y.; Swift, M. Mortality rates among carriers of ataxia-telangiectasia mutant alleles. *Ann. Intern. Med.* **2000**, *133*, 770–778. [CrossRef] [PubMed]
111. Pilié, P.G.; Johnson, A.M.; Hanson, K.L.; Dayno, M.E.; Kapron, A.L.; Stoffel, E.M.; Cooney, K.A. Germline genetic variants in men with prostate cancer and one or more additional cancers. *Cancer* **2017**, *123*, 3925–3932. [CrossRef] [PubMed]
112. Li, Z.; Yu, J.; Zhang, T.; Li, H.; Ni, Y. rs189037, a functional variant in ATM gene promoter, is associated with idiopathic nonobstructive azoospermia. *Fertil. Steril.* **2013**, *100*, 1536–1541. [CrossRef]
113. Li, S.; Peng, Q.; Chen, Y.; You, J.; Chen, Z.; Deng, Y.; Lao, X.; Wu, H.; Qin, X.; Zeng, Z. DNA repair gene XRCC1 polymorphisms, smoking, and bladder cancer risk: A meta-analysis. *PLoS ONE* **2013**, *8*, e73448. [CrossRef]
114. Gu, A.H.; Liang, J.; Lu, N.X.; Wu, B.; Xia, Y.K.; Lu, C.C.; Song, L.; Wang, S.L.; Wang, X.R. Association of XRCC1 gene polymorphisms with idiopathic azoospermia in a Chinese population. *Asian J. Androl.* **2007**, *9*, 781–786. [CrossRef] [PubMed]
115. Zheng, L.R.; Wang, X.F.; Zhou, D.X.; Zhang, J.; Huo, Y.W.; Tian, H. Association between XRCC1 single-nucleotide polymorphisms and infertility with idiopathic azoospermia in northern Chinese Han males. *Reprod. Biomed. Online* **2012**, *25*, 402–407. [CrossRef]
116. Yi, L.; Xiao-Feng, H.; Yun-Tao, L.; Hao, L.; Ye, S.; Song-Tao, Q. Association between the XRCC1 Arg399Gln polymorphism and risk of cancer: Evidence from 297 case-control studies. *PLoS ONE* **2013**, *8*, e78071. [CrossRef] [PubMed]
117. Singh, V.; Bansal, S.K.; Sudhakar, D.V.; Neelabh; Chakraborty, A.; Trivedi, S.; Gupta, G.; Thangaraj, K.; Rajender, S.; Singh, K. SNPs in ERCC1, ERCC2, and XRCC1 genes of the DNA repair pathway and risk of male infertility in the Asian populations: Association study, meta-analysis, and trial sequential analysis. *J. Assist. Reprod. Genet.* **2019**, *36*, 79–90. [CrossRef] [PubMed]
118. Akbas, H.; Balkan, M.; Binici, M.; Gedik, A. The Possible Role of XRCC1 Gene Polymorphisms with Idiopathic Non-obstructive Azoospermia in Southeast Turkey. *Urol. J.* **2019**, *16*, 380–385. [CrossRef] [PubMed]
119. Ji, G.; Gu, A.; Xia, Y.; Lu, C.; Liang, J.; Wang, S.; Ma, J.; Peng, Y.; Wang, X. ERCC1 and ERCC2 polymorphisms and risk of idiopathic azoospermia in a Chinese population. *Reprod. Biomed. Online* **2008**, *17*, 36–41. [CrossRef]
120. Xu, Z.; Ma, W.; Gao, L.; Xing, B. Association between ERCC1 C8092A and ERCC2 K751Q polymorphisms and risk of adult glioma: A meta-analysis. *Tumour Biol.* **2014**, *35*, 3211–3221. [CrossRef]
121. Ding, Y.W.; Gao, X.; Ye, D.X.; Liu, W.; Wu, L.; Sun, H.Y. Association of ERCC1 polymorphisms (rs3212986 and rs11615) with the risk of head and neck carcinomas based on case-control studies. *Clin. Transl. Oncol.* **2015**, *17*, 710–719. [CrossRef]
122. Guo, X.G.; Wang, Q.; Xia, Y.; Zheng, L. The C8092A polymorphism in the ERCC1 gene and breast carcinoma risk: A meta-analysis of case-control studies. *Int. J. Clin. Exp. Med.* **2015**, *8*, 3691–3699. [PubMed]
123. Bonduelle, M.; Legein, J.; Derde, M.P.; Buysse, A.; Schietecatte, J.; Wisanto, A.; Devroey, P.; Van Steirteghem, A.; Liebaers, I. Comparative follow-up study of 130 children born after intracytoplasmic sperm injection and 130 children born after in-vitro fertilization. *Hum. Reprod.* **1995**, *10*, 3327–3331. [CrossRef] [PubMed]
124. In't Veld, P.; Brandenburg, H.; Verhoeff, A.; Dhont, M.; Los, F. Sex chromosomal abnormalities and intracytoplasmic sperm injection. *Lancet* **1995**, *346*, 773. [CrossRef]
125. Tournaye, H.; Liu, J.; Nagy, Z.; Joris, H.; Wisanto, A.; Bonduelle, M.; Van der Elst, J.; Staessen, C.; Smitz, J.; Silber, S. Intracytoplasmic sperm injection (ICSI): The Brussels experience. *Reprod. Fertil. Dev.* **1995**, *7*, 269–279. [CrossRef]
126. Foresta, C.; Rossato, M.; Garolla, A.; Ferlin, A. Male infertility and ICSI: Are there limits? *Hum. Reprod.* **1996**, *11*, 2347–2348. [CrossRef] [PubMed]

127. Pang, M.G.; Hoegerman, S.F.; Cuticchia, A.J.; Moon, S.Y.; Doncel, G.F.; Acosta, A.A.; Kearns, W.G. Detection of aneuploidy for chromosomes 4, 6, 7, 8, 9, 10, 11, 12, 13, 17, 18, 21, X and Y by fluorescence in-situ hybridization in spermatozoa from nine patients with oligoasthenoteratozoospermia undergoing intracytoplasmic sperm injection. *Hum. Reprod.* **1999**, *14*, 1266–1273. [CrossRef]
128. Moosani, N.; Pattinson, H.A.; Carter, M.D.; Cox, D.M.; Rademaker, A.W.; Martin, R.H. Chromosomal analysis of sperm from men with idiopathic infertility using sperm karyotyping and fluorescence in situ hybridization. *Fertil. Steril.* **1995**, *64*, 811–817. [CrossRef]
129. Esteves, S.C.; Roque, M.; Bedoschi, G.; Haahr, T.; Humaidan, P. Intracytoplasmic sperm injection for male infertility and consequences for offspring. *Nat. Rev. Urol.* **2018**, *15*, 535–562. [CrossRef] [PubMed]
130. Wen, J.; Jiang, J.; Ding, C.; Dai, J.; Liu, Y.; Xia, Y.; Liu, J.; Hu, Z. Birth defects in children conceived by in vitro fertilization and intracytoplasmic sperm injection: A meta-analysis. *Fertil. Steril.* **2012**, *97*, 1331–1337.e4. [CrossRef]
131. Lacamara, C.; Ortega, C.; Villa, S.; Pommer, R.; Schwarze, J.E. Are children born from singleton pregnancies conceived by ICSI at increased risk for congenital malformations when compared to children conceived naturally? A systematic review and meta-analysis. *JBRA Assist. Reprod.* **2017**, *21*, 251–259. [CrossRef] [PubMed]
132. Foresta, C.; Ferlin, A. Offspring conceived by intracytoplasmic sperm injection. *Lancet* **2001**, *358*, 1270. [CrossRef]
133. Massaro, P.A.; MacLellan, D.L.; Anderson, P.A.; Romao, R.L. Does intracytoplasmic sperm injection pose an increased risk of genitourinary congenital malformations in offspring compared to in vitro fertilization? A systematic review and meta-analysis. *J. Urol.* **2015**, *193*, 1837–1842. [CrossRef] [PubMed]
134. Halliday, J. Outcomes for offspring of men having ICSI for male factor infertility. *Asian J. Androl.* **2012**, *14*, 116–120. [CrossRef] [PubMed]
135. Rumbold, A.R.; Sevoyan, A.; Oswald, T.K.; Fernandez, R.C.; Davies, M.J.; Moore, V.M. Impact of male factor infertility on offspring health and development. *Fertil. Steril.* **2019**, *111*, 1047–1053. [CrossRef] [PubMed]
136. Sandin, S.; Nygren, K.G.; Iliadou, A.; Hultman, C.M.; Reichenberg, A. Autism and mental retardation among offspring born after in vitro fertilization. *JAMA* **2013**, *310*, 75–84. [CrossRef]
137. Hvidtjørn, D.; Schieve, L.; Schendel, D.; Jacobsson, B.; Svaerke, C.; Thorsen, P. Cerebral palsy, autism spectrum disorders, and developmental delay in children born after assisted conception: A systematic review and meta-analysis. *Arch. Pediatr. Adolesc. Med.* **2009**, *163*, 72–83. [CrossRef]
138. Bay, B.; Mortensen, E.L.; Hvidtjørn, D.; Kesmodel, U.S. Fertility treatment and risk of childhood and adolescent mental disorders: Register based cohort study. *BMJ* **2013**, *347*, f3978. [CrossRef] [PubMed]
139. Kissin, D.M.; Zhang, Y.; Boulet, S.L.; Fountain, C.; Bearman, P.; Schieve, L.; Yeargin-Allsopp, M.; Jamieson, D.J. Association of assisted reproductive technology (ART) treatment and parental infertility diagnosis with autism in ART-conceived children. *Hum. Reprod.* **2015**, *30*, 454–465. [CrossRef]
140. Sutcliffe, A.G.; Saunders, K.; McLachlan, R.; Taylor, B.; Edwards, P.; Grudzinskas, G.; Leiberman, B.; Thornton, S. A retrospective case-control study of developmental and other outcomes in a cohort of Australian children conceived by intracytoplasmic sperm injection compared with a similar group in the United Kingdom. *Fertil. Steril.* **2003**, *79*, 512–516. [CrossRef]
141. Bonduelle, M.; Ponjaert, I.; Van Steirteghem, A.; Derde, M.P.; Devroey, P.; Liebaers, I. Developmental outcome at 2 years of age for children born after ICSI compared with children born after IVF. *Hum. Reprod.* **2003**, *18*, 342–350. [CrossRef]
142. Wennerholm, U.B.; Bonduelle, M.; Sutcliffe, A.; Bergh, C.; Niklasson, A.; Tarlatzis, B.; Kai, C.M.; Peters, C.; Victorin Cederqvist, A.; Loft, A. Paternal sperm concentration and growth and cognitive development in children born with a gestational age more than 32 weeks after assisted reproductive therapy. *Hum. Reprod.* **2006**, *21*, 1514–1520. [CrossRef] [PubMed]
143. Belva, F.; Henriet, S.; Liebaers, I.; Van Steirteghem, A.; Celestin-Westreich, S.; Bonduelle, M. Medical outcome of 8-year-old singleton ICSI children (born ≥32 weeks' gestation) and a spontaneously conceived comparison group. *Hum. Reprod.* **2007**, *22*, 506–515. [CrossRef]
144. Belva, F.; Painter, R.; Bonduelle, M.; Roelants, M.; Devroey, P.; De Schepper, J. Are ICSI adolescents at risk for increased adiposity? *Hum. Reprod.* **2012**, *27*, 257–264. [CrossRef]
145. Belva, F.; Roelants, M.; De Schepper, J.; Roseboom, T.J.; Bonduelle, M.; Devroey, P.; Painter, R.C. Blood pressure in ICSI-conceived adolescents. *Hum. Reprod.* **2012**, *27*, 3100–3108. [CrossRef]
146. Belva, F.; Bonduelle, M.; Provyn, S.; Painter, R.C.; Tournaye, H.; Roelants, M.; De Schepper, J. Metabolic Syndrome and Its Components in Young Adults Conceived by ICSI. *Int. J. Endocrinol.* **2018**, *2018*, 8170518. [CrossRef] [PubMed]
147. Kettner, L.O.; Matthiesen, N.B.; Ramlau-Hansen, C.H.; Kesmodel, U.S.; Bay, B.; Henriksen, T.B. Fertility treatment and childhood type 1 diabetes mellitus: A nationwide cohort study of 565,116 live births. *Fertil. Steril.* **2016**, *106*, 1751–1756. [CrossRef] [PubMed]
148. Sonntag, B.; Eisemann, N.; Elsner, S.; Ludwig, A.K.; Katalinic, A.; Kixmüller, J.; Ludwig, M. Pubertal development and reproductive hormone levels of singleton ICSI offspring in adolescence: Results of a prospective controlled study. *Hum. Reprod.* **2020**, *35*, 968–976. [CrossRef] [PubMed]
149. Katagiri, Y.; Neri, Q.V.; Takeuchi, T.; Schlegel, P.N.; Megid, W.A.; Kent-First, M.; Rosenwaks, Z.; Palermo, G.D. Y chromosome assessment and its implications for the development of ICSI children. *Reprod. Biomed. Online* **2004**, *8*, 307–318. [CrossRef]
150. Palermo, G.D.; Neri, Q.V.; Takeuchi, T.; Squires, J.; Moy, F.; Rosenwaks, Z. Genetic and epigenetic characteristics of ICSI children. *Reprod. Biomed. Online* **2008**, *17*, 820–833. [CrossRef]
151. Belva, F.; Bonduelle, M.; Roelants, M.; Michielsen, D.; Van Steirteghem, A.; Verheyen, G.; Tournaye, H. Semen quality of young adult ICSI offspring: The first results. *Hum. Reprod.* **2016**, *31*, 2811–2820. [CrossRef] [PubMed]

152. Krausz, C.; Giachini, C.; Lo Giacco, D.; Daguin, F.; Chianese, C.; Ars, E.; Ruiz-Castane, E.; Forti, G.; Rossi, E. High Resolution X Chromosome-Specific Array-CGH Detects New CNVs in Infertile Males. *PLoS ONE* **2012**, *7*, e44887. [CrossRef] [PubMed]
153. Lopes, A.M.; Aston, K.I.; Thompson, E.; Carvalho, F.; Gonçalves, J.; Huang, N.; Matthiesen, R.; Noordam, M.J.; Quintela, I.; Ramu, A.; et al. Human Spermatogenic Failure Purges Deleterious Mutation Load from the Autosomes and Both Sex Chromosomes, including the Gene DMRT1. *PLoS Genet.* **2013**, *9*, e1003349. [CrossRef] [PubMed]
154. Tüttelmann, F.; Simoni, M.; Kliesch, S.; Ledig, S.; Dworniczak, B.; Wieacker, P.; Röpke, A. Copy Number Variants in Patients with Severe Oligozoospermia and Sertoli-Cell-Only Syndrome. *PLoS ONE* **2011**, *6*, e19426. [CrossRef]
155. Krausz, C. Editorial for the special issue on the molecular genetics of male infertility. *Hum. Genet.* **2021**, *140*, 1–5. [CrossRef]

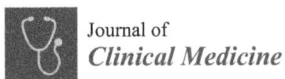

Review

Prediction Models for Successful Sperm Retrieval in Patients with Non-Obstructive Azoospermia Undergoing Microdissection Testicular Sperm Extraction: Is There Any Room for Further Studies?

Ettore Caroppo [1,*] and Giovanni Maria Colpi [2]

1. Andrology Outpatients Clinic, Asl Bari, PTA "F Jaia", Conversano, 70014 Bari, Italy
2. Andrology Unit, Procrea Institute, 6900 Lugano, Switzerland; gmcolpi@yahoo.com
* Correspondence: ecaroppo@teseo.it

Abstract: Several prediction models for successful sperm retrieval (SSR) in patients with azoospermia due to spermatogenic dysfunction (also termed non-obstructive azoospermia—NOA) have been developed and published in the past years, however their resulting prediction accuracy has never been strong enough to translate their results in the clinical practice. This notwithstanding, the number of prediction models being proposed in this field is growing. We have reviewed the available evidence and found that, although patients with complete AZFc deletion or a history of cryptorchidism may have better probability of SSR compared to those with idiopathic NOA, no clinical or laboratory marker is able to determine whether a patient with NOA should or should not undergo microdissection testicular sperm extraction (mTESE) to have his testicular sperm retrieved. Further research is warranted to confirm the utility of evaluating the expression of noncoding RNAs in the seminal plasma, to individuate patients with NOA with higher probability of SSR.

Keywords: non-obstructive azoospermia; sperm retrieval; male infertility; microTESE; prediction model

1. Introduction

Prediction models are widely used in the clinic to estimate the risk (or probability) of existing disease or outcome for an individual, determined by the possible values of one or more predictors. In the case of patients with azoospermia due to spermatogenetic dysfunction (also termed non-obstructive azoospermia—NOA), the probability of surgically retrieving sperm from one or both testes represents the outcome that needs to be estimated. Since the ability to predict such an outcome would allow the urologist to individuate those patients who are suited for microdissection testicular sperm extraction (mTESE), several prediction models have been developed to date, however their resulting prediction accuracy was never strong enough to translate their results to the clinical practice. Few candidate predictors have been proposed to be associated with better chances of successful sperm retrieval (SSR), but a consensus has not been reached about them. As a result, actually no clinical or laboratory factor may be used to counsel patients with NOA about their chances of mTESE success.

Indeed, there are some issues that may explain these findings. The most important one is that, in patients with NOA, the testicular parenchyma is not rarely characterized by a highly heterogeneous distribution of histologically and functionally distinct seminiferous tubules (STs), so that the retrieval of sperm is mostly dependent upon the skill and experience of the urologist, his/her learning curve being strictly correlated with the outcome of mTESE [1–3], rather than upon the severity of the spermatogenic dysfunction. In addition, the definition of SSR is not homogeneous among groups: ideally, SSR is defined as the retrieval of an adequate number and quality of sperm for intracytoplasmic sperm injection

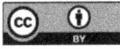

(ICSI); however, at least in some cases, the difference between successful (positive outcome) and failed sperm retrieval (negative outcome) may not always be as sharp as it should be to avoid the risk of misclassification.

This notwithstanding, the number of prediction models being evaluated in this field is growing. To establish whether the current knowledge about prediction of mTESE success may justify further studies, in the present article, we will review the evidence about the predictive ability of the clinical and laboratory factors that have been previously proposed as candidate predictors of mTESE outcome.

2. Clinical Factors

Some prediction models of successful sperm retrieval have evaluated the predictive ability of clinical conditions that may be involved in the etiology of NOA (Klinefelter's syndrome, Y chromosome microdeletions, cryptorchidism, varicocele), or may represent putative prognostic factors of mTESE success (testicular volume).

2.1. Klinefelter Syndrome

Klinefelter syndrome (KS) is the most common chromosomal abnormality in men, and is found in about 3–4% of infertile men and in more than 10% of azoospermic men [4]. KS men have typically small, atrophic testes and hypergonadotropic hypogonadism, with tubular hyalinization as the prevalent histopathological pattern. Their genetic profile is characterized in 85–90% of cases by the presence of a supernumerary X chromosome (47, XXY karyotype), while the remaining patients show a mosaic karyotype (46, XY/47, XXY), or rarely, a super-numerous sex chromosome [5]. Despite the severe spermatogenic dysfunction, 8% of patients may have sperm in the ejaculate [6], while testicular sperm may be retrieved in 20–66% of KS men by means of mTESE (see Table 1). Such a wide range of sperm retrieval rates (SRR) may be explained by the unique testicular architecture found in men with KS, who may have sperm in focal enlargements of otherwise sclerotic tubules, instead of having sperm throughout a uniformly dilated tubule [7], so that only a meticulous search within these very small testes may be successful. In addition, as summarized in Table 1, some studies suggest that SRRs may be affected by age (younger patients have better SRRs) or preoperative testosterone level (normal testosterone level is associated with better SRRs).

The predictive role of KS on SSR is still debated. A neural computational model built on 1026 men with NOA demonstrated that KS significantly predicted SSR (OR 3.07 (1.84–5.03), $p < 0.001$) [8]. On the other hand, a meta-analysis evaluating 117 studies enrolling 21,404 patients showed that SSR decreased as a function of the number of KS subjects included in the population of NOA (S = $-0.02(-0.04; -0.01)$; $p < 0.01$) [9]. Still, different surgical methods of sperm retrievals, different surgeons and embryologists' skill and experience, and heterogeneities in patients' characteristics may explain such conflicting results. Further studies should clearly provide information about patients' ages, as well as surgeon's learning curve, to allow the correct interpretation of data.

2.2. Y Chromosome Microdeletions

The global prevalence of AZF microdeletions in infertile men is estimated to be 7% (95% CL 6.74–6.79) [10]. The most frequently deleted locus in infertile men is AZFc (60–70%), followed by AZFa (0.5–4%), AZFb (1–5%) and AZFb+c (1–3%) deletion [10]. Men with complete AZFa and AZFb deletions are azoospermic, and sperm cannot be surgically retrieved [11]. A study reported that 3 out of 15 patients with AZFb deletions had sperm on mTESE [12]; however, the Authors defined the AZFb deletions using sY127 and sY134 marker, while classically, the AZFb locus is proximally defined by sY108 and distally characterized by sY134 or sY135; therefore, a partial AZFb deletion could not be excluded in such cases. Men with complete AZFc deletions may have sperm in the ejaculate or be azoospermic, but with good chances of SSR: a recent review reporting the results of 32 studies found that sperm could be retrieved in 13 to 100% of cases, particularly when mTESE was used [11]. Thus, AZFc deletion may confer better chances of SSR to patients with NOA.

2.3. Cryptorchidism

Cryptorchidism is considered as a reliable predictor factor of SSR in patients with NOA. A study utilizing an artificial neural network (ANN) to model the chance of SSR of 1026 men with NOA (770 training set, 256 test set) undergoing microTESE found that cryptorchidism was significant to the model [OR 2.29 (1.47–3.57), $p < 0.0001$] [8]. Sperm retrieval rates vary from 52.6% to 75% [12–15]. There is no consensus about the predictive ability of age at surgery, side (unilateral vs. bilateral) or testicular volume on SRR. Ozan and coworkers evaluated 148 patients with NOA and history of cryptorchidism undergoing mTESE, and found that SSR did not vary with age at surgery (65.1% vs. 55.4% in patients undergoing orchidopexy before or after 10 years of age respectively) or side (62.9% vs. 59.3% in patients, with unilateral of bilateral cryptorchidism, respectively) [13]. Okada et al. found that only testicular volume was predictive of SSR in a cohort of 36 formerly cryptorchid patients with NOA (OR 1.328, 95% CI 1.089–1619, $p = 0.045$) [14], while Cayan and collaborators evaluated a cohort of 327 azoospermic men with previous cryptorchidism, and found that SRR was higher in patients with total testicular volume > 13.75 mL (65.3% vs. 45.5%, $p = 0.001$), serum testosterone > 300.5 ng/dL (65.9% vs. 40.5%), serum FSH level > 17.25 mIU/mL (72.7% vs. 44.3%, $p < 0.0001$), and age at surgery < 9.5 years (70.8% vs. 42.1%, $p < 0.0001$) [15]. Well designed, multicentric studies are warranted to clarify the impact of age at surgery on the chances of SSR of formerly cryptorchid patients with NOA.

2.4. Varicocele

Varicocele is found in 5–10% of men with NOA [16]. Although several pathophysiological hypotheses have been proposed about the link between varicocele and NOA, no definite conclusions can be drawn [17]. Despite this, varicocele repair has been proposed to be beneficial in patients with NOA: a meta-analysis evaluating 16 studies for a total cohort of 344 azoospermic men who had undergone varicocele repair reported that 43.9% (151/344) of them had sperm in the ejaculate (sperm count was 1.82 ± 1.58 million/mL (95% CI: 0.98–2.77 millions/mL), sperm motility was $22.9\% \pm 15.5\%$ (95% CI: 12.5–33.2%) 4.5 to 11 months after surgery; testicular biopsies were obtained in 8 out of 16 studies, histopathology demonstrating that the chance of having sperm in the ejaculate was significantly higher in patients with hypospermatogenesis (HS) compared to maturation arrest (MA) (OR: 2.35; 95% CI: 1.04–5.29; $p = 0.04$), and to Sertoli cell only syndrome (SCO) (OR: 12.0; 95% CI: 4.34–33.17; $p < 0.001$) [18]. However, since positive changes in the semen parameters following varicocele repair may not last forever, sperm cryopreservation is recommended [17]. The same meta-analysis reports the results of three studies evaluating the SRR in patients with varicocele, which was significantly greater in men with prior varicocele repair, compared to untreated patients (OR 2.65, 95% CI 1.69–4.14). Still, such studies were not devoid of selection bias. On the other hand, Schlegel and Kaufmann evaluated 138 patients with NOA and varicocele, 68 with a prior varicocelectomy, and 70 who did not undergo surgery: SRR was comparable in both groups (41/68 (60%) vs. 42/70 (60%), and did not vary with histopathological subcategories (26 vs. 38% in SCO, 53 vs. 47% in MA, and 96 vs. 96% in HS in patients with prior varicocelectomy or no treatment, respectively) [19]. Similarly, a study evaluating 860 patients with NOA, of whom 169 had prior history of varicocele repair, by means of a predictive model with varicocelectomy, age, prior sperm retrieval, testis volume, FSH, LH, testosterone level and diagnosis of KS as candidate predictors (all found to be predictive of SSR in univariate logistic regression), found that prior varicocelectomy was not predictive of SSR in multivariate logistic regression [20]. Given the conflicting results as above, well-designed randomized clinical trials are warranted to clarify whether varicocele repair may help in the management of patients with NOA.

2.5. Testis Volume

Since seminiferous tubules contribute to approximately 80% of testis volume, this clinical parameter has been classically correlated with spermatogenesis. Indeed, a large sample size study (2.672 patients) demonstrated that testis volume correlates with sperm parameters and serum gonadotrophins levels [21], and men with testicular long axis 4.6 cm or less have been found to be more likely to have azoospermia, due to spermatogenic dysfunction [22]. Nevertheless, the correlation between testis volume and SSR in mTESE is not as intuitive as one would expect. On one hand, sperm may be retrieved even in patients with testis volume lower than 2 mL, with SRR being comparable to that of patients with larger testes (sample size = 1127 patients) [23]; on the other hand, patients with NOA due to early maturation arrest usually display normal testis volume, but have the worst chance of sperm retrieval [24].

Still, a meta-analysis evaluating 117 studies enrolling 21,404 patients found that testis volume significantly predicted SRR, specifically a mean volume higher than 12.5 mL predicted a SRR > 60%, with an accuracy of 86.2 ± 0.01% ($p < 0.0001$) and a specificity and sensitivity of 73% and 74% respectively; notably, the study design of the studies included in the analysis was heterogeneous with regard to patients' clinical characteristics and the surgical procedure applied (cTESE or mTESE) [9]. Indeed, a meta-analysis that included only studies evaluating patients with NOA who had undergone mTESE (5 studies with a total of 1764 cases) found that testis volume had limited value in predicting positive sperm retrieval in patients with NOA (AUC 0.63), mostly due to low specificity (sensitivity 80%, 95% CI: 0.78–0.83, specificity 35%, 95% CI: 0.32–0.39) [25]. It may be concluded, therefore, that patients with NOA with small testes should not be discouraged from attempting mTESE in the hand of skilled urologists.

Table 1. Comparison of sperm retrieval rates in patients with NOA with normal karyotype or Klinefelter syndrome.

Author	Sample Size	Sperm Retrieval Rate	Predictive Factors
Ramasamy 2009 [26]	68 KS undergoing 91 mTESE	66%	Younger age associated with higher SRRs; normal T levels associated with better SRR (86%)
Bakircioglu 2011 [27]	106 KS vs. 379 nkNOA	47% in KS and 50% in nkNOA	
Sabbaghian 2014 [28]	134 KS, 537 nkNOA	28.4 in KS, 22.2% in nkNOA	T level significantly higher in patients with successful sperm retrieval
Rohayem J 2015 [29]	50 adolescent KS (13–19 years) and 85 adult KS (20–61 years)	45% in adolescent vs. 31% in adults.	LH < 17.5 and T > 7.5 nmol/L associated with the best SRR (54%)
Donker 2017 [30]	176 KS, 1423 nkNOA	28% in KS, 60% in nkNOA	
Ozer 2018 [31]	110 KS	20%	
Kizilcan 2019 [20]	81 KS, 231 nkNOA	19.7% in KS, 36.8% nkNOA ($p = 0.006$)	
Chen 2019 [32]	66 KS, 529 nkNOA	45% in KS, 44.9% in nkNOA	
Huang 2020 [33]	66 KS	36.4%	
Guo F 2020 [34]	184 KS	43.5%	Preoperative T levels affected the SRR; 134 out of 184 patients received hCG
Zhang 2021 [35]	284 KS, 485 nkNOA	44.7 in KS, 46.8% in nkNOA	
Kocamanoglu F 2021 [36]	121 KS vs. 178 nkNOA	38% vs. 55.6% ($p = 0.012$) in KS and nkNOA respectively	

hCG, human chorionic gonadotropin, nkNOA, patients with NOA with normal karyotype, KS, patients with Klinefelter syndrome, SRR, sperm retrieval rate, T, serum testosterone level.

3. Hormonal Parameters

Follicle-stimulating hormone (FSH) and testosterone (T) are both required to promote full spermatogenesis; in addition, their serum levels reflect both the pituitary and testicular function in physiological and pathological conditions. Indeed, the measurement of FSH and T serum levels represents the minimal initial hormonal evaluation of the azoospermic men, to distinguish between primary and secondary testicular failure [37]. Their role as predictors of spermatogenesis in patients with NOA is, however, questionable.

3.1. Follicle-Stimulating Hormone (FSH)

Elevated serum FSH levels are usually found in patients with non-obstructive azoospermia; however, a normal or near-normal serum FSH concentration does not always guarantee normal spermatogenesis [37]. Indeed, patients with NOA due to early maturation arrest may have low normal serum FSH level, despite having the worst chance of sperm retrieval [24]. The poor predictive ability of FSH on the chance of sperm retrieval was shown by a study on 792 men undergoing mTESE, which provided the counterintuitive demonstration that higher FSH levels were associated with greater chances of SSR [38]; a neural computational model built on 1026 men with NOA confirmed that relying on serum FSH level to counsel patients with NOA is no more accurate than flipping a coin [8]. Other studies challenged these results, but their sample size was not large enough to detect a true association.

Since FSH level correlates with the number of spermatogonia and, to a lesser extent, primary spermatocytes [39], relying on its serum levels to counsel patients with NOA about their probability of SSR may be misleading: patients with MA and HS, as well as those with SCO with or without foci of hypospermatogenesis (focal SCO), may have comparable FSH levels, but their probability of SSR differs significantly. Indeed, a prediction model built on a development ($N = 558$) and a validation set ($N = 695$) of patients with NOA demonstrated that serum FSH level is unable to predict histopathological subcategories such as MA and focal SCO, and has low sensitivity (40.9%) and specificity (46.8%) in predicting HS and SCO, respectively [40]. These data reinforce older data against the use of basal FSH level as a predictor of SSR in patients with NOA, and should discourage further evaluation of serum FSH as marker of residual spermatogenesis in these patients.

3.2. Testosterone

Testosterone (T) signaling is required for spermatogenesis to proceed beyond meiosis. Consequently, it has been postulated that patients with hypogonadism (serum T < 300 ng/dL) may have lower chances of SSR compared to patients with normal serum T levels. Indeed, a pooled estimate of six studies evaluating 2029 patients with NOA undergoing mTESE demonstrated that patients with normal T levels had a significantly higher chance of SSR compared to those with subnormal T levels (OR 1.63, 95% CI 1.08–2.45, $p = 0.02$) [41]. However, the available evidence has provided conflicting results. Reifsnyder et al. evaluated 736 men undergoing mTESE; 348 (47.3%) with baseline T level < 300 ng/dL and 388 (53%) with baseline testosterone levels greater than 300 ng/dL. Among patients with hypogonadism, 88% received hormonal treatment. SRR did not vary among men with low vs. normal baseline T levels; yet, the mean presurgical T level was normal in patients with previous low baseline T levels as the effect of hormonal treatment. Moreover, 18% of patients receiving hormonal treatment did not respond to treatment, but their SRR was comparable to that of responders to treatment [42]. Enatsu et al. evaluated 329 patients, of whom 65 had KS, and found that serum T levels did not differ among men with SSR (97) and SRF (232) (420 + 180 vs. 430 + 190 ng/dL; $p = 0.42$) [43]. Althakafi et al. evaluated 421 patients, of whom 181 had low baseline T levels, and found no difference in SRR between those with normal and low T levels (SRR 38.6% vs. 40.3%, $p = 0.718$). Fifty patients received hormonal treatment with clomiphene citrate (CC) or human chorionic gonadotropin (hCG) due to subnormal T levels: their SRR was comparable to that of patients with normal baseline T levels (36% vs. 38%, $p = 0.736$) [44]. Kizilkan et al. evaluated 860 patients and found that T levels were predictive of SSR in univariate, but not in multivariate, logistic regression [20]. On the other hand, Mehmood et al. and Çayan et al., evaluating 264 and 327 patients respectively, found that SRR was significantly lower in men with low baseline T levels compared to those with normal baseline T levels (40.6 vs. 57.25, $p = 0.0068$, and 40.5% vs. 65.9%, $p < 0.0001$

respectively) [15,45]. Accumulating evidence suggests that higher baseline T levels may be associated with a higher probability of SSR in men with KS [26,34].

It has been suggested that intratesticular testosterone (ITT) measurement could represent a more reliable way of assessing the role of testosterone on the probability of SSR in men with NOA. Due to the inherent risks of performing testicular aspiration to obtain a direct assessment of ITT level, a measurement of the circulating levels of 17-hydroxyprogesterone (17OHP) has been proposed as an indirect biomarker of ITT levels, since 17 OHP is likely to be of testicular and not adrenal origin in men. Indeed, serum 17 OHP levels were found to be undetectable in men receiving exogenous testosterone replacement therapy, and to increase after CC and hCG treatment [46]. Studies evaluating the predictive ability of serum 17 OHP on the probability of SSR in patients with NOA are needed to provide evidence in support or against such a hypothesis.

4. Testis Histology

There is great consensus about the close relationship between different histopathological categories and mTESE outcome: patients with SCO have the lowest probability of SSR (22.5–41%), while patients with HS have the best chances of sperm retrieval (73–100%), and patients with late MA have better prognosis (SRR 27–86%) compared to those with early MA (SRR 27–40%) [47]. Indeed, a meta-analysis evaluating 19 articles showed that HS predicted SSR (pooled diagnostic odds ratio (DOR) 16.49, 95% CI: 9.63–28.23) with a sensitivity of 30% and specificity of 98%, AUC 0.6758; SCO had a negative predictive ability on SSR (AUC 0.27), while MA had a poor predictive accuracy (AUC 0.55) [25].

To obtain a realistic picture of the severity of spermatogenic dysfunction, the testicular specimen sent to the pathologist should be representative of the overall appearance of the testicular parenchyma. However, it is not uncommon for men with NOA to have more than one histopathological report. Very recently, Punjani et al. demonstrated that these patients may display up to four distinct histopathological subcategories, the increasing histopathological variety being associated with a higher probability of SSR (SRR was 33% in men with one histopathological subtype, compared to 94% in men with 4 subtypes) [48].

Testis histology has been found to be predictive of SRR also in men undergoing salvage mTESE after a failed surgical attempt. Despite previous surgery possibly harming the blood supply of the testis with a potential risk of testicular tissue damage, Tsujimura [49] and Kalsi et al. [50] found comparable SRRs in patients undergoing salvage mTESE after failed cTESE stratified according to testis histology (39% and 40% in SCO, 41.7% and 36% in MA, and 100% and 75% in HS, respectively). Data from Xu et al. [51] confirmed that HS associates with high SRR (85%) even in patients with previous sperm retrieval attempts, but found lower SRR in patients with SCO (5.5%) and MA (25%) compared to previous reports. Very recently, our group found that early and late MA were associated with the lowest probability of SSR (8.7 and 11.1%, respectively), while sperm was retrieved in 85% of men with HS; SRRs in patients with SCO differed significantly according to the presence (focal SCO) or not (complete SCO) of residual areas of HS (SRR 100% vs. 24.4%, respectively) [52].

The obvious limit of testis histology is that it may be obtained only after surgery, therefore it may be used to counsel patients about the probability of having their testicular sperm retrieved in further surgical attempts. In occasional situations, however, testicular histology may be available when a diagnostic testicular biopsy has been done prior to microTESE, and there may be of help in the counselling of patients with NOA.

5. Molecular Markers Expression in the Seminal Plasma

Given the limited accuracy of hormonal and clinical parameters in predicting the probability of SSR in patients with NOA prior to surgery, researchers have sought to evaluate the feasibility of using the expression of some molecular markers in the seminal plasma as markers of residual spermatogenesis in such patients.

The evaluation of germ cell-specific mRNAs as predictors of SSR in patients with NOA has brought conflicting results. Following the demonstration that the testicular expression of ESX1, an X-linked homeobox gene, was restricted to germ cells, particularly the spermatogonia/preleptotene spermatocytes and round spermatids, and correlated with SSR [53], a group of researchers found that the seminal plasma levels of ESXI were significantly lower in men with NOA compared to normozoospermic subjects ($p < 0.0001$), and predicted SSR in men with NOA with a sensitivity of 84%, but with a specificity of 28% [54]. However, in a further study, the seminal plasma of ESXI was found to be comparable among men with NOA and normozoospermic men [55]; on the other hand, the seminal plasma levels of protamine-1 (PRM1) were found to predict SSR with a sensitivity of 89%, and a specificity of 90%. In another study, however, seminal plasma of PRM1, together with PRM2, DAZ and AKAP4, although being undetectable in patients with SCO, could not predict SSR [56]. Finally, several studies have evaluated the predictive ability of seminal DDX4 mRNA expression on SSR, but again, with conflicting results [reviewed in [57].

Seminal plasma also contains high concentrations of extracellular vesicles that are consistent with exosomes, which originate from the male reproductive tract, and contain coding and noncoding RNAs that vary according to their origin, enabling them to (hypothetically) reflect the pathophysiological conditions of the organ of origin. Some microRNAs (miRNAs) have been found to be preferentially expressed and localized to spermatocytes and spermatids (miR-34b/c and miR-449) or late-stage male germ cells (miR-122), and to be differentially expressed in testis biopsies of patients with and without elongated spermatids (miR-449a, miR-34c-5p and miR-122) [58]. A study evaluated the expression of exosomal miRNAs in the seminal plasma of infertile men with NOA or obstructive azoospermia, demonstrating that three miRNAs, miR-31-5p, miR-539-5p and miR-941, were downregulated in patients with obstructive azoospermia compared to men with NOA. The further evaluation of 12 patients with NOA with ($N = 8$) or without ($N = 4$) SSR showed that the association of the expression values of miR-539-5p and the miR-941 was predictive of SSR [59]. However, due to the very small sample size of such a study, further studies are warranted to provide conclusive results. Indeed, another study found that miR-539-5p was not predictive of SSR, nor could it discriminate normozoospermic, oligozoospermic, and azoospermic men from each other [60].

Long noncoding RNAs (lncRNAs) have been found to play a critical role in spermatogenesis: specifically, they have been implicated in regulating protein-coding genes at the epigenetic level, and it has been speculated that these germ-specific lncRNAs may be involved in epigenetic regulation during spermatogenesis [61]. Many of them display restricted expression in the testis, thus enabling their use as noninvasive biomarkers of spermatogenesis in men with NOA. A recent study investigated the predictive ability of extracellular vesicle long noncoding RNAs (exlncRNAs) in patients with NOA: after having selected 16 exlncRNAs on the basis of their different expression in normozoospermic and azoospermic patients, the Authors evaluated their diagnostic accuracy in predicting SSR in 30 patients with NOA who had ($N = 18$) or not ($N = 12$) their testicular sperm retrieved by mTESE. The Authors built a prediction model based on 9 exlncRNAs (LOC100505685, SPATA42, CCDC37-DT, GABRG3-AS1, LOC440934, LOC101929088, LOC101929088, LINC00343 and LINC00301) and found that it predicted the probability of SSR with a sensitivity of 88.9% and a specificity of 100%, AUC 0.986. The model was then validated on 66 patients with NOA, with a resulting AUC of 0.960 [60]. Further studies are, however, warranted to validate the findings of the present study, and to confirm or challenge the predictive ability of other molecular markers expressed in the seminal plasma.

6. Conclusions

The available evidence suggests that no patient with NOA should be discouraged from attempting mTESE, based on the clinical and laboratory parameters that have been tested to date as candidate predictors of SSR. Azoospermic men with complete AZFc deletions and history of cryptorchidism may have better chances of SSR compared to those with idiopathic NOA, while the predictive role of KS on SSR is still debated. While serum

FSH level and testis volume are hardly informative about the presence of residual foci of spermatogenesis in patients with NOA, it could be interesting to assess the predictive role of markers of intratesticular testosterone level (such as serum 17 OHP) on SSR. Future studies are also required to evaluate the feasibility of molecular markers in the seminal plasma, particularly non-coding RNAs, as markers of residual spermatogenesis in patients with NOA.

Author Contributions: E.C. drafted the manuscript; G.M.C. critically revised the manuscript. All authors have read and agreed to the published version of the manuscript.

Funding: This research received no external funding.

Institutional Review Board Statement: Not applicable.

Informed Consent Statement: Not applicable.

Data Availability Statement: Not applicable.

Conflicts of Interest: The authors declare no conflict of interest.

References

1. Ishikawa, T.; Nose, R.; Yamaguchi, K.; Chiba, K.; Fujisawa, M. Learning curves of microdissection testicular sperm extraction for nonobstructive azoospermia. *Fertil. Steril.* **2010**, *94*, 1008–1011. [CrossRef] [PubMed]
2. Dabaja, A.A.; Schlegel, P.N. Microdissection testicular sperm extraction: An update. *Asian J. Androl.* **2013**, *15*, 35–39. [CrossRef]
3. Colpi, G.M.; Caroppo, E. Performing Microdissection Testicular Sperm Extraction: Surgical Pearls from a High-Volume Infertility Center. *J. Clin. Med.* **2021**, *10*, 4296. [CrossRef] [PubMed]
4. Krausz, C.; Cioppi, F. Genetic Factors of Non-Obstructive Azoospermia: Consequences on Patients' and Offspring Health. *J. Clin. Med.* **2021**, *10*, 4009. [CrossRef] [PubMed]
5. Bojesen, A.; Juul, S.; Gravholt, C. Prenatal and Postnatal Prevalence of Klinefelter Syndrome: A National Registry Study. *J. Clin. Endocrinol. Metab.* **2003**, *88*, 622–626. [CrossRef]
6. Masterson, T.A., III; Nassau, D.E.; Ramasamy, R. A clinical algorithm for management of fertility in adolescents with the Klinefelter syndrome. *Curr. Opin. Urol.* **2020**, *30*, 324–327. [CrossRef]
7. Kang, C.; Punjani, N.; Schlegel, P. Reproductive Chances of Men with Azoospermia Due to Spermatogenic Dysfunction. *J. Clin. Med.* **2021**, *10*, 1400. [CrossRef]
8. Ramasamy, R.; Padilla, W.O.; Osterberg, E.C.; Srivastava, A.; Reifsnyder, J.E.; Niederberger, C.; Schlegel, P.N. A Comparison of Models for Predicting Sperm Retrieval before Microdissection Testicular Sperm Extraction in Men with Nonobstructive Azoospermia. *J. Urol.* **2013**, *189*, 638–642. [CrossRef]
9. Corona, G.; Minhas, S.; Giwercman, A.; Bettocchi, C.; Dinkelman-Smit, M.; Dohle, G.; Fusco, F.; Kadioglou, A.; Kliesch, S.; Kopa, Z.; et al. Sperm recovery and ICSI outcomes in men with non-obstructive azoospermia: A systematic review and meta-analysis. *Hum. Reprod. Update* **2019**, *25*, 733–757. [CrossRef]
10. Colaco, S.; Modi, D. Genetics of the human Y chromosome and its association with male infertility. *Reprod. Biol. Endocrinol.* **2018**, *16*, 1–24. [CrossRef]
11. Yuen, W.; Golin, A.P.; Flannigan, R.; Schlegel, P.N. Histology and sperm retrieval among men with Y chromosome microdeletions. *Transl. Androl. Urol.* **2021**, *10*, 1442–1456. [CrossRef]
12. Zhang, F.; Li, L.; Wang, L.; Yang, L.; Liang, Z.; Li, J.; Jin, F.; Tian, Y. Clinical characteristics and treatment of azoospermia and severe oligospermia patients with Y-chromosome microdeletions. *Mol. Reprod. Dev.* **2013**, *80*, 908–915. [CrossRef]
13. Ozan, T.; Karakeci, A.; Kaplancan, T.; Pirincci, N.; Firdolas, F.; Orhan, I. Are predictive fators in sperm retrieval and pregnancy rates present in nonobstructive azoospermia patients by microdissection testicular sperm extraction on testicle with a history of orchidopexy operation? *Andrologia* **2019**, *51*, e12430. [CrossRef] [PubMed]
14. Osaka, A.; Iwahata, T.; Kobori, Y.; Shimomura, Y.; Yoshikawa, N.; Onota, S.; Yamamoto, A.; Ide, H.; Sugimoto, K.; Okada, H. Testicular volume in non-obstructive azoospermia with a history of bilateral cryptorchidism may predict successful sperm retrieval by testicular sperm extraction. *Reprod. Med. Biol.* **2020**, *19*, 372–377. [CrossRef] [PubMed]
15. Ayan, S.; Orhan, I.; Altay, B.; Aşci, R.; Akbay, E.; Ayas, B.; Yaman, Ő. Fertility outcomes and predictors for successful sperm retrieval and pregnancy in 327 azoospermic men with a history of cryptorchidism who underwent microdissection testicular sperm extraction. *Andrology* **2021**, *9*, 253–259.
16. Elznaty, S. Varicocele repair in non-obstructive azoospermic men: Diagnostic value of testicular biopsy—A meta-analysis. *Scand. J. Urol.* **2014**, *48*, 494–498. [CrossRef]
17. Practice Committee of the American Society for Reproductive Medicine. Management of nonobstructive azoospermia: A committee opinion. *Fertil. Steril.* **2018**, *110*, 1239–1245. [CrossRef]
18. Esteves, S.C.; Miyaoka, R.; Roque, M.; Agarwal, A. Outcome of varicocele repair in men with nonobstructive azoospermia: Systematic review and meta-analysis. *Asian J. Androl.* **2016**, *18*, 246–253. [CrossRef] [PubMed]

19. Schlegel, P.N.; Kaufmann, J. Role of varicocelectomy in men with nonobstructive azoospermia. *Fertil. Steril.* **2004**, *81*, 1585–1588. [CrossRef]
20. Kizilkan, Y.; Toksoz, S.; Turunc, T.; Ozkardes, H. Parameters predicting sperm retrieval rates during microscopic testicular sperm extraction in nonobstructive azoospermia. *Andrologia* **2019**, *51*, e13441. [CrossRef]
21. Ehala-Aleksejev, K.; Punab, M. Relationship between total testicular volume, reproductive parameters and surrogate measures of adiposity in men presenting for couple's infertility. *Andrologia* **2018**, *50*, e12952. [CrossRef]
22. Schoor, R.A.; Elhanbly, S.; Niederberger, C.; Ross, L.S. The role of testicular biopsy in the modern management of male infertility. *J. Urol.* **2002**, *167*, 197–200. [CrossRef]
23. Bryson, C.F.; Ramasamy, R.; Sheehan, M.; Palermo, G.D.; Rosenwaks, Z.; Schlegel, P.N. Severe Testicular Atrophy does not Affect the Success of Microdissection Testicular Sperm Extraction. *J. Urol.* **2014**, *191*, 175–178. [CrossRef] [PubMed]
24. Bernie, A.M.; Shah, K.; Halpern, J.A.; Scovell, J.; Ramasamy, R.; Robinson, B.; Schlegel, P.N. Outcomes of microdissection testicular sperm extraction in men with nonobstructive azoospermia due to maturation arrest. *Fertil. Steril.* **2015**, *104*, 569–573. [CrossRef] [PubMed]
25. Wang, T.; Li, H.; Chen, L.-P.; Yang, J.; Li, M.-C.; Chen, R.-B.; Lan, R.-Z.; Wang, S.; Liu, J.-H. Predictive value of FSH, testicular volume, and histopathological findings for the sperm retrieval rate of microdissection TESE in nonobstructive azoospermia: A meta-analysis. *Asian J. Androl.* **2018**, *20*, 30–36. [CrossRef] [PubMed]
26. Ramasamy, R.; Ricci, J.A.; Palermo, G.D.; Gosden, L.V.; Rosenwaks, Z.; Schlegel, P.N. Successful fertility treatment for Klinefelter's syndrome. *J. Urol.* **2009**, *182*, 1108–1113. [CrossRef]
27. Bakircioglu, M.E.; Ulug, U.; Erden, H.F.; Tosun, S.; Bayram, A.; Ciray, N.; Bahceci, M. Klinefelter syndrome: Does it confer a bad prognosis in treatment of nonobstructive azoospermia? *Fertil. Steril.* **2011**, *95*, 1696–1699. [CrossRef]
28. Sabbaghian, M.; Modarresi, T.; Hosseinifar, H.; Hosseini, J.; Farrahi, F.; Dadkhah, F.; Chehrazi, M.; Khalili, G.; Gilani, M.A.S. Comparison of Sperm Retrieval and Intracytoplasmic Sperm Injection Outcome in Patients with and without Klinefelter Syndrome. *Urology* **2014**, *83*, 107–110. [CrossRef] [PubMed]
29. Rohayem, J.; Fricke, R.; Czeloth, K.; Mallidis, C.; Wistuba, J.; Krallmann, C.; Zitzmann, M.; Kliesch, S. Age and markers of Leydig cell function, but not of Sertoli cell function predict the success of sperm retrieval in adolescents and adults with Klinefelter's syndrome. *Andrology* **2015**, *3*, 868–875. [CrossRef]
30. Donker, R.B.; Vloeberghs, V.; Groen, H.; Tournaye, H.; van Ravenswaaij-Arts, C.M.A.; Land, J.A. Chromosomal abnormal-ities in 1663 infertile men with azoospermia: The clinical consequences. *Hum. Reprod.* **2017**, *32*, 2574–2580. [CrossRef]
31. Ozer, C.; Caglar Aytac, P.; Goren, M.R.; Toksoz, S.; Gul, U.; Turunc, T. Sperm retrieval by microdissection testicular sperm extraction and intracytoplasmic sperm injection outcomes in nonobstructive azoospermic patients with *Klinefelter syndrome*. *Andrologia* **2018**, *50*, e12983. [CrossRef]
32. Chen, X.; Ma, Y.; Zou, S.; Wang, S.; Qiu, J.; Xiao, Q.; Zhou, L.; Ping, P. Comparison and outcomes of nonobstructive azoo-spermia patients with different etiology undergoing MicroTESE and ICSI treatments. *Transl. Androl. Urol.* **2019**, *8*, 366–373. [CrossRef] [PubMed]
33. Huang, I.-S.; Fantus, R.; Chen, W.-J.; Wren, J.; Kao, W.-T.; Huang, E.Y.-H.; Bennett, N.E.; Brannigan, R.E.; Huang, W.J. Do partial AZFc deletions affect the sperm retrieval rate in non-mosaic Klinefelter patients undergoing microdissection testicular sperm extraction? *BMC Urol.* **2020**, *20*, 1–8. [CrossRef] [PubMed]
34. Guo, F.; Fang, A.; Fan, Y.; Fu, X.; Lan, Y.; Liu, M.; Cao, S.; An, G. Role of treatment with human chorionic gonadotropin and clinical parameters on testicular sperm recovery with microdissection testicular sperm extraction and intracytoplasmic sperm injection outcomes in 184 Klinefelter syndrome patients. *Fertil. Steril.* **2020**, *114*, 997–1005. [CrossRef]
35. Zhang, H.L.; Zhao, L.M.; Mao, J.M.; Liu, D.F.; Tang, W.H.; Lin, H.C.; Zhang, L.; Lian, Y.; Hong, K.; Jiang, H. Sperm retrieval rates and clinical outcomes for patients with different causes of azoospermia who undergo microdissection testicular sperm extraction-intracytoplasmic sperm injection. *Asian J. Androl.* **2021**, *23*, 59–63. [CrossRef]
36. Kocamanoglu, F.; Ayas, B.; Bolat, M.S.; Abur, U.; Bolat, R.; Asci, R. Endocrine, sexual and reproductive functions in patients with Klinefelter syndrome compared to non-obstructive azoospermic patients. *Int. J. Clin. Pract.* **2021**, *75*, e14294. [CrossRef] [PubMed]
37. Practice Committee of the American Society for Reproductive Medicine in collaboration with the Society for Male Reproduction and Urology. Evaluation of the azoospermic male: A committee opinion. *Fertil. Steril.* **2018**, *109*, 777–782. [CrossRef] [PubMed]
38. Ramasamy, R.; Lin, K.; Gosden, L.V.; Rosenwaks, Z.; Palermo, G.D.; Schlegel, P.N. High serum FSH levels in men with nonobstructive azoospermia does not affect success of microdissection testicular sperm extraction. *Fertil. Steril.* **2009**, *92*, 590–593. [CrossRef]
39. De Kretser, D.M.; Burger, H.G.; Hudson, B. The relationship between germinal cells and serum FSH levels in males with infertility. *J. Clin. Endocrinol. Metab.* **1974**, *38*, 787–793. [CrossRef]
40. Caroppo, E.; Colpi, E.M.; D'Amato, G.; Gazzano, G.; Colpi, G.M. Prediction model for testis histology in men with non-obstructive azoospermia: Evidence for a limited predictive role of serum follicle-stimulating hormone. *J. Assist. Reprod. Genet.* **2019**, *36*, 2575–2582. [CrossRef]
41. Caroppo, E.; Colpi, G.M. Hormonal treatment of men with nonobstructive azoospermia: What does the evidence suggest? *J. Clin. Med.* **2021**, *10*, 387. [CrossRef]
42. Reifsnyder, J.E.; Ramasamy, R.; Husseini, J.; Schlegel, P.N. Role of Optimizing Testosterone Before Microdissection Testicular Sperm Extraction in Men with Nonobstructive Azoospermia. *J. Urol.* **2012**, *188*, 532–537. [CrossRef]

43. Enatsu, N.; Miyake, H.; Chiba, K.; Fujisawa, M. Predictive factors of successful sperm retrieval on microdissection testicular sperm extraction in Japanese men. *Reprod. Med. Biol.* **2015**, *15*, 29–33. [CrossRef]
44. Althakafi, S.A.; Mustafa, O.M.; Seyam, R.M.; Al-Hathal, N.; Kattan, S. Serum testosterone levels and other determinants of sperm retrieval in microdissection testicular sperm extraction. *Transl. Androl. Urol.* **2017**, *6*, 282–287. [CrossRef] [PubMed]
45. Mehmood, S.; Alhathal, N.; Aldaweesh, S.; Junejo, N.N.; Altaweel, W.M.; Kattan, S.A. Microdissection testicular sperm extraction: Overall results and impact of preoperative testosterone level on sperm retrieval rate in patients with nonobstructive azoospermia. *Urol. Ann.* **2019**, *11*, 287–293. [CrossRef]
46. Lima, T.F.N.; Patel, P.; Blachman-Braun, R.; Madhusoodanan, V.; Ramasamy, R. Serum 17-Hydroxyprogesterone is a Potential Biomarker for Evaluating Intratesticular Testosterone. *J. Urol.* **2020**, *204*, 551–556. [CrossRef] [PubMed]
47. Flannigan, R.; Back, P.V.; Schlegel, P.N. Microdissection testicular sperm extraction. *Transl. Urol.* **2017**, *6*, 745–752. [CrossRef] [PubMed]
48. Punjani, N.; Flannigan, R.; Kang, C.; Khani, F.; Schlegel, P.N. Quantifying Heterogeneity of Testicular Histopathology in Men with Nonobstructive Azoospermia. *J. Urol.* **2021**, *206*, 1268–1275. [CrossRef] [PubMed]
49. Tsujimura, A.; Miyagawa, Y.; Takao, T.; Takada, S.; Koga, M.; Takeyama, M.; Matsumiya, K.; Fujioka, H.; Okuyama, A. Salvage Microdissection Testicular Sperm Extraction After Failed Conventional Testicular Sperm Extraction in Patients With Nonobstructive Azoospermia. *J. Urol.* **2006**, *175*, 1446–1449. [CrossRef]
50. Kalsi, J.S.; Shah, P.; Thum, Y.; Muneer, A.; Ralph, D.J.; Minhas, S. Salvage micro-dissection testicular sperm extraction; Outcome in men with Non obstructive azoospermia with previous failed sperm retrievals. *BJU Int.* **2015**, *116*, 460–465. [CrossRef]
51. Xu, T.; Peng, L.; Lin, X.; Li, J.; Xu, W. Predictors for successful sperm retrieval of salvage microdissection testicular sperm extraction (TESE) following failed TESE in nonobstructive azoospermia patients. *Andrologia* **2016**, *49*, e12642. [CrossRef]
52. Caroppo, E.; Castiglioni, F.; Campagna, C.; Colpi, E.M.; Piatti, E.; Gazzano, G.; Colpi, G.M. Intrasurgical parameters associated with successful sperm retrieval in patients with non-obstructive azoospermia undergoing salvage microdissection testicular sperm extraction. *Andrology* **2021**, *9*, 1864–1871. [CrossRef]
53. Bonaparte, E.; Moretti, M.; Colpi, G.M.; Nerva, F.; Contalbi, G.; Vaccalluzzo, L.; Tabano, S.M.; Grati, F.R.; Gazzano, G.; Sirchia, S.M.; et al. ESX1 gene expression as a robust marker of residual spermatogenesis in azoospermic men. *Hum. Reprod.* **2010**, *25*, 1398–1403. [CrossRef]
54. Pansa, A.; Sirchia, S.M.; Melis, S.; Giacchetta, D.; Castiglioni, M.; Colapietro, P.; Fiori, S.; Falcone, R.; Paganini, L.; Bonaparte, E.; et al. ESX1 mRNA expression in seminal fluid is an indicator of residual spermatogenesis in non-obstructive azoospermic men. *Hum. Reprod.* **2014**, *29*, 2620–2627. [CrossRef]
55. Hashemi, M.-S.; Mozdarani, H.; Ghaedi, K.; Nasr-Esfahani, M.H. Could analysis of testis-specific genes, as biomarkers in seminal plasma, predict presence of focal spermatogenesis in non-obstructive azoospermia? *Andrologia* **2020**, *52*, e13483. [CrossRef] [PubMed]
56. Aslani, F.; Modarresi, M.H.; Soltanghoraee, H.; Akhondi, M.M.; Shabani, A.; Lakpour, N.; Sadeghi, M.R. Seminal molecular markers as a non-invasive diagnostic tool for the evaluation of spermatogenesis in non-obstructive azoospermia. *Syst. Biol. Reprod. Med.* **2011**, *57*, 190–196. [CrossRef]
57. Zarezadeh, R.; Nikanfar, S.; Oghbaei, H.; Rezaei, Y.R.; Jafari-Gharabaghlou, D.; Ahmadi, Y.; Nouri, M.; Fattahi, A.; Dittrich, R. Omics in Seminal Plasma: An Effective Strategy for Predicting Sperm Retrieval Outcome in Non-obstructive Azoospermia. *Mol. Diagn. Ther.* **2021**, *25*, 315–325. [CrossRef] [PubMed]
58. Muñoz, X.; Mata, A.; Bassas, L.; Larriba, S. Altered miRNA Signature of Developing Germ-cells in Infertile Patients Relates to the Severity of Spermatogenic Failure and Persists in Spermatozoa. *Sci. Rep.* **2015**, *5*, 17991. [CrossRef] [PubMed]
59. Barceló, M.; Mata, A.; Bassas, L.; Larriba, S. Exosomal microRNAs in seminal plasma are markers of the origin of azoospermia and can predict the presence of sperm in testicular tissue. *Hum. Reprod.* **2018**, *33*, 1087–1098. [CrossRef]
60. Xie, Y.; Yao, J.; Zhang, X.; Chen, J.; Gao, Y.; Zhang, C.; Chen, H.; Wang, Z.; Zhao, Z.; Chen, W.; et al. A panel of extracellular vesicle long noncoding RNAs in seminal plasma for predicting testicular spermatozoa in nonobstructive azoospermia patients. *Hum. Reprod.* **2020**, *35*, 2413–2427. [CrossRef]
61. Hong, S.H.; Kwon, J.T.; Kim, J.; Jeong, J.; Kim, J.; Lee, S.; Cho, C. Profiling of testis-specific long noncoding RNAs in mice. *BMC Genom.* **2018**, *19*, 539. [CrossRef] [PubMed]

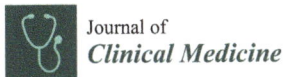

Review

Hormonal Treatment of Men with Nonobstructive Azoospermia: What Does the Evidence Suggest?

Ettore Caroppo [1],* and Giovanni M. Colpi [2]

[1] Asl Bari, PTA "F Jaia", Andrology Outpatients Clinic, 70014 Conversano (BA), Italy
[2] Andrology Unit, ProCrea Institute, 6900 Lugano, Switzerland; gmcolpi@yahoo.com
* Correspondence: ecaroppo@teseo.it

Abstract: Hormonal stimulation of spermatogenesis prior to surgery has been tested by some authors to maximize the sperm retrieval yield in patients with nonobstructive azoospermia. Although the rationale of such an approach is theoretically sound, studies have provided conflicting results, and there are unmet questions that need to be addressed. In the present narrative review, we reviewed the current knowledge about the hormonal control of spermatogenesis, the relationship between presurgical serum hormones levels and sperm retrieval rates, and the results of studies investigating the effect of hormonal treatments prior to microdissection testicular sperm extraction. We pooled the available data about sperm retrieval rate in patients with low vs. normal testosterone levels, and found that patients with normal testosterone levels had a significantly higher chance of successful sperm retrieval compared to those with subnormal T levels (OR 1.63, 95% CI 1.08–2.45, $p = 0.02$). These data suggest that hormonal treatment may be justified in patients with hypogonadism; on the other hand, the available evidence is insufficient to recommend hormonal therapy as standard clinical practice to improve the sperm retrieval rate in patients with nonobstructive azoospermia.

Keywords: nonobstructive azoospermia; micro-TESE; FSH treatment; hormonal treatment; testosterone level

1. Introduction

Azoospermia, defined as the absence of sperm in the ejaculate, affects about 10–15% of infertile men, and in about two-third of cases is due to severe spermatogenic dysfunction [1]: such a clinical condition is termed nonobstructive azoospermia (NOA) to differentiate it from the less severe (in terms of spermatogenesis impairment) form of azoospermia due to obstruction of the seminal tract. Men with NOA may still have residual focal areas of spermatogenesis that could enable them to father children genetically of their own if mature sperm are surgically retrieved and used for intracytoplasmic sperm injection (ICSI): however, sperm retrieval is successful in up to 58% of cases, even when the most effective surgical technique, namely, microdissection testicular sperm extraction (micro-TESE), is used [2]. Among the strategies sought to maximize the sperm retrieval yield, hormonal stimulation of spermatogenesis prior to surgery has been tested by several authors. Although the rationale of such an approach is theoretically sound, studies in the field have provided conflicting results, so that the beneficial effect of hormonal optimization of spermatogenesis is yet to be demonstrated. The present narrative review is intended to discuss the evidence in the field and to offer some points for reflection for further studies. To provide unbiased results and avoid the possible impact of less effective surgical procedure on the sperm retrieval rates, only studies evaluating patients undergoing the gold-standard surgical technique for sperm retrieval (micro-TESE) [2] have been included in the present review.

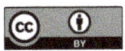

2. Hormonal Control of Spermatogenesis

The role of follicle-stimulating hormone (FSH) in the modulation of spermatogenesis has been a matter of debate since a study on five men with inactivating mutation of the FSH receptor (FSHR) gene showed that none was azoospermic and that two had children [3]. This finding prompted some researchers to hypothesize that FSH was not necessary for spermatogenesis, but the finding that men with inactivating mutations in FSH beta subunit were completely azoospermic [4] challenged that hypothesis. Further studies clarified that the mutant FSHR is not completely inactive [5], so that a residual FSH action could be able to promote spermatogenesis and that mutations in the FSH gene are more severe than those of the FSHR [6].

Studies in mice lacking FSH (FSHKO) or FSHR (FSHRKO) clearly demonstrated that FSH is required to increase the number of spermatogonia and spermatocytes [7] and that FSH treatment was found to increase spermatogonial and spermatocyte number in hypophysectomized or gonadotropin-releasing hormone (GnRH)-immunized adult rats [8]. FSH acts also as a survival factor for spermatogonia, since acute FSH suppression induces spermatogonial apoptosis [9] and is required to stimulate the prenatal and prepubertal proliferation of Sertoli cell, an effect which is totally independent from luteinizing hormone (LH) action, as demonstrated in hypogonadal LH receptor null mice [10], as well as from testosterone action, as demonstrated in mice lacking Sertoli cell androgen receptor (SCARKO) and FSHR, which had a Sertoli cell number comparable to that of FSHRKO mice [7]. In the absence of FSH or FSHR, the Sertoli cell number is decreased by about 30–45% in comparison to normal testicular development: since the Sertoli cell is able to support a certain number of germ cells, the number of Sertoli cells determines the quantity of sperm produced. This may explain why FSHRKO mice present with complete spermatogenesis, but the amount of germ cells is lower than in wild-type animals [7].

Studies in men with congenital hypogonadotropic hypogonadism suggest that pretreatment with FSH alone prior to combined gonadotropin treatment enhances spermatogenesis [11]. However, FSH alone is not able to promote spermatogenesis beyond the pachytene spermatocytes: a recent study on SCARKO mice demonstrated that Sertoli cell androgen receptor (AR) signaling is required for the survival of meiotic prophase spermatocytes, since SCARKO mice exhibited loss of meiotic germ cells and failure of surviving spermatocytes to progress. Early meiotic prophase events are not dependent upon androgen signaling, therefore, chromosome synapsis and recombination occurred normally in surviving spermatocytes that entered meiotic prophase; however, SCARKO pachytene spermatocytes were found to acquire aberrant transcriptomic attributes (leptotene or zygotene transcriptome state) and failed to progress to subsequent transcriptomic signatures [12].

FSH alone has been also found to maintain spermatogenesis independently from testosterone; this is the case of transgenic male mice with activating FSHR mutation that enabled strong FSH activation (cAMP response > 10-fold above basal). Use of the antiandrogen flutamide to interfere the binding of androgens to the AR had no effect on spermatogenesis [13].

In normal conditions, however, testosterone signaling is required for spermatogenesis to proceed beyond meiosis. Testosterone signaling contributes also to maintaining tight junctions between adjacent Sertoli cells (essential for the blood-testis barrier) and a specialized environment for germ cells, mainly through its modulation of micro-RNAs that target genes essential for cell junction restructuring and Sertoli-germ cell adhesion. The absence of T results in disruption of blood–testis barrier, premature detachment of developing spermatid germ cells from Sertoli cells, and block of the release of mature spermatozoa from Sertoli cells, with consequent germ cells phagocytosis by Sertoli cells [14].

Testosterone (T) is produced by Leydig cells in response to LH, and mediates its effects by the AR expressed by the Sertoli cells via classical and nonclassical pathways. In the classical (genomic) pathway, T diffuses through the plasma membrane and interacts with AR and the complex T/AR translocates to the nucleus to bind to androgen response elements

(AREs) in gene promoter regions and regulates gene transcription, while in the nonclassical (nongenomic) pathway, T/AR rapidly phosphorylates the SRC kinase, resulting in the stimulation of the epithelial growth factor (EGF) receptor and the fast (within 1 min) activation of MAP-kinase cascade and the CREB transcription factor, with a resulting sustained (for at least 12 h) increased protein phosphorylation and long-term gene expression changes that are mediated by increased kinase activity [15]. Both pathways are essential for spermatogenesis: a study performed on testis explants of male Sprague Dawley rats containing intact seminiferous tubules and accompanying interstitial cells, using inhibitors to specifically block each pathway in vitro, demonstrated that both pathways are able to activate transcription of the Sertoli cell-specific Rhox5 mRNA, which is dramatically upregulated in the presence of T in vivo, and that activation of either T signaling pathway in Sertoli cells can differentially modulate germ cells gene expression [15].

It has been classically demonstrated that intratesticular testosterone (ITT) concentration are much higher (50–100-fold) than circulating levels, however, spermatogenesis may be maintained by very low ITT concentration: mice with inactivation of the LH receptor (LuRKO mice) had intact spermatogenesis despite very low ITT levels (2% of control level), but administration of the antiandrogen flutamide halted sperm maturation at the round spermatid stage [16]. In addition, a more recent study demonstrated that spermatogenesis in LuRKO mice could be normalized with exogenous testosterone that achieved a serum T concentration comparable to that of WT mice, but an ITT level less than 1.5% of the WT concentration [17]. The relationship between serum and intratesticular T levels is, therefore, far to have been clearly established, so that further studies are needed.

It has been proposed that testosterone alone could induce complete spermatogenesis without the need of FSH action; indeed, subcutaneous testosterone supplementation in male mice with hypogonadotropic hypogonadism due to Kiss1 knockout was able to restore serum and intratesticular testosterone levels, promote testicular descent, and induce complete spermatogenesis from spermatocytes to elongated spermatids, but the resultant testicular weight reached only 40% of wild-type controls, similarly to what was found in hypogonadal or GnRH KO mice treated with testosterone supplementation. [18]. Such a quantitative deficit of spermatogenesis is likely to be due to the lack of FSH.

Both FSH and testosterone are, therefore, required to promote full spermatogenesis; in addition, both hormones have synergistic effects upon spermatogenesis. FSH regulates transcripts required for normal testicular function, including StAR gene, which is essential for steroid synthesis [14], and stimulates the Sertoli cell production of androgen binding globulin, which helps maintain a high T concentration within the testes. On the other hand, testosterone is thought to modulate the oligosaccharide complexity of pituitary FSH; castration induces changes in the oligosaccharide composition of pituitary FSH both in prepubertal and adult animals, and administration of flutamide, able to interfere the binding of androgens to the AR both peripherally and at hypothalamic-pituitary level, lead to a predominance of circulating FSH glycosylation variants bearing incomplete oligosaccharides [19]. Administration of testosterone enanthate to pubertal patients does not modify the serum FSH levels, but lead to a significant increase in the proportion of FSH bearing complex oligosaccharides [20].

3. Relationship between Serum Hormones Levels and Sperm Retrieval

It has been clearly established that preoperative FSH levels are poorly or not predictive of successful sperm retrieval in men with NOA undergoing micro-TESE [21,22]. FSH serum levels are usually high in men with NOA, and although lower levels can be found in those patients who may theoretically benefit from hormonal treatment, such as those with testis histology revealing hypospermatogenesis (HYPO) or maturation arrest (MA) [23], they cannot be used to reliably predict these conditions before surgery [24]. Lower FSH levels are not always predictive of intact spermatogenesis in patients with NOA; on the contrary, micro-TESE has been found to be more successful in patients with higher serum FSH (>15 mIU/mL) compared to those with lower serum FSH [25], and in the subset of

NOA patients with MA, normal serum FSH level was associated with the lowest chance of sperm retrieval [26]. Since basal FSH serum level is not related to spermatogenesis nor to the chance of retrieving sperm in patients with NOA, it is unlikely that it may be used to predict which patient with NOA could respond to hormonal treatment. High or very high FSH serum levels should not prevent the use of exogenous FSH to stimulate spermatogenesis; although it has been classically demonstrated that such a condition could induce desensitization of the Sertoli cell signaling [27], a more recent in vitro study using KK-1 mouse granulosa cells demonstrated that FSH receptor recycling promotes the maintenance of cell surface receptors and preserves hormonal responsiveness during exogenous FSH stimulation [28].

The situation is quite different for the predictive role of serum T on the chances of sperm retrieval, since studies in the field have reported conflicting results. We were able to individuate 14 studies [29–42] who clearly reported the relationship between serum T levels and sperm retrieval rates (SRR) (Table 1). Studies differed for study design, inclusion criteria, and patients' characteristics. Some studies were designed to compare the SRRs of conventional TESE vs. micro-TESE, while others were sought to assess presurgical markers of sperm retrieval. In 8 out of 14 studies, the cohorts included patients with Klinefelter syndrome (KS) (1.7–36.2% of the total sample), who have been found to have better chances of successful sperm retrieval (SSR) when their presurgical T levels are normal [43,44]. In 3 studies, patients received presurgical hormonal treatment (hCG, clomiphene citrate—CC, or aromatase inhibitors—AI), while in other 3, no treatment was used; in the remainders, it is not clear whether patients received any hormonal treatment before micro-TESE.

Seven studies included patients with subnormal presurgical T levels, and six of them [34,37,38,40–42] provided the sperm retrieval rates in patients with low vs. normal T levels. We pooled these latter data to compute the resulting odds ratio (OR), using random-effects models to comply with the high heterogeneity in study design, as detected by I^2 and by Cochran's Q. Computations and forest plot were obtained using Review Manager (RevMan, Version 5.3. Copenhagen: The Nordic Cochrane Centre, The Cochrane Collaboration, 2014). The pooled estimate, as displayed in Figure 1, showed that patients with normal T levels had a significantly higher chance of SSR compared to those with subnormal T levels (OR 1.63, 95% CI 1.08–2.45, p = 0.02). Notably, in the study with the largest sample size included in the analysis [34], 88% of patients with low T received hormonal treatment, but their post-treatment T levels remained still below the normal cut-off level of 300 ng/dL. However, as illustrated in the previous paragraph, the relationship between serum and intratesticular T levels needs to be fully clarified.

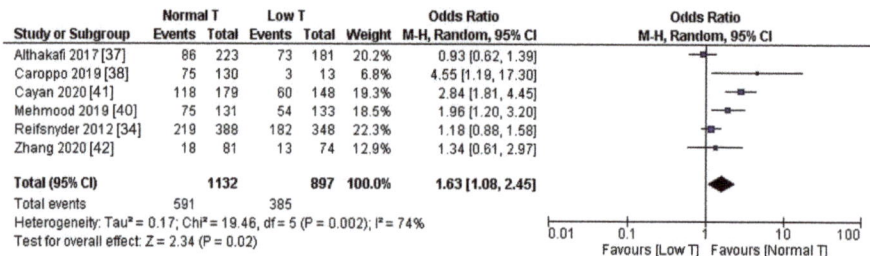

Figure 1. Pooled estimation of the sperm retrieval rate in patients with subnormal vs. normal testosterone level.

Table 1. Testosterone level and sperm retrieval in patients with nonobstructive azoospermia (NOA) undergoing microdissection testicular sperm extraction (micro-TESE).

Study	Patients Characteristics	KS	Subnormal T Levels	Main Results	Hormonal Treatment
[29]	74 patients SRR 44.4%	Yes (11/74; 14.8%)	Not shown	No relationship was found between serum T levels and SSR. Data about T serum level in patients with SSR and SRF are not provided	NS
[30]	100 patients SRR 41%	No	Not shown	T was significantly higher in men with SSR than in those with SRF (410 ± 170 vs. 320 ± 110 ng/dL. p = 0.0036). On multivariate logistic regression. T was predictive of SSR (OR 1.57; 95% CI 1.02–2.42; p = 0.042). Patients with SRF had also significantly higher FSH level and smaller testis size compared to those with SSR	NS
[31]	100 patients SRR 41%	No	Not shown	T predicted SSR at univariate logistic analysis (p = 0.0008) but not at multivariate logistic analysis. Data about T serum level in patients with SSR and SRF are not provided	NS
[32]	56 patients with previous failed TESA/TESE SRR 57%	Yes (1/56; 1.7%)	13 patients (23%) with T < 280 ng/dL	T was significantly higher in patients with SSR (32) compared to those with SRF (24) (458.3 ± 254.2 vs. 378.5 ± 257.3; p = 0.021).	NS
[33]	65 patients. SRR 56.9%	No	Not shown	T levels did not affect SSR (OR 1.06; 95% CI 0.84–1.33; p = 0.64). Data about T serum level in patients with SSR and SRF are not provided	NS
[34]	736 patients SRR 54.4%	Yes (88/736; 12%)	348 patients (47%) had low T levels (<300 ng/dL) before hormonal treatment. Post-treatment T levels are not provided	SRR was 52% of patients with low T vs. 56% of patients with normal T (p = 0.29). No difference in terms of SSR in patients with low basal T who did or did not receive hormonal treatment post-treatment T levels are not displayed.	Yes (307/348 patients with low basal T levels)
[35]	191 patients SRR 54.5%	Yes (7/191; 3%)	Not shown	Testosterone level was significantly higher in men with SSR compared to those with SRF (468 ± 263 vs. 367 ± 258; p = 0.023). The testosterone serum cut-off-level of 400 ng/mL significantly predicted SSR with a sensitivity of 55.2 and a specificity of 60%. AUC 0.648	NS
[36]	329 patients SRR 29.5%	Yes (65/329; 19.7%)	Not shown	T levels did not differ among men with SSR (97) and SRF (232) (420 ± 180 vs. 430 ± 190 ng/dL; p = 0.42)	NS
[37]	421 patients SSR 39.4%	Yes (13/431; 3%)	181 patients (43%) had low T (≤9.9 nmol/L).	SRR did not differ in patients with low T (40.3%) compared to those with normal T (38.6%) (p = 0.718); Mean serum T was 11.51 ± 7.40 nmol/L in patients with SSR and 11.67 ± 6.42 nmol/L in patients with SRF. SRR did not differ between patients with normal T vs. untreated low T (42%. p = 0.526) and normal vs. pretreated low T normalized with hormonal treatment (36%; p = 0.736)	Yes (50/421)
[38]	143 patients SRR 55.2%	Yes (6/143; 4.1%)	13 patients (9%) had low T (300 ng/dL)	Testosterone serum level was significantly lower in patients with SRF compared to those with SSR (380 vs. 422 ng/dL; p = 0.007). Sperm retrieval was 23% in patients with low T and 58% in those with normal T (p = 0.014). However. T was not predictive of SSR in multivariate logistic analysis.	No
[39]	860 patients SSR 45.8%	Yes (312/860; 36.2%)	Not shown	Testosterone level was predictive of SSR in univariate but not in multivariate logistic regression	Yes (54/860)
[40]	264 patients 89 (33.9%) had previous surgery SRR 48.86%	NS	133 with low T (<10 nmol/L = 288 ng/dL)	SSR was 40.6 in low T vs. 57.25 in normal T (p = 0.0068)	No
[41]	327 patients with history of cryptorchidism SSR 52.6%	No	148 (45.2%) patients had low T (<300 ng/dL)	SSR was 40.5% in low T and 65.9% in normal T (p < 0.0001).	No
[42]	155 patients with idiopathic NOA SSR 20%	No	74 patients (48%) had T < 9.9 nmol/L.	SSR was 17.6 in low T and 22.2 in normal T (p = NS)	NS

AUC, Area under curve; KS, Klinefelter syndrome; NS, not specified; SRR, sperm retrieval rate; SSR, successful sperm retrieval; SRF, sperm retrieval failure; T, testosterone.

This is the reason why it has been suggested that ITT measurement, more than serum T level assay, could add to the evaluation of patients with NOA. Testicle aspiration is not always feasible and advisable, due to the possible inherent risks of such a procedure (pain, bleeding, infection, and testis injury), so that attempts have been made to individuate serum biomarker able to identify men with insufficient ITT and to serve for ITT levels monitoring following hormonal treatment. Since most of the circulating 17-hydroxyprogesterone (17OH-P) in men is likely of testicular and not adrenal origin, as demonstrated in orchiectomized men [45], it has been postulated that serum 17 OHP may reflect the ITT levels. Unfortunately, only a few studies tried to address this issue. Amory and coworkers evaluated 29 healthy men who received testosterone enanthate to suppress endogenous secretion before being randomly assigned to three hCG doses (125, 250, or 500 IU every other day for 3 weeks) or placebo. ITT levels were assessed by fine needle aspiration of testicular fluid; serum 17 OHP did not correlate with ITT at baseline, but following hCG treatment, a strong relationship between ITT and 17 OHP was found in men who received 250 or 500 IU hCG [46]. Very recently, Lima et al. evaluated the serum 17 OHP levels in 30 men receiving CC and/or hCG, 21 men under exogenous testosterone replacement therapy, and 42 fertile men with normal serum testosterone; despite serum T level was in the normal range in all men, serum 17-OHP was undetectable in men who received exogenous testosterone replacement therapy compared to the other two groups, and increased after CC and hCG treatment [47].

A possible role for serum insulin-like factor 3 (INSL3) as marker of ITT has been also postulated; gonadotropin suppression with exogenous testosterone and progestin resulted in decline of serum INSL3 levels compared to baseline, which was partially reversed by hCG or FSH plus hCG administration; following long-term gonadotropin suppression, serum T recovered significantly better (80% baseline) compared to serum INSL3 (38.9% baseline) [48]. In a subsequent randomized placebo-controlled clinical trial, serum INSL3 concentrations in normal men were found to dramatically decrease following acute gonadotropin suppression, and to increase in a dose–response relationship with low-dose hCG stimulation, correlating highly with ITT and serum T concentration [49].

Although intriguing, the diagnostic accuracy of 17 OHP and/or INSL3 assay as marker of ITT should be verified in larger sample studies before their introduction in the clinical practice.

4. Hormonal Treatment before Micro-TESE

Administration of exogenous gonadotropins has been classically found to be effective in restoring spermatogenesis in azoospermic men with hypogonadotropic hypogonadism. Consequently, hormonal treatment in men with NOA has been pursued with the aim of improving spermatogenesis before surgery, despite these patients may display high FSH and LH levels. It has been demonstrated, in fact, that in these patients Leydig cells respond to high dose hCG stimulation with increased amounts of testosterone production, even under a hypergonadotropic condition [23]. The authors demonstrated that patients with NOA display an altered gonadotrophin pulse amplitude and hypothesized that this weak endogenous gonadotrophin activity could be due to the desensitization of target cells (e.g., Sertoli and Leydig cells). Indeed, other studies demonstrated that men with NOA display abnormalities in gonadotropins pulse frequency and amplitude [50], however, these findings are presumably the consequence of an altered hypothalamus–pituitary–gonadal axis due to reduced testosterone and inhibin B feedback signaling, rather than to desensitization of target cells. As a matter of fact, it has demonstrated that desensitization of Sertoli cells does not occur, but hormonal responsiveness during FSH treatment is preserved, thanks to FSH receptor recycling [28]. Consequently, it may be hypothesized that at least a subset of men with NOA, e.g., those with subnormal T serum levels and inhibin B levels may have an altered endogenous gonadotropin secretion that justifies the use of exogenous gonadotropins or selective estrogen receptors modulators (SERMs) like CC.

Indeed, Shinjo et al. [51] found that hCG treatment significantly increased the ITT levels in patients with NOA; although ITT did not differ among those with SSR or sperm retrieval failure (SRF), men with SSR had significantly lower basal ITT levels compared to men who experienced SRF. This may reinforce the hypothesis that hormonal stimulation is required for men with subnormal T levels to optimize the sperm recovery. However, the administration of hCG alone, although being effective in improving SSR, may be not sufficient to promote spermatogenesis in men with NOA; in the same study, only men who received FSH had an increased spermatogonial proliferating cell nuclear antigen (PCNA) expression, a protein involved in nucleotide excision repair mechanisms prominently expressed in the nuclei of mitotic active spermatogonia, which has been proposed as a marker of normally active spermatogonia [52]. Furthermore, it has been demonstrated that the expression of AR on Sertoli cells increased following FSH plus hCG stimulation rather than after hCG alone [53], supporting the previous demonstration about the role of FSH in regulating Sertoli cell AR expression [54].

The results of the few studies available in this field, however, are not fully able to demonstrate a beneficial effect of hormonal treatment on the SRR in men with NOA. As displayed in Table 2, five studies [34,55–58] were carried in NOA men who underwent micro-TESE for the first time, while four [23,51,53,59] enrolled men undergoing salvage micro-TESE. The first two studies evaluated a well-selected cohort of patients, e.g., normogonadotropic men [55] and men with well-defined testis histology (MA and HYPO) [56], therefore, their results have poor generalizability, while the results of Amer and coworkers [58] are weakened by the relatively low overall SRR (32,2%), probably due to differences in skill and experience among the 15 urologists who performed micro-TESE. The two largest sample studies [34,57] provided conflicting results, i.e., in the study of Reifsnyder et al. [34], SRR did not differed among men with subnormal T levels receiving hormonal treatment (N = 307) or no treatment (N = 41), while in the study of Hussein et al. [57], SRR was significantly higher in men receiving hormonal treatment (N = 496) compared to those receiving no treatment (N = 112), and 10.9% of treated patients had sperm in the ejaculate after treatment. It has to be remarked that the post-treatment T levels differed significantly among studies, since in the study of Reifsnyder, 82% of treated patients responded to hormonal treatment with a serum T level of at least 250 ng, while in the study of Hussein, treatment was titrated to reach a target T level of 600–800 ng/dL; still, the SRR in the study of Reifsnyder in both treated and untreated patients (51 and 61%, respectively) was comparable to that obtained by patients undergoing hormonal treatment in the study of Hussein, while the SRR of untreated patients in this latter study was too low compared to the average SRR reported by studies in the micro-TESE setting.

On the other hand, the two out of four studies evaluating the results of salvage micro-TESE in treated vs. untreated patients [23,59] agreed in demonstrating the beneficial effect of hormonal treatment on SRR, however, the small number of subjects (48 treated vs. 40 untreated overall) does not allow to draw firm conclusions about that.

Another indication to hormonal treatment in men with NOA has been proposed to be their testicular histological pattern. Kato and coworkers observed that men with early MA had a lower AR index compared to those with late MA [53]; indeed, SCARKO mice have been found to display pachytene spermatocytes with aberrant transcriptomic attributes (leptotene or zygotene transcriptome state) that fail to progress to subsequent transcriptomic signatures [12]. Based on these results, Shiraishi hypothesized that only patients with late MA may respond to hormonal treatment [23]. Indeed, Aydos and coworkers did not observe improvements in SRR in patients with early MA undergoing hormonal treatment [55]. Other groups demonstrated that men with MA or HYPO respond to hormonal treatment with either the appearance of sperm in the ejaculate [57] or with improved SSR [56] even in the case of salvage micro-TESE [51]. However, also in this case, larger sample size studies are needed to confirm these findings.

The results of the available studies, although promising, are insufficient to recommend the hormonal treatment for every patient with NOA before surgery. Therefore, as stated by the recent AUA/ASRM guidelines on the diagnosis and management of infertility in men [60], patients with NOA should be informed of the limited data supporting pharmacologic prior to surgical intervention (Conditional Recommendation; Evidence Level; Grade C).

Table 2. Hormonal treatment and successful sperm retrieval (SSR) in patients with NOA undergoing micro-TESE.

Study	Patients Characteristics	Treatment	Results
[55]	108 men. 16 with SCO. 36 with focal SCO. 19 with MA. 37 with HYPO. All had serum FSH level below 8 mIU/mL	63 men received FSH 75 IU 3 times/week. 45 received no treatment	SSR 64% (40/63) in FSH treated and 33% (15/45) in controls ($p < 0.01$) SCO 2/7 (28% controls) vs. 4/9 (44% treated) p = NS FSCO 4/16 (25%) vs. 13/20 (65% treated) ($p < 0.01$) MA 3/8 (37%) vs. 5/11 (45% treated) p = NS HYPO 6/14 (42%) vs. 18/23 (78% treated) $p < 0.05$
[56]	42 men with MA (42.9%) and HYPO (57.1%)	CC 25–75 mg/day to achieve T 600–800 ng/dL (study target)	27/42 (64.3%) had sperm in the ejaculate; SSR 100% (15/15)
[34]	348 out of 736 patients had subnormal T. 307 out of 348 received hormonal therapy. 41 (12%) received no treatment	348 (47%) with low T (<300) and 388 with normal T (>300). 307 out of 348 (88%) were treated with hormonal therapy. 41 (12%) were not treated.	SSR in 52% of patients with low T and in 56% of patients with normal T. SSR 51% in treated vs. 61% in untreated
[23]	48 men with failed micro-TESE	28 hCG/hCG plus FSH if FSH levels decreased during treatment. 20 received no treatment. T did not differ among groups	Sperm retrieval 21% (treatment) vs. 0 (no treatment).
[57]	608 men	496 received CC, then hCG, and, eventually, hMG according to their response to CC, while 112 received no treatment. Target T level = 600–800 ng/dL	10.9% of patients had sperm in the ejaculate; SSR was 57% in treated and 33% in controls
[51]	20 men with failed micro-TESE	hCG followed by FSH if serum FSH < 2	SSR 3/20 (15%). T did not differ among patients with SSR and SRF Spermatogonial PCNA expression increased in patients receiving FSH Patients with SSR had significantly lower basal ITT compared to those with SRF. Post-treatment ITT increased in all patients
[53]	22 men with failed micro-TESE	All received hCG 5000 3 times a week; 12 patients received also FSH 150 thrice/week since FSH level dropped below 2	SSR 4/22 (18%). A significant increase in the AR index was observed in 12 patients receiving FSH + hCG. AR index was significantly higher in men with SSR compared to SRF. T levels did not correlate with AR index
[58]	1395 patients evaluated by different surgeons	SSR 450/1395 (32.2%) Hormonal therapy (CC or hCG or HMG or FSH or T or AI combination of drugs) in 426 patients	SSR was 27.6% (118/426) in treated vs. 31.7% (308/969) in untreated. No data about T levels in treated vs. untreated.
[59]	40 men with failed micro-TESE.	20 received testosterone for 1 month. then FSH plus testosterone, while 20 received no treatment	SSR in salvage micro-TESE was 10% in treated vs. 0 in controls. No data about T levels in treated vs. untreated.

FSCO, focal Sertoli cell only syndrome; HYPO, hypospermatogenesis; ITT, intratesticular testosterone level; MA, maturation arrest; PCNA, proliferating cell nuclear antigen; NA, not applicable; SCO, Sertoli cell only syndrome; SRF, sperm retrieval failure; SSR, successful sperm retrieval.

5. Unmet Needs and Future Directions

The management of patients with NOA is to a large extent knowledge based. Thanks to the evidence produced by the literature of the past 20 years, we know with a good approximation that about 57–60% of patients with NOA may be successful in having their testicular sperm retrieved, what clinical conditions are predictive of SSR, that SRR may vary significantly according to testis histology and that micro-TESE provides better results in terms of SRR compared to the other available surgical techniques [61]. What we do not know, due to the inconclusive data provided by the literature, is whether and how should we treat these patients before surgery to maximize the chance of sperm retrieval.

The pooled estimation of studies reporting the SRRs in patients with subnormal T compared to those with normal T levels (Figure 1) suggests that optimization of serum T levels may be indicated in hypogonadal men before micro-TESE, since it may improve the SRR. However, due to the demonstrated poor relationship between serum and intratesticular T levels [17], and to the relatively low ITT required for spermatogenesis [16], the target serum T levels to be achieved to improve spermatogenesis is not clear. Relevantly, two large sample studies [34,57] reported similar SRRs despite significantly different post-treatment T levels (230 vs. 600–800 ng/dL). To improve our knowledge in this field, it could be helpful to identify serum biomarker that could reliably predict ITT levels and serve for post-treatment ITT levels monitoring. In this perspective, the demonstration that serum 17 OHP and INSL3 levels are, to some extent, related to ITT levels, may pave the way for a new line of research. In addition, the possible predictive role of bioactive T level (computed by the formula (Bio T= free T + albumin-bound T)) on SRR would deserve further studies.

Optimization of testosterone and, possibly, ITT levels, may require also FSH, since the expression of AR on Sertoli cells increases following FSH stimulation but not with hCG [53]. In addition, since FSH is essential to promote spermatogonial proliferation in men with NOA [51], many authors added FSH to hCG or CC when falling serum FSH levels were observed following hormonal treatment (Table 2). Interestingly, although the feasibility of FSH as treatment of infertile men with oligozoospermia has been investigated by many studies, with a recent one even proposing that possible responders to FSH treatment may be identified by means of epigenetic biomarkers [62], very few studies sought to evaluate the effect of FSH alone to improve the chance of SRR in patients with NOA. Indeed, the finding that FSH may maintain spermatogenesis independently from testosterone, as found in transgenic male mice with activating FSHR mutation that enabled strong FSH activation, may prompt further studies on high dose FSH treatment of men with NOA.

Although we know with a good approximation the chance of SSR in men with different testis histology, we need more data to establish whether a specific histological pattern may be considered an indication or a contraindication to hormonal treatment. It would be helpful, therefore, for further studies in this field to report the response to hormonal treatment as stratified by testis histology. It is reminded here that, to obtain reliable testis histology pictures, the fragments of seminiferous tubules sent to the pathologist should be representative of the predominant tissue as observed at high magnification during micro-TESE.

In conclusion, to establish whether hormonal treatment may be of help in improving the reproductive potential of men with NOA, it is of the utmost importance to design studies with large sample size and well-defined entry criteria and outcome measures: in this view, collaborative multicentric studies could provide valuable data. The actual evidence is insufficient to support the indiscriminate use of hormonal treatment prior to surgery in patients with NOA.

Author Contributions: Drafted the manuscript, E.C.; critically revised the manuscript, G.M.C. All authors have read and agreed to the published version of the manuscript.

Funding: This research received no external funding

Data Availability Statement: No new data were created or analyzed in this study. Data sharing is not applicable to this article.

Conflicts of Interest: The authors declare no conflict of interest.

Abbreviations

17OHP	17 hydroxyprogesterone
AI	aromatase inhibitors
AR	androgen receptor
ARE	androgen response elements
ARKO	AR knock out animals
cAMP	cyclic adenosine monophosphate
CC	clomiphene citrate
CI	confidence interval
CREB	cAMP response element-binding protein
EGF	epithelial growth factor
FSH	follicle-stimulating hormone
FSHKO	FSH knock out animals
FSHR	FSH receptor
FSHRKO	FSHR knock out animals
GNRH	gonadotropin-releasing hormone
HCG	human chorionic gonadotropin
HYPO	hypospermatogenesis
INSL3	insulin-like factor 3
ITT	intratesticular testosterone
KS	Klinefelter syndrome
LH	luteinizing hormone
LHR	LH receptor
LuRKO	LHR knock out animals
MA	maturation arrest
MAP kinase	mitogen-activated protein kinase
Micro-TESE	microdissection testicular sperm extraction
NOA	nonobstructive azoospermia
OR	odds ratio
SCARKO	Sertoli cell AR knock out animals
SCO	Sertoli-cell only syndrome
SERM	selective estrogen receptors modulators
SRF	sperm retrieval failure
SRR	sperm retrieval rate
SSR	successful sperm retrieval
STAR	steroidogenic acute regulatory protein
T	testosterone

References

1. Esteves, S.C. Clinical management of infertile men with nonobstructive azoospermia. *Asian J. Androl.* **2015**, *17*, 459–470. [CrossRef] [PubMed]
2. Bernie, A.M.; Mata, D.A.; Ramasamy, R.; Schlegel, P.N. Comparison of microdissection testicular sperm extraction, conventional testicular sperm extraction, and testicular sperm aspiration for nonobstructive azoospermia: A systematic review and meta-analysis. *Fertil. Steril.* **2015**, *104*, 1099–1103. [CrossRef] [PubMed]
3. Tapanainen, J.S.; Aittomäki, K.; Min, J.; Vaskivuo, T.; Huhtaniemi, I.T. Men homozygous for an inactivating mutation of the follicle-stimulating hormone (FSH) receptor gene present variable suppression of spermatogenesis and fertility. *Nat. Genet.* **1997**, *15*, 205–206. [CrossRef] [PubMed]
4. Zheng, J.; Mao, J.; Cui, M.; Liu, Z.; Wang, X.; Xiong, S.; Nie, M.; Wu, X. Novel FSHβ mutation in a male patient with isolated FSH deficiency and infertility. *Eur. J. Med Genet.* **2017**, *60*, 335–339. [CrossRef] [PubMed]
5. Rannikko, A.; Pakarinen, P.; Manna, P.R.; Beau, I.; Misrahi, M.; Aittomäki, K. Functional characterization of the human FSH receptor with an inactivating Ala189Val mutation. *Mol. Hum. Reprod.* **2002**, *8*, 311–317. [CrossRef]
6. Siegel, E.T.; Kim, H.G.; Nishimoto, H.K.; Layman, L.C. The molecular basis of impaired follicle-stimulating hormone action: Evidence from human mutations and mouse models. *Reprod. Sci.* **2013**, *20*, 211–233. [CrossRef]

7. Abel, M.H.; Baker, P.J.; Charlton, H.M.; Monteiro, A.; Verhoeven, G.; De Gendt, K.; Guillou, F.; O'Shaughnessy, P.J. Spermatogenesis and sertoli cell activity in mice lacking sertoli cell receptors for follicle-stimulating hormone and androgen. *Endocrinology* **2008**, *149*, 3279–3285. [CrossRef]
8. McLachlan, R.I.; Wreford, N.G.; de Kretser, D.M.; Robertson, D.M. The effects of recombinant follicle-stimulating hormone on the restoration of spermatogenesis in the gonadotropin-releasing hormone-immunized adult rat. *Endocrinology* **1995**, *136*, 4035–4043. [CrossRef]
9. Ruwanpura, S.M.; McLachlan, R.I.; Meachem, S.J. Hormonal regulation of male germ cell development. *J. Endocrinol.* **2010**, *205*, 117–131. [CrossRef]
10. Allan, C.M.; Garcia, A.; Spaliviero, J.; Zhang, F.P.; Jimenez, M.; Huhtaniemi, I.; Handelsman, D.J. Complete Sertoli cell proliferation induced by follicle-stimulating hormone (FSH) independently of luteinizing hormone activity: Evidence from genetic models of isolated FSH action. *Endocrinology* **2004**, *145*, 1587–1593. [CrossRef]
11. Dwyer, A.A.; Sykiotis, G.P.; Hayes, F.J.; Boepple, P.A.; Lee, H.; Loughin, K.R.; Dym, M.; Sluss, P.M.; Crowley, W.F.; Pitteloud, N. Trial of recombinant follicle-stimulating hormone pretreatment for GnRH-induced fertility in patients with congenital hypogonadotropic hypogonadism. *J. Clin. Endocrinol. Metab.* **2013**, *98*, E1790–E1795. [CrossRef] [PubMed]
12. Larose, H.; Kent, T.; Ma, Q.; Shami, A.N.; Harerimana, N.; Li, J.Z.; Hammoud, S.S.; Handel, M.A. Regulation of meiotic progression by Sertoli-cell androgen signaling. *Mol. Biol. Cell* **2020**, *31*, 2841–2862. [CrossRef] [PubMed]
13. Oduwole, O.O.; Peltoketo, H.; Poliandri, A.; Vengadabady, L.; Chrusciel, M.; Doroszko, M.; Samanta, L.; Owen, L.; Keevil, B.; Rahman, N.A.; et al. Constitutively active follicle-stimulating hormone receptor enables androgen-independent spermatogenesis. *J. Clin. Invest.* **2018**, *128*, 1787–1792. [CrossRef] [PubMed]
14. Smith, L.B.; Walker, W.H. Hormone signaling in the testis. In *Knobil and Neil's Physiology of Reproduction*, 4th ed.; Academic Press: Cambridge, MA, USA, 2015; pp. 637–690.
15. Toocheck, C.; Clister, T.; Shupe, J.; Crum, C.; Ravindranathan, P.; Lee, T.K.; Ahn, J.M.; Raj, G.V.; Sukhwani, M.; Orwig, K.E.; et al. Mouse spermatogenesis requires classical and nonclassical testosterone signaling. *Biol. Reprod.* **2016**, *94*, 11. [CrossRef]
16. Zhang, F.P.; Pakarainen, T.; Poutanen, M.; Toppari, J.; Huhtaniemi, I. The low gonadotropin-independent constitutive production of testicular testosterone is sufficient to maintain spermatogenesis. *Proc. Natl. Acad. Sci. USA* **2003**, *100*, 13692–13697. [CrossRef]
17. Oduwole, O.O.; Vydra, N.; Wood, N.E.; Samanta, L.; Owen, L.; Keevil, B.; Donaldson, M.; Naresh, K.; Huhtaniemi, I.T. Overlapping dose responses of spermatogenic and extragonadal testosterone actions jeopardize the principle of hormonal male contraception. *FASEB J.* **2014**, *28*, 2566–2576. [CrossRef]
18. Goto, T.; Hirabayashi, M.; Watanabe, Y.; Sanbo, M.; Tomita, K.; Inoue, N.; Tsukamura, H.; Uenoyama, Y. Testosterone supplementation rescues spermatogenesis and in vitro fertilizing ability of sperm in Kiss1 knockout mice. *Endocrinology* **2020**, *161*, bqaa092. [CrossRef]
19. Campo, S.; Andreone, L.; Ambao, V.; Urrutia, M.; Calandra, R.S.; Rulli, S.B. Hormonal regulation of follicle-stimulating hormone glycosylation in males. *Front. Endocrinol.* **2019**, *10*, 17. [CrossRef]
20. Campo, S.; Ambao, V.; Creus, S.; Gottlieb, S.; Fernandez Vera, G.; Benencia, H.; Bergadà, C. Carbohydrate complexity and proportions of serum FSH isoforms in the male: Lectin-based studies. *Mol. Cell. Endocrinol.* **2007**, *260–262*, 197–204. [CrossRef]
21. Li, H.; Chen, L.P.; Yang, J.; Li, M.C.; Chen, R.B.; Lan, R.Z.; Wang, S.G.; Liu, J.H.; Wang, T. Predictive value of FSH, testicular volume, and histopathological findings for the sperm retrieval rate of microdissection TESE in nonobstructive azoospermia: A meta-analysis. *Asian J. Androl.* **2018**, *20*, 30–36.
22. Ramasamy, R.; Padilla, W.O.; Osterberg, C.; Srivastava, A.; Reifsnyder, J.E.; Niederberger, C.; Schlegel, P.N. A comparison of models for predicting sperm retrieval before microdissection testicular sperm extraction in men with nonobstructive azoospermia. *J. Urol.* **2013**, *189*, 638–642. [CrossRef] [PubMed]
23. Shiraishi, K.; Ohmi, C.; Shimabukuro, T.; Matsuyama, H. Human chorionic gonadotrophin treatment prior to microdissection testicular sperm extraction in nonobstructive azoospermia. *Hum. Reprod.* **2012**, *27*, 331–339. [CrossRef] [PubMed]
24. Caroppo, E.; Colpi, E.M.; D'Amato, G.; Gazzano, G.; Colpi, G.M. Prediction model for testis histology in men with nonobstructive azoospermia: Evidence for a limited predictive role of serum follicle-stimulating hormone. *J. Assist. Reprod. Genet.* **2019**, *36*, 2575–2582. [CrossRef] [PubMed]
25. Ramasamy, R.; Lin, K.; Gosden, L.V.; Rosenwaks, Z.; Palermo, G.D.; Schlegel, P.N. High serum FSH levels in men with nonobstructive azoospermia does not affect success of microdissection testicular sperm extraction. *Fertil. Steril.* **2009**, *92*, 590–593. [CrossRef] [PubMed]
26. Bernie, A.M.; Shah, K.; Halpern, J.A.; Scovell, J.; Ramasamy, R.; Robinson, B.; Schlegel, P.N. Outcomes of microdissection testicular sperm extraction in men with nonobstructive azoospermia due to maturation arrest. *Fertil. Steril.* **2015**, *104*, 569–573. [CrossRef]
27. Themmen, A.P.; Blok, L.J.; Post, M.; Baarends, W.M.; Hoogerbrugge, J.W.; Parmentier, M.; Vassart, G.; Grootegoed, J.A. Follitropin receptor down-regulation involves a cAMP-dependent post-transcriptional decrease of receptor mRNA expression. *Mol. Cell. Endocrinol.* **1991**, *78*, R7–R13. [CrossRef]
28. Bhaskaran, R.S.; Ascoli, M. The post-endocytotic fate of the gonadotropin receptors is an important determinant of the desensitization of gonadotropin responses. *J. Mol. Endocrinol.* **2005**, *34*, 447–457. [CrossRef]
29. Okada, H.; Dobashi, M.; Yamazaki, T.; Hara, I.; Fujisawa, M.; Arakawa, S.; Kamidono, S. Conventional versus microdissection testicular sperm extraction for nonobstructive azoospermia. *J. Urol.* **2002**, *168*, 1063–1067. [CrossRef]

30. Tsujimura, A.; Matsumiya, K.; Miyagawa, Y.; Takao, S.; Fujita, K.; Koga, M.; Takeyama, M.; Fujioka, H.; Okuyama, A. Prediction of successful outcome of microdissection testicular sperm extraction in men with idiopathic nonobstructive azoospermia. *J. Urol.* **2004**, *172*, 1944–1947. [CrossRef]
31. Tusjiimura, A.; Miyagawa, Y.; Takao, T.; Fujita, K.; Komori, K.; Matsuoka, Y.; Takada, S.; Koga, M.; Takeyama, M.; Fujioka, H.; et al. Impact of age, follicle stimulating hormone and Johnsen's score on successful sperm retrieval by microdissection testicular sperm extraction. *Reprod. Med. Biol.* **2005**, *4*, 53–57.
32. Ravizzini, P.; Carizza, C.; Abdelmassih, V.; Abdelmassih, S.; Azevedo, M.; Abdelmassih, R. Microdissection testicular sperm extraction and IVF-ICSI outcome in nonobstructive azoospermia. *Andrologia* **2008**, *40*, 219–226. [CrossRef] [PubMed]
33. Ghalayini, I.F.; Al-Ghazo, M.A.; Hani, O.B.; Al-Azab, R.; Bani-Hani, I.; Zayed, F.; Haddad, Y. Clinical comparison of conventional testicular sperm extraction and microdissection techniques for non-obstructive azoospermia. *J. Clin. Med. Res.* **2011**, *3*, 124–131. [CrossRef] [PubMed]
34. Reifsnyder, J.E.; Ramasamy, R.; Husseini, J.; Schlegel, P.N. Role of optimizing testosterone before microdissection testicular sperm extraction in men with nonobstructive azoospermia. *J. Urol.* **2012**, *188*, 532–537. [CrossRef] [PubMed]
35. Cetinkaya, M.; Onem, K.; Zorba, O.U.; Ozkara, H.; Alici, B. Evaluation of microdissection testicular sperm extraction results in patients with non-obstructive azoospermia: Independent predictive factors and best cutoff values for sperm retrieval. *Urol. J.* **2015**, *12*, 2436–2443. [PubMed]
36. Enatsu, N.; Miyake, H.; Chiba, K.; Fujisawa, M. Predictive factors of successful sperm retrieval on microdissection testicular sperm extraction in Japanese men. *Reprod. Med. Biol.* **2015**, *15*, 29–33. [CrossRef] [PubMed]
37. Althakafi, S.A.; Mustafa, O.M.; Seyam, R.M.; Al-Hathal, N.; Kattan, S. Serum testosterone levels and other determinants of sperm retrieval in microdissection testicular sperm extraction. *Transl. Androl. Urol.* **2017**, *6*, 282–287. [CrossRef]
38. Caroppo, E.; Colpi, E.M.; Gazzano, G.; Vaccalluzzo, L.; Piatti, E.; D'Amato, G.; Colpi, G.M. The seminiferous tubule caliber pattern as evaluated at high magnification during microdissection testicular sperm extraction predicts sperm retrieval in patients with non-obstructive azoospermia. *Andrology* **2019**, *7*, 8–14. [CrossRef]
39. Kizilkan, Y.; Toksoz, S.; Turunc, T.; Ozkardes, H. Parameters predicting sperm retrieval rates during microscopic testicular sperm extraction in nonobstructive azoospermia. *Andrologia* **2019**, *51*, e13441. [CrossRef]
40. Mehmood, S.; Aldaweesh, S.; Junejo, N.N.; Altaweel, W.M.; Kattan, S.A.; Alhathal, N. Microdissection testicular sperm extraction: Overall results and impact of preoperative testosterone level on sperm retrieval rate in patients with nonobstructive azoospermia. *Urol. Ann.* **2019**, *11*, 287–293. [CrossRef]
41. Çayan, S.; Orhan, İ.; Altay, B.; Aşcı, R.; Akbay, E.; Ayas, B.; Yaman, Ö. Fertility outcomes and predictors for successful sperm retrieval and pregnancy in 327 azoospermic men with a history of cryptorchidism who underwent microdissection testicular sperm extraction. *Andrology* **2020**. [CrossRef]
42. Zhang, H.; Xi, Q.; Zhang, X.; Zhang, H.; Jiang, Y.; Liu, R.; Yu, Y. Prediction of microdissection testicular sperm extraction outcome in men with idiopathic nonobstructive azoospermia. *Medicine* **2020**, *99*, e19934. [CrossRef] [PubMed]
43. Guo, F.; Fang, A.; Fan, Y.; Fu, X.; Lan, Y.; Liu, M.; Cao, S.; An, G. Role of treatment with human chorionic gonadotropin and clinical parameters on testicular sperm recovery with microdissection testicular sperm extraction and intracytoplasmic sperm injection outcomes in 184 Klinefelter syndrome patients. *Fertil. Steril.* **2020**, *114*, 997–1005. [CrossRef] [PubMed]
44. Ramasamy, R.; Ricci, J.A.; Palermo, G.D.; Gosden, L.V.; Rosenwaks, Z.; Schlegel, P.N. Successful fertility treatment for Klinefelter's syndrome. *J. Urol.* **2009**, *182*, 1108–1113. [CrossRef]
45. Huhtaniemi, I.; Nikula, H.; Rannikko, S. Pituitary-testicular function of prostatic cancer patients during treatment with a gonadotropin-releasing hormone agonist analog. I. Circulating hormone levels. *J. Androl.* **1987**, *8*, 355–362. [CrossRef] [PubMed]
46. Amory, J.K.; Coviello, A.D.; Page, S.T.; Anawalt, B.D.; Matsumoto, A.M.; Bremner, W.J. Serum 17-hydroxyprogesterone strongly correlates with intratesticular testosterone in gonadotropin-suppressed normal men receiving various dosages of human chorionic gonadotropin. *Fertil. Steril.* **2008**, *89*, 380–386. [CrossRef]
47. Lima, T.F.N.; Patel, P.; Blachman-Braun, R.; Madhusoodanan, V.; Ramasamy, R. Serum 17-hydroxyprogesterone is a potential biomarker for evaluating intratesticular testosterone. *J. Urol.* **2020**, *204*, 551–556. [CrossRef]
48. Bay, K.; Matthiesson, K.; McLachlan, R.; Andersson, A.M. The effects of gonadotropin suppression and selective replacement on insulin-like factor 3 secretion in normal adult men. *J. Clin. Endocrinol. Metab.* **2006**, *91*, 1108–1111. [CrossRef]
49. Roth, M.Y.; Lin, K.; Bay, K.; Amory, J.K.; Anawalt, B.D.; Matsumoto, A.M.; Marck, B.T.; Bremner, W.J.; Page, S.T. Serum insulin-like factor 3 is highly correlated with intratesticular testosterone in normal men with acute, experimental gonadotropin deficiency stimulated with low-dose human chorionic gonadotropin: A randomized, controlled trial. *Fertil. Steril.* **2013**, *99*, 132–139. [CrossRef]
50. Levalle, O.A.; Zylbersztein, C.; Aszpis, S.; Mariani, V.; Ponzio, R.; Aranda, C.; Guitelman, A.; Scaglia, H.E. Serum luteinizing hormone pulsatility and intratesticular testosterone and oestradiol concentrations in idiopathic infertile men with high and normal follicle stimulating hormone serum concentrations. *Hum. Reprod.* **1994**, *9*, 781–787. [CrossRef]
51. Shinjo, E.; Shiraishi, K.; Matsuyama, H. The effect of human chorionic gonadotropin-based hormonal therapy on intratesticular testosterone levels and spermatogonial DNA synthesis in men with nonobstructive azoospermia. *Andrology* **2013**, *1*, 929–935. [CrossRef]

52. Bar-Shira Maymon, B.; Yogev, L.; Yavetz, H.; Lifschitz-Mercer, B.; Schreiber, L.; Kleiman, S.E.; Botchan, A.; Hauser, R.; Paz, G. Spermatogonial proliferation patterns in men with azoospermia of different etiologies. *Fertil. Steril.* **2003**, *80*, 1175–1180. [CrossRef]
53. Kato, Y.; Shiraishi, K.; Matsuyama, H. Expression of testicular androgen receptor in non-obstructive azoospermia and its change after hormonal therapy. *Andrology* **2014**, *2*, 734–740. [CrossRef] [PubMed]
54. Blok, L.J.; Mackenbach, P.; Trapman, J.; Themmen, A.P.; Brinkmann, A.O.; Grootegoed, J.A. Follicle-stimulating hormone regulates androgen receptor mRNA in Sertoli cells. *Mol. Cell. Endocrinol.* **1989**, *63*, 267–271. [CrossRef]
55. Aydos, K.; Unlü, C.; Demirel, L.C.; Evirgen, O.; Tolunay, O. The effect of pure FSH administration in non-obstructive azoospermic men on testicular sperm retrieval. *Eur. J. Obstet. Gynecol. Reprod. Biol.* **2003**, *108*, 54–58. [CrossRef]
56. Hussein, A.; Ozgok, Y.; Ross, L.; Niederberger, C. Clomiphene administration for cases of nonobstructive azoospermia: A multi-center study. *J. Androl.* **2005**, *26*, 787–791. [CrossRef]
57. Hussein, A.; Ozgok, Y.; Ross, L.; Rao, P.; Niederberger, C. Optimization of spermatogenesis-regulating hormones in patients with nonobstructive azoospermia and its impact on sperm retrieval: A multicentre study. *BJU Int.* **2013**, *111*, E110–E114. [CrossRef]
58. Amer, M.K.; Ahmed, A.R.; Abdel Hamid, A.A.; Gamal El Din, S.F. Can spermatozoa be retrieved in non-obstructive azoospermic patients with high FSH level? A retrospective cohort study. *Andrologia* **2019**, *51*, e13176. [CrossRef]
59. Amer, M.K.; Ahmed, H.E.H.; Gamal El Din, S.F.; Fawzy Megawer, A.; Ahmed, A.R. Evaluation of neoadjuvant gonadotropin administration with downregulation by testosterone prior to second time microsurgical testicular sperm extraction: A prospective case-control study. *Urologia* **2020**, *87*, 185–190. [CrossRef]
60. Schlegel, P.N.; Sigman, M.; Collura, B.; De Jonge, C.J.; Eisenberg, M.L.; Lamb, D.J.; Mulhall, J.P.; Niederberger, C.; Sandlow, J.I.; Sokol, R.Z.; et al. Diagnosis and treatment of infertility in men: AUA/ASRM guideline. Part II. *Fertil. Steril.* **2020**, *115*, 62–69. [CrossRef]
61. Colpi, G.M.; Caroppo, E. Re: Predictors of surgical sperm retrieval in non-obstructive azoospermia: Summary of current literature. *Int. Urol. Nephrol.* **2020**, *52*, 2039–2041. [CrossRef]
62. Luján, S.; Caroppo, E.; Niederberger, C.; Arce, J.C.; Sadler-Riggleman, I.; Beck, D.; Nilsson, E.; Skinner, M.K. Sperm DNA methylation epimutation biomarkers for male infertility and FSH therapeutic responsiveness. *Sci. Rep.* **2019**, *9*, 16786. [CrossRef] [PubMed]

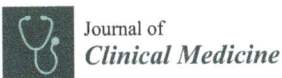

Review

Two Decades from the Introduction of Microdissection Testicular Sperm Extraction: How This Surgical Technique Has Improved the Management of NOA

Nahid Punjani [†], Caroline Kang [†] and Peter N. Schlegel *

Department of Urology, Weill Cornell Medical College, New York, NY 10065, USA; nap4001@med.cornell.edu (N.P.); cak4005@med.cornell.edu (C.K.)
* Correspondence: pnschleg@med.cornell.edu
† Equal contribution.

Abstract: The treatment of men with non-obstructive azoospermia (NOA) has improved greatly over the past two decades. This is in part due to the discovery of in vitro fertilization (IVF) and intracytoplasmic sperm injection (ICSI), but also significantly due to improvements in surgical sperm retrieval methods, namely the development of microdissection testicular sperm extraction (mTESE). This procedure has revolutionized the field by allowing for identification of favorable seminiferous tubules while simultaneously limiting the amount of testicular tissue removed. Improving sperm retrieval rates is imperative in this cohort of infertile men as there are a limited number of factors that are predictive of successful sperm retrieval. Currently, sperm retrieval in NOA men remains dependent on surgeon experience, preoperative patient optimization and teamwork with laboratory personnel. In this review, we discuss the evolution of surgical sperm retrieval methods, review predictors of sperm retrieval success, compare and contrast the data of conventional versus mTESE, share tips for optimizing sperm retrieval outcomes, and discuss the future of sperm retrieval in men with NOA.

Keywords: microdissection testicular sperm extraction; non-obstructive azoospermia; management

1. Introduction

Infertility affects up to 15% of couples attempting to conceive globally, with a male factor implicated in up to 50% of cases [1]. While the precise etiology remains unclear in many of these cases, azoospermia, or the lack of sperm in the ejaculate, occurs in 1% of all males and 10–15% of infertile males and is often considered the most severe phenotype of male infertility classified as either obstructive azoospermia (30–40% of azoospermia cases) or non-obstructive azoospermia (NOA) (60–70% of azoospermia cases) [2–6]. NOA remains a particularly challenging condition to treat as the majority of cases are idiopathic, with only a subset attributable to an identifiable genetic (i.e., Klinefelter Syndrome, Y-chromosome microdeletion or mutations in individual genes) or acquired (i.e., chemotherapy, radiation, cryptorchidism/prior orchiopexy or malignancy) condition [7,8]. NOA men have spermatogenic failure with a range of histopathologic changes that include hypospermatogenesis, maturation arrest, and Sertoli cell only syndrome [7]. Currently, NOA men require surgical retrieval of sperm with assisted reproductive technology to father children. This review highlights milestones in the evolution of surgical sperm retrieval methods, summarizes predictors of sperm retrieval success, evaluates the data of conventional microdissection testicular sperm extraction (cTESE) versus microdissection testicular sperm extraction (mTESE), discusses tips for optimizing sperm retrieval, and comments on the future of sperm retrieval in men with NOA.

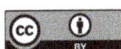

2. History of Surgical Sperm Retrieval

While NOA men currently rely on surgical sperm retrieval with assisted reproductive technology to father biological children, these men were historically relegated to using adoption or use of donor sperm to have a family [9]. The first successful in vitro fertilization (IVF), the process by which a sperm and oocyte are fertilized outside of the body and then later implanted, was performed in 1978 utilizing ejaculated sperm from a fertile man, and resulted in the birth of Louise Brown (Figure 1) [10]. Sperm was surgically retrieved for the use of IVF for the first time in the 1980s, utilizing motile sperm from the epididymis of man with obstructive azoospermia [11]. Intracytoplasmic sperm injection (ICSI), a process where only a single sperm is injected into an oocyte using a micropipette, was then introduced in 1992, thereby potentially providing an opportunity for men with severe spermatogenic dysfunction (i.e., men with NOA) to father children [12]. The first description of testicular sperm for use in assisted reproduction occurred in 1993 [13]. Successful fertilization, embryo development, implantation and pregnancy was considered to be an unanticipated result by some reproductive experts given the expected need for additional maturation by sperm that was known to occur during epididymal transit [14].

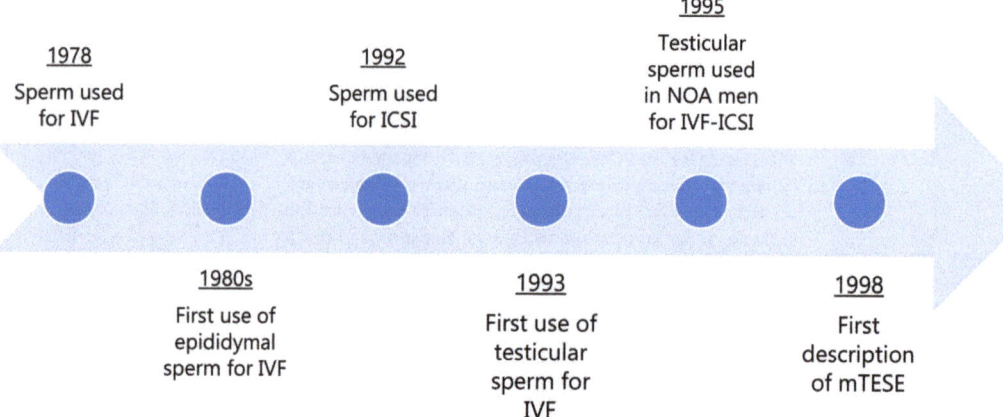

Figure 1. Timeline of the history of surgical sperm retrieval prior to the discovery of mTESE. IVF: in vitro fertilization; ICSI: intracytoplasmic sperm injection; NOA: non-obstructive azoospermia; mTESE: microdissection testicular sperm extraction.

It was not until 1995 that testicular sperm extraction (TESE), an open surgical procedure to directly extract testicular tissue, was performed on a man with NOA and testicular sperm utilized for successful IVF-ICSI [15]. This success was revolutionary for the treatment of men with NOA, but certain challenges remained given the sporadic, almost anecdotal, success of initial efforts to treat men with NOA who were previously considered to be sterile [16]. Based on observations that limited sperm was retrieved during simple biopsy, it was originally thought that multiple testis biopsies would increase the chance of retrieval as sperm production was believed to occur in isolated areas in the testis of men with NOA and spermatogenic failure [14]. In reality, multiple open biopsies resulted in removal of large quantities of testicular tissue and created a new risk, namely of harm to the blood supply of the testis from multiple incisions on the tunica albuginea. These incisions threatened to divide the vessels under the surface of the tunica vaginalis, with a potential risk of testis devascularization [17]. Percutaneous needle aspiration of the testis provided a minimally invasive alternative to sperm retrieval in NOA, but the lower sperm yield often did not provide enough sperm to inject all oocytes during an attempted ICSI attempt [18]. Given the risk of vascular injury, an approach to widely opening the testis and identifying individual tubules with the aid of an operating microscope was initiated. With this additional magnification, differences in seminiferous tubules could be visualized and appreciated, in particular differences shown to reflect potential focal sites of sperm production in an otherwise highly dysfunctional testis. Additional considerations of the intratesticular blood supply that runs parallel to seminiferous tubules within the testis allowed the development of microdissection testicular sperm extraction (mTESE) by Schlegel et al. in 1998 [19]. Additional studies have documented enhanced sperm retrieval rates with this technique, as well as the additional safety of mTESE, by eliminating the need for multiple biopsies or incisions of the tunica albuginea, reducing the impact to the testicular blood supply [20,21].

3. Surgical Testicular Sperm Extraction

TESE is the surgical removal of tissue from the testicle in order to retrieve sperm, and can be completed with or without a standard operating microscope. cTESE may be completed with local anesthetic or sedation, but is commonly completed under general anesthesia. A skin incision may be made in the scrotal midline or through a unilaterally transverse or longitudinal incision over the selected hemiscrotum. Dissection is carried through subcutaneous dartos tissue down towards the tunica vaginalis which is then opened to reveal the testis. If delivered, the testis should be examined to identify and avoid areas of prominent vascularity, commonly seen in the midline and lower poles of the testis. An ultra-sharp or ophthalmic blade is used to sharply enter the tunica albuginea. Gentle pressure is applied around the tunical incision to extrude a sample of seminiferous tubules (Figure 2A). The tubules are sharply excised with scissors and processed in sperm-appropriate media by mincing the tissue with scissors and passage through a 24-gauge angiocatheter. The specimen is then examined by a trained andrologist, under light or phase-contrast microscopy at 20× magnification, for the presence of sperm.

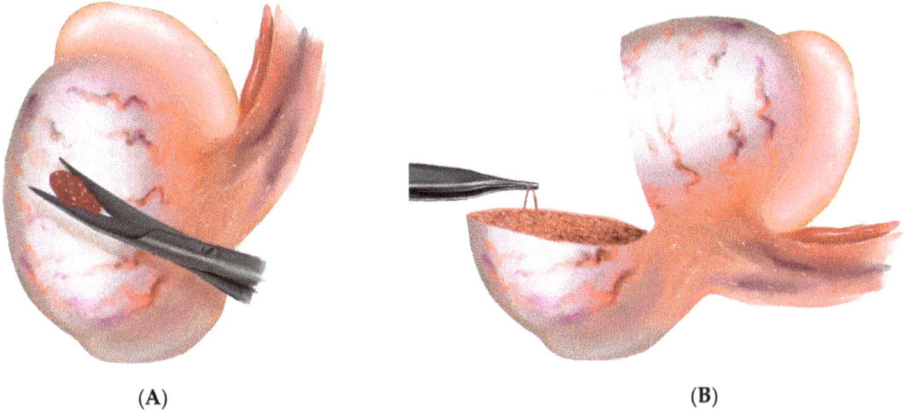

(A)   (B)

Figure 2. Graphical representation of a (**A**) conventional testicular sperm extraction with or without an operating microscope and (**B**) microdissection testicular sperm extraction using an operating microscope.

mTESE is now considered the gold standard procedure for sperm retrieval in men with NOA [22]. Under general anesthesia, a dissection identical to cTESE is performed, and the testis is delivered through an opening in the parietal tunica vaginalis. After delivery of the testicle, adhesions on the visceral tunica vaginalis should be released to ensure optimal visualization and location of vasculature. The tunica vaginalis is then sharply incised with an ultra-sharp or ophthalmic blade, but bi-valved equatorially (Figure 2B). The tunical edges are secured with clamps to prevent avulsion of the tunica from the underlying tubules. The seminiferous tubules are then examined carefully and systematically prior to manipulation. Bipolar cautery should be used to limit postoperative bleeding as well as tissue damage. The tissue should be manipulated with care to avoid disruption of individual seminiferous tubules or the vessels which run parallel to the tubules in a radial pattern from the center to the periphery of the testicular parenchyma. Once an optimal tubule is identified, the tubule should be taken in its entirety, whenever possible. Optimal tubules (i.e., those likely to contain sperm) are generally larger and more opaque [20]. Once an adequate number of tubules are selected, processing should occur as previously described using sharp scissors and aspiration through a 24-gauge angiocatheter. This mechanical disruption of testicular tissue can allow detection of rare sperm within the tissue that may not be identifiable in a sample that has not been similarly processed. Note that sperm, when present, are inside the seminiferous tubules, so the tubules must be broken open to release sperm into the tissue suspension. As previously described, a limited part of this dispersed tissue specimen can then be examined by an experienced andrologist using 20× phase contrast microscopy on a simple slide with cover slip.

4. Predictors of Sperm Retrieval in mTESE

Although many studies have been conducted examining sperm retrieval rates in men with NOA undergoing mTESE, limited definitive predictors of sperm retrieval exist.

4.1. Histopathology

Histopathology is one of the strongest predictors of sperm retrieval as it provides a direct snapshot of the testicular architecture [23]. However, performance of a testicular biopsy solely for diagnostic purposes is not routinely recommended because of its invasiveness. In addition, a diagnostic biopsy samples only a small section of the testicular tissue, so its predictive value is limited. Diagnostic biopsy is suggested at the time of retrieval attempt to document the condition treated and rule out pathologic processes such as intratubular germ cell neoplasia. Additionally, testis biopsy may also be performed to differentiate maturation arrest from normal production in men with normal volume azoospermia, normal serum follicle stimulating hormone (FSH) concentrations, palpable vas deferens, and normal testicular volume [24].

Histopathologic subtype has been correlated to sperm retrieval rate, and those with Sertoli cell only syndrome histopathology have lower sperm retrieval rates compared to those with maturation arrest or hypospermatogenesis patterns [25]. As expected, the presence of mature spermatozoa is a strong predictor of sperm retrieval [26]. Unfortunately, despite the utility of testicular histopathology, it often is not available prior to sperm retrieval procedures, and is of limited value when no spermatozoa are seen [27]. For example, men with a diagnostic biopsy showing Sertoli cell only syndrome are expected to have sperm production elsewhere in the testis in at least 37% of cases. At our institution it is standard that pathology reports include all histologic patterns present in a testis biopsy, as even small foci of spermatogenesis are correlated with successful sperm retrieval. Pathology reports that state only the predominant or most severe histopathology are highly unlikely to reflect the likelihood of sperm retrieval in men with NOA.

4.2. Testis Size

In a meta-analysis by Corona et al., men with testis size >12 cc had higher rates of sperm retrieval, however, sperm retrieval was still possible in small volume testes (<8 cc) [28]. Our observations are the opposite; that men with larger testes are more likely to have obstructive azoospermia, as suggested by Schoor et al., and that men with NOA have similar sperm retrieval chances, regardless of testis volume [27]. With an effective mTESE search for rare foci of sperm, the testis volume or FSH level (which reflects overall testicular function) cannot predict the region of best function/sperm production inside the testis. Other meta-analyses have demonstrated limited predictive value of testicular volume even when testis biopsy histopathologic patterns were also used in the analysis [29]. Overall, these data suggest that testis size should not be considered a factor to exclude a patient from an attempt at sperm retrieval. In fact, in our experience, sperm can be routinely retrieved even in testes less than 2 cc in volume [30].

4.3. Serum Follicle Stimulating Hormone Levels

Serum FSH concentrations have been suggested, in some isolated reports, to predict sperm retrieval in conventional TESE [31]. Other studies have reported FSH levels to inversely correlate with the number of germ cells present and stages of spermatogenesis [32]. However, while high serum FSH levels may provide a more global representation of the level of spermatogenic dysfunction within a testis, there still may be small foci of spermatogenesis that can be identified and retrieved during mTESE [33]. Therefore, we do not recommend using baseline serum FSH concentrations as a preoperative predictor of sperm retrieval in NOA men.

4.4. Age

Male age has been correlated with deterioration in ejaculated semen parameters and increased serum FSH concentrations [34]. It has been proposed that FSH increases secondary to decreased androgen production associated with aging [35]. However, since FSH is not predictive of sperm retrieval, as discussed above, age also should not be a predictive factor [28]. Age has been suggested to be a predictive factor in certain patient subsets, such as those men with Klinefelter Syndrome, but at our center, sperm retrieval rates for Klinefelter Syndrome patients in the oldest age group (>35 years) are still 50%. These observations do not provide compelling evidence for early sperm retrieval [36]. It has been our uncontrolled observation that in many men with severe oligozoospermia followed longitudinally using repeated semen analyses that it is rare for these men to progress to azoospermia during our observation period. Finally, while advanced paternal age has reported negative impact on outcomes in offspring (increased genetic risks), our experience has demonstrated no upper age limit (even men in their 80s) for successful sperm retrieval [37].

4.5. Genetics

The genetic makeup of a man with NOA may provide insight into his chances of successful sperm retrieval and can aid greatly in preoperative counseling. As per guidelines from the American Society of Reproductive Medicine and American Urologic Association, men with NOA or severe oligozoospermia (<5 million sperm/mL) should undergo karyotype analysis and screening for Y chromosome microdeletions [22,24]. It is well-known that the presence and location of a Y chromosome microdeletion in a man with NOA is helpful in predicting the chance of sperm retrieval [38]. Men with complete AZFa and AFZb deletions have sperm retrieval rates of zero, whereas men with AZFc deletions have reported sperm retrieval rates of up to 70% [38,39]. Furthermore, detection of Klinefelter Syndrome (47,XXY) provides favorable prognostic information, as these men tend to have similar or better rates of sperm retrieval as compared to other NOA men (ranging from 65–70% retrieval rates at our center over time) [9,37]. Moving forward, improved diagnostics such as whole exome sequencing may identify specific genetic abnormalities that may provide further prognostic information related to sperm retrieval success [40,41].

4.6. History of Cryptorchidism/Orchiopexy

Most men with a history of cryptorchidism have sperm in their ejaculate and nearly normal fertility (unilateral cryptorchidism) or mildly impaired fertility (bilateral cryptorchidism). Therefore, men who are azoospermic with a history of cryptorchidism are relatively unique. Our experience has demonstrated that men with azoospermia and a history of cryptorchidism/orchiopexy have unique anatomic features. These men often have a testis that is in a different anatomic configuration with the epididymis anterior, and the caput epididymis that may be inferior within the scrotum. Taken together with the lack of tunica vaginalis that is typically present after orchiopexy, exploration of the scrotum in these men can be difficult. Care must be taken to identify each anatomic structure, with special care taken to identify the testicular blood supply. The surface of the testis in these patients often has very prominent vessels that course in a longitudinal fashion, almost suggesting a pattern of neovascularity. In some cases, the primary testicular blood supply does not enter in the standard location just medial to the caput epididymis.

Since most pexed testes have good sperm production, the azoospermic man with cryptorchidism/orchiopexy has a very different spermatogenic picture. Given the intraoperative observations we have made, it is possible that some of these men are azoospermic because of an alteration in testicular blood supply that occurred during, or as a consequence of, surgical orchiopexy.

Only limited reports of sperm retrieval success after orchiopexy for cryptorchidism have been published to-date, as of 2020 [42–46]. In these studies, combinations of testicular volume, unilateral and bilateral cryptorchidism have been debated as potential factors affecting the chance of sperm retrieval. Overall, a history of cryptorchidism has been suggested to be a favorable factor for sperm retrieval, with retrieval rates of 55–74% reported in these studies. We have typically found that most of the testis will be replaced with sclerotic tubules, with small distinct foci of sperm production, often in areas with Leydig cell hyperplasia (notable by the yellow color around the enlarged seminiferous tubules in these sites.)

4.7. Other Factors

Various studies have attempted to explore other factors including inhibin B levels, various gene products or transcripts in the ejaculate as well as anti-Müllerian hormone levels as predictors of successful sperm retrieval, but none have shown adequate association to warrant clinical application as predictors of sperm retrieval [37,47,48].

5. Outcomes of cTESE vs. mTESE

Numerous studies have endeavored to compare cTESE to mTESE. One of the first reviews summarized seven studies between 1999 and 2013 and reported sperm retrieval rates of 16.7–45.0% in the cTESE group and 42.9–63.0% in the mTESE group [49]. Shortly after, a meta-analysis of 15 studies with almost 2000 patients demonstrated that mTESE had a 1.5× greater likelihood of successful sperm retrieval compared to cTESE [47]. The strength of this meta-analysis was that it included only comparative studies, i.e., publications where the same selection of patients and same surgical/laboratory expertise was applied to compare patient outcomes in these settings. These data remain the most robust comparisons of testicular fine needle aspiration (TESA) with cTESE, showing a two-fold improvement in sperm retrieval rates with cTESE vs. TESA, as well as a higher rate of sperm retrieval with mTESE vs. cTESE (1.5× higher).

The review by Corona et al. published in 2019, included over 21,000 patients [28]. Since the authors included data from different patient cohorts with varying underlying etiologies for NOA, it is not possible to rely on the results tabulated as being a valid comparison of different sperm retrieval techniques. They did note a randomized trial which reported a retrieval rate of 42% (29/69 testicles) in the cTESE group versus 52% (36/69 testicles) in the mTESE group who had sperm retrieved at the time of surgery [48]. The authors suggest that this difference was due to an ability to view larger tubules, obtain tubules from more vascularized areas, and the ability to map the testicle during mTESE. The findings of this one prospective RCT (randomized control trial) should be considered strongly as the randomized study design reduces confounding and affords the greatest exchangeability between study groups. The quality of a meta-analysis is only as good as the studies for which it summarizes, and in this case consisted almost entirely of observational data with many possible sources of bias.

6. Optimizing Success

Since NOA men may have focal areas of sperm production within their testis, preoperative optimization is a key strategy for successful sperm retrieval during TESE. As spermatogenesis takes approximately 74 days, it is important to ensure that patients do not have surgical intervention to the testicle including biopsy for at least 6 months prior to their procedure [9]. Men with varicocele warrant consideration of possible varicocele repair, and may be considered in certain selected patients, especially couples with a younger female partner and lower FSH (less risk of Sertoli cell only syndrome) as well as those with previously documented sperm in the ejaculate or those with ample time to benefit from a return of sperm in their ejaculate. The caveat to varicocele repair is that it may take >6 months for return of sperm to the ejaculate, and only a small subset (<10%) may have adequate numbers of sperm to negate the need for surgical retrieval [9]. Again, of concern in these studies is the lack of a control group to compare to the patients who had varicocele repair for NOA. Some men with previously documented azoospermia will have rare sperm detected in a repeat semen analysis, especially if the concentrated pellet is more carefully examined ("extended sperm search") [50].

Hormonally, men with NOA typically have elevated gonadotropins (i.e., FSH), low serum testosterone (and subsequently low intratesticular testosterone), and mildly elevated estradiol levels [51]. This hormone profile lends itself to possible manipulation in an effort to increase intratesticular testosterone levels and spermatogenesis. Those with low serum testosterone and elevated estradiol (abnormal ratio of testosterone to estradiol) may have increased levels of aromatase, and therefore off-label use of aromatase inhibitors may increase serum testosterone levels, decrease estradiol, support spermatogenesis and increase intratesticular testosterone [52]. Other strategies for hormone optimization in NOA men include the use of selective estrogen receptor modulators (SERMs) and human chorionic gonadotrophic (hCG). Clomiphene citrate is a SERM that promotes gonadotropin release secondary to competitive binding of the estrogen receptor resulting in increased androgen production, and hCG works to directly stimulate luteinizing hormone (LH) receptors on Leydig cells in the testicle for androgen production [4]. Although normalizing serum testosterone levels (and thereby enhancing intratesticular sperm production) makes sense for men with low testosterone, the proof that such medical intervention helps sperm retrieval rates is limited. Most studies have been non-comparator trials, with the same limitations as noted for varicocele repair prior to TESE. Indeed, our non-randomized results showed that men with low T who were treated had a sperm retrieval rate of 51%, but the men with low T who were not treated had sperm found in 61% of cases ($p = 0.3$) [53].

Sperm processing, as previously described, is also a key aspect for optimization and identification of sperm. Using sharp scissors to finely mince the harvested tissue, followed by repeated aspiration of the tissue homogenate through a 24-gauge angiocath ensures that surgically retrieved tissue is adequately disrupted, and results in up to a 300-fold increase in detectable sperm within minutes of analysis in the operating room [9].

7. The Future of Sperm Retrieval in NOA Men

mTESE has been a revolutionary procedure for the treatment of men with NOA. However, there are relatively limited preoperative factors at this time that help to predict sperm retrieval. Therefore, there is ongoing reliance on dedicated surgical examination of testicular tissue in these patients as well as surgeon experience, preoperative optimization (hormone levels and varicocele repair), and teamwork with reliable and experienced laboratory personnel to increase success. Unfortunately, further processing of tissue in the laboratory rarely identifies sperm that was not detected on preliminary examination of a well-digested testicular tissue specimen in the operating room. Moving forward, new technologies for assisted reproduction, including microfluidics, cell sorting, or other micro-identification techniques could permit identification of rare sperm and possibly selection of optimal sperm from a limited pool to improve the likelihood of pregnancy success and live birth rate. Although testicular sperm have 0% normal morphology and are often qualitatively seen to be grossly abnormal, even immotile, from men with NOA, the 43% clinical pregnancy rate obtained with such sperm remains a remarkable reflection of the ability of sperm to contribute to a normal pregnancy with ICSI. Little further improvement in sperm retrieval rates is likely to occur with current surgical techniques, but the learning curve for finding rare sperm is difficult to master, and the care taken to maintain testicular function is critical. Advanced imaging techniques to identify sites of sperm production preoperatively could greatly enhance the application of surgical sperm retrieval. Furthermore, a better understanding of the likely genetic components of NOA may allow non-surgical interventions to enhance sperm production, especially for men with maturation arrest as the presentation of NOA.

Author Contributions: Conceptualization: P.N.S.; writing: N.P., C.K. and P.N.S.; writing—review and editing: N.P., C.K. and P.N.S.; supervision P.N.S. All authors have read and agreed to the published version of the manuscript.

Funding: N.P. and C.K. are supported in part by the Frederick J. and Theresa Dow Wallace Fund of the New York Community Trust.

Institutional Review Board Statement: Not applicable.

Informed Consent Statement: Not applicable.

Data Availability Statement: Not applicable.

Acknowledgments: The authors would like to thank Vanessa Dudley for her excellent illustrations.

Conflicts of Interest: The authors have no conflicts of interest to declare.

References

1. Agarwal, A.; Mulgund, A.; Hamada, A.; Chyatte, M.R. A unique view on male infertility around the globe. *Reprod. Biol. Endocrinol.* **2015**, *13*, 1–9. [CrossRef]
2. Schlegel, P.N. Causes of azoospermia and their management. *Reprod. Fertil. Dev.* **2004**, *16*, 561. [CrossRef]
3. Kumar, R. Medical management of non-obstructive azoospermia. *Clinics* **2013**, *68*, 75–79. [CrossRef]
4. Esteves, S.C. Clinical management of infertile men with nonobstructive azoospermia. *Asian J. Androl.* **2015**, *17*, 459–470. [CrossRef]
5. Fedder, J.; Crüger, D.; Oestergaard, B.; Petersen, G.B. Etiology of azoospermia in 100 consecutive nonvasectomized men. *Fertil. Steril.* **2004**, *82*, 1463–1465. [CrossRef]
6. Matsumiya, K.; Namiki, M.; Takahara, S.; Kondoh, N.; Takada, S.; Kiyohara, H.; Okuyama, A. Clinical study of azoospermia. *Int. J. Androl.* **1994**, *17*, 140–142. [CrossRef] [PubMed]
7. Das, A.; Halpern, J.A.; Darves-Bornoz, A.L.; Patel, M.; Wren, J.; Keeter, M.K.; Brannigan, R.E. Sperm retrieval success and testicular histopathology in idiopathic nonobstructive azoospermia. *Asian J. Androl.* **2020**, *22*, 555–559. [CrossRef] [PubMed]
8. Krausz, C.; Riera-Escamilla, A.; Moreno-Mendoza, D.; Holleman, K.; Cioppi, F.; Algaba, F.; Pybus, M.; Friedrich, C.; Wyrwoll, M.J.; Casamonti, E.; et al. Genetic dissection of spermatogenic arrest through exome analysis: Clinical implications for the management of azoospermic men. *Genet. Med.* **2020**, *22*, 1956–1966. [CrossRef] [PubMed]
9. Schlegel, P.N. Nonobstructive Azoospermia: A Revolutionary Surgical Approach and Results. *Semin. Reprod. Med.* **2009**, *27*, 165–170. [CrossRef] [PubMed]
10. Wang, J.; Sauer, M.V. In vitro fertilization (IVF): A review of 3 decades of clinical innovation and technological advancement. *Ther. Clin. Risk Manag.* **2006**, *2*, 355–364. [CrossRef]
11. Temple-Smith, P.D.; Southwick, G.J.; Yates, C.A.; Trounson, A.O.; De Kretser, D.M. Human pregnancy by in vitro fertilization (IVF) using sperm aspirated from the epididymis. *J. Assist. Reprod. Genet.* **1985**, *2*, 119–122. [CrossRef]
12. Palermo, G.; Joris, H.; Devroey, P.; Van Steirteghem, A.C. Pregnancies after intracytoplasmic injection of single spermatozoon into an oocyte. *Lancet* **1992**, *340*, 17–18. [CrossRef]
13. Craft, I.; Bennett, V.; Nicholson, N. Fertilising ability of testicular spermatozoa. *Lancet* **1993**, *342*, 864. [CrossRef]
14. Enatsu, N.; Chiba, K.; Fujisawa, M. The development of surgical sperm extraction and new challenges to improve the outcome. *Reprod. Med. Biol.* **2015**, *15*, 137–144. [CrossRef]
15. Devroey, P.; Liu, J.; Nagy, Z.; Goossens, A.; Tournaye, H.; Camus, M.; Van Steirteghem, A.; Silber, S. Pregnancies after testicular sperm extraction and intracytoplasmic sperm injection in non-obstructive azoospermia. *Hum. Reprod.* **1995**, *10*, 1457–1460. [CrossRef]
16. Schlegel, P.N.; Palermo, G.D.; Goldstein, M.; Menendez, S.; Zaninovic, N.; Veeck, L.L.; Rosenwaks, Z. Testicular sperm ex-traction with intracytoplasmic sperm injection for nonobstructive azoospermia. *Urology* **1997**, *49*, 435–440. [CrossRef]
17. Tash, J.A.; Schlegel, P.N. Histologic effects of testicular sperm extraction on the testicle in men with nonobstructive azoo-spermia. *Urology* **2001**, *57*, 334–337. [CrossRef]
18. Lewin, A.; Weiss, D.B.; Friedler, S.; Ben-Shachar, I.; Porat-Katz, A.; Meirow, D.; Schenker, J.G.; Safran, A. Delivery following intracytoplasmic injection of mature sperm cells recovered by testicular fine needle aspiration in a case of hypergonadotropic azoospermia due to maturation arrest. *Hum. Reprod.* **1996**, *11*, 769–771. [CrossRef] [PubMed]
19. Schlegel, P.N.; Li, P.S. Microdissection tese: Sperm retrieval in non-obstructive azoospermia. *Hum. Reprod. Update* **1998**, *4*, 439. [CrossRef] [PubMed]

20. Schlegel, P.N. Testicular sperm extraction: Microdissection improves sperm yield with minimal tissue excision. *Hum. Reprod.* **1999**, *14*, 131–135. [CrossRef] [PubMed]
21. Ramasamy, R.; Yagan, N.; Schlegel, P.N. Structural and functional changes to the testis after conventional versus microdis-section testicular sperm extraction. *Urology* **2005**, *65*, 1190–1194. [CrossRef] [PubMed]
22. Schlegel, P.N.; Sigman, M.; Collura, B.; De Jonge, C.J.; Eisenberg, M.L.; Lamb, D.J.; Mulhall, J.P.; Niederberger, C.; Sandlow, J.I.; Sokol, R.Z.; et al. Diagnosis and treatment of infertility in men: AUA/ASRM guideline part II. *Fertil. Steril.* **2021**, *115*, 62–69. [CrossRef] [PubMed]
23. Tournaye, H.; Verheyen, G.; Nagy, P.; Ubaldi, F.; Goossens, A.; Silber, S.; Van Steirteghem, A.C.; Devroey, P. Are there any predictive factors for successful testicular sperm recovery in azoospermic patients? *Hum. Reprod.* **1997**, *12*, 80–86. [CrossRef]
24. Schlegel, P.N.; Sigman, M.; Collura, B.; De Jonge, C.J.; Eisenberg, M.L.; Lamb, D.J.; Mulhall, J.P.; Niederberger, C.; Sandlow, J.I.; Sokol, R.Z.; et al. Diagnosis and Treatment of Infertility in Men: AUA/ASRM Guideline Part I. *J. Urol.* **2021**, *205*, 36–43. [CrossRef] [PubMed]
25. Seo, J.T.; Ko, W.-J. Predictive factors of successful testicular sperm recovery in non-obstructive azoospermia patients. *Int. J. Androl.* **2001**, *24*, 306–310. [CrossRef] [PubMed]
26. Raheem, A.A.; Garaffa, G.; Rushwan, N.; De Luca, F.; Zacharakis, E.; Raheem, T.A.; Freeman, A.; Serhal, P.; Harper, J.C.; Ralph, D. Testicular histopathology as a predictor of a positive sperm retrieval in men with non-obstructive azoospermia. *BJU Int.* **2013**, *111*, 492–499. [CrossRef]
27. Schoor, R.A.; Elhanbly, S.; Niederberger, C.S.; Ross, L.S. The role of testicular biopsy in the modern management of male in-fertility. *J. Urol.* **2002**, *167*, 197–200. [CrossRef]
28. Corona, G.; Minhas, S.; Giwercman, A.; Bettocchi, C.; Dinkelman-Smit, M.; Dohle, G.; Fusco, F.; Kadioglou, A.; Kliesch, S.; Kopa, Z.; et al. Sperm recovery and icsi outcomes in men with non-obstructive azoospermia: A systematic review and meta-analysis. *Hum. Reprod. Update* **2019**, *25*, 733–757. [CrossRef]
29. Wang, T.; Li, H.; Chen, L.-P.; Yang, J.; Li, M.-C.; Chen, R.-B.; Lan, R.-Z.; Wang, S.-G.; Liu, J.-H. Predictive value of FSH, testicular volume, and histopathological findings for the sperm retrieval rate of microdissection TESE in nonobstructive azoospermia: A meta-analysis. *Asian J. Androl.* **2018**, *20*, 30–36. [CrossRef]
30. Bryson, C.F.; Ramasamy, R.; Sheehan, M.; Palermo, G.D.; Rosenwaks, Z.; Schlegel, P.N. Severe Testicular Atrophy does not Affect the Success of Microdissection Testicular Sperm Extraction. *J. Urol.* **2014**, *191*, 175–178. [CrossRef]
31. Ishikawa, T. Surgical recovery of sperm in non-obstructive azoospermia. *Asian J. Androl.* **2011**, *14*, 109–115. [CrossRef]
32. Silber, S.J.; Van Steirteghem, A.; Nagy, Z.; Liu, J.; Tournaye, H.; Devroey, P. Normal pregnancies resulting from testicular sperm extraction and intracytoplasmic sperm injection for azoospermia due to maturation arrest. *Fertil. Steril.* **1996**, *66*, 110–117. [CrossRef]
33. Ramasamy, R.; Lin, K.; Gosden, L.V.; Rosenwaks, Z.; Palermo, G.D.; Schlegel, P.N. High serum fsh levels in men with nonob-structive azoospermia does not affect success of microdissection testicular sperm extraction. *Fertil. Steril.* **2009**, *92*, 590–593. [CrossRef]
34. Grunewald, S.; Glander, H.-J.; Paasch, U.; Kratzsch, J. Age-dependent inhibin B concentration in relation to FSH and semen sample qualities: A study in 2448 men. *Reproduction* **2013**, *145*, 237–244. [CrossRef] [PubMed]
35. Chen, B.; Yang, Q.; Huang, Y.-P.; Wang, H.-X.; Hu, K.; Wang, Y.-X.; Huang, Y.-R. Follicle-stimulating hormone as a predictor for sperm retrieval rate in patients with nonobstructive azoospermia: A systematic review and meta-analysis. *Asian J. Androl.* **2015**, *17*, 281–284. [CrossRef] [PubMed]
36. Bakircioglu, M.E.; Erden, H.F.; Kaplancan, T.; Ciray, N.; Bener, F.; Bahceci, M. Aging may adversely affect testicular sperm recovery in patients with Klinefelter syndrome. *Urology* **2006**, *68*, 1082–1086. [CrossRef] [PubMed]
37. Bernie, A.M.; Ramasamy, R.; Schlegel, P.N. Predictive factors of successful microdissection testicular sperm extraction. *Basic Clin. Androl.* **2013**, *23*, 1–7. [CrossRef] [PubMed]
38. Hopps, C.V.; Mielnik, A.; Goldstein, M.; Palermo, G.D.; Rosenwaks, Z.; Schlegel, P.N. Detection of sperm in men with Y chromosome microdeletions of the AZFa, AZFb and AZFc regions. *Hum. Reprod.* **2003**, *18*, 1660–1665. [CrossRef]
39. Stahl, P.J.; Masson, P.; Mielnik, A.; Marean, M.B.; Schlegel, P.N.; Paduch, D.A. A decade of experience emphasizes that testing for Y microdeletions is essential in American men with azoospermia and severe oligozoospermia. *Fertil. Steril.* **2010**, *94*, 1753–1756. [CrossRef]
40. A Fakhro, K.; ElBardisi, H.; Arafa, M.; Robay, A.; Rodriguez-Flores, J.L.; Al-Shakaki, A.; Syed, N.; Mezey, J.G.; Khalil, C.A.; A Malek, J.; et al. Point-of-care whole-exome sequencing of idiopathic male infertility. *Genet. Med.* **2018**, *20*, 1365–1373. [CrossRef]
41. Ramasamy, R.; Bakircioglu, M.E.; Cengiz, C.; Karaca, E.; Scovell, J.; Jhangiani, S.N.; Akdemir, Z.C.; Bainbridge, M.; Yu, Y.; Huff, C.; et al. Whole-exome sequencing identifies novel homozygous mutation in npas2 in family with nonobstructive azoo-spermia. *Fertil. Steril.* **2015**, *104*, 286–291. [CrossRef]
42. Osaka, A.; Iwahata, T.; Kobori, Y.; Shimomura, Y.; Yoshikawa, N.; Onota, S.; Yamamoto, A.; Ide, H.; Sugimoto, K.; Okada, H. Testicular volume in non-obstructive azoospermia with a history of bilateral cryptorchidism may predict successful sperm re-trieval by testicular sperm extraction. *Reprod. Med. Biol.* **2020**, *19*, 372–377. [CrossRef]
43. Ozan, T.; Karakeci, A.; Kaplancan, T.; Pirincci, N.; Firdolas, F.; Orhan, I. Are predictive factors in sperm retrieval and preg-nancy rates present in nonobstructive azoospermia patients by microdissection testicular sperm extraction on testicle with a history of orchidopexy operation? *Andrologia* **2019**, *51*, e13430. [CrossRef]
44. Glina, S.; Vieira, M. Prognostic factors for sperm retrieval in non-obstructive azoospermia. *Clinics* **2013**, *68*, 121–124. [CrossRef]

45. Ramasamy, R.; Padilla, W.O.; Osterberg, E.C.; Srivastava, A.; Reifsnyder, J.E.; Niederberger, C.; Schlegel, P.N. A comparison of models for predicting sperm retrieval before microdissection testicular sperm extraction in men with nonobstructive azoo-spermia. *J. Urol.* **2013**, *189*, 638–642. [CrossRef]
46. Raman, J.D.; Schlegel, P.N. Testicular Sperm Extraction with Intracytoplasmic Sperm Injection is Successful for the Treatment of Nonobstructive Azoospermia Associated with Cryptorchidism. *J. Urol.* **2003**, *170*, 1287–1290. [CrossRef] [PubMed]
47. Bernie, A.M.; Mata, D.A.; Ramasamy, R.; Schlegel, P.N. Comparison of microdissection testicular sperm extraction, conventional testicular sperm extraction, and testicular sperm aspiration for nonobstructive azoospermia: A systematic review and meta-analysis. *Fertil. Steril.* **2015**, *104*, 1099–1103.e3. [CrossRef]
48. Colpi, G.M.; Colpi, E.M.; Piediferro, G.; Giacchetta, D.; Gazzano, G.; Castiglioni, F.M.; Magli, M.C.; Gianaroli, L. Microsurgical TESE versus conventional TESE for ICSI in non-obstructive azoospermia: A randomized controlled study. *Reprod. Biomed. Online* **2009**, *18*, 315–319. [CrossRef]
49. Deruyver, Y.; Vanderschueren, D.; Van Der Aa, F. Outcome of microdissection TESE compared with conventional TESE in non-obstructive azoospermia: A systematic review. *Andrology* **2014**, *2*, 20–24. [CrossRef] [PubMed]
50. Ron-El, R.; Strassburger, D.; Friedler, S.; Komarovski, D.; Bern, O.; Soffer, Y.; Raziel, A. Extended sperm preparation: An al-ternative to testicular sperm extraction in non-obstructive azoospermia. *Hum. Reprod.* **1997**, *12*, 1222–1226. [CrossRef]
51. Practice Committee of the American Society for Reproductive Medicine in Collaboration with the Society for Male Reproduction and Urology. Evaluation of the azoospermic male: A committee opinion. *Fertil. Steril.* **2018**, *109*, 777–782. [CrossRef] [PubMed]
52. Schlegel, P.N. Aromatase inhibitors for male infertility. *Fertil. Steril.* **2012**, *98*, 1359–1362. [CrossRef] [PubMed]
53. Reifsnyder, J.E.; Ramasamy, R.; Husseini, J.; Schlegel, P.N. Role of Optimizing Testosterone Before Microdissection Testicular Sperm Extraction in Men with Nonobstructive Azoospermia. *J. Urol.* **2012**, *188*, 532–537. [CrossRef] [PubMed]

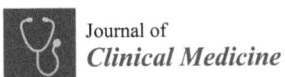

Review

Reproductive Chances of Men with Azoospermia Due to Spermatogenic Dysfunction

Caroline Kang [†], Nahid Punjani [†] and Peter N. Schlegel *

Department of Urology, Weill Cornell Medical College, New York, NY 10021, USA; cak4005@med.cornell.edu (C.K.); nap4001@med.cornell.edu (N.P.)
* Correspondence: pnschleg@med.cornell.edu
† Equal contribution.

Abstract: Non-obstructive azoospermia (NOA), or lack of sperm in the ejaculate due to spermatogenic dysfunction, is the most severe form of infertility. Men with this form of infertility should be evaluated prior to treatment, as there are various underlying etiologies for NOA. While a significant proportion of NOA men have idiopathic spermatogenic dysfunction, known etiologies including genetic disorders, hormonal anomalies, structural abnormalities, chemotherapy or radiation treatment, infection and inflammation may substantively affect the prognosis for successful treatment. Despite the underlying etiology for NOA, most of these infertile men are candidates for surgical sperm retrieval and subsequent use in intracytoplasmic sperm injection (ICSI). In this review, we describe common etiologies of NOA and clinical outcomes following surgical sperm retrieval and ICSI.

Keywords: non-obstructive azoospermia; infertility; intracytoplasmic sperm injection

1. Introduction

Infertility affects up to 15% of couples worldwide, with up to 50% of cases attributable to male factor infertility [1]. In a majority of cases, the precise etiology underlying infertility in the male partner remains unclear. A subset of men with infertility have no sperm in the ejaculate, known as azoospermia, which may further be classified into obstructive (OA) or non-obstructive azoospermia (NOA). The majority of cases of NOA are idiopathic, however some known etiologies include genetic disorders, chemotherapy or radiation, developmental or structural abnormalities, and hormonal imbalances (Table 1). Despite the etiology underlying the spermatogenic dysfunction resulting in NOA, sperm often can be surgically extracted from the testis for use in assisted reproductive technology (ART) with varying success. Intracytoplasmic sperm injection (ICSI) requires only a single spermatozoon for injection into an oocyte, and thus has improved the chances for men with NOA to conceive biological children. In this review, we discuss common etiologies for NOA and the reproductive outcomes for NOA men after surgical sperm retrieval and ICSI.

Table 1. Etiologies of non-obstructive azoospermia.

Etiology	Example
Idiopathic	
Genetic/Chromosomal	Klinefelter syndrome, Y-chromosome microdeletions
Iatrogenic/Surgical	Chemotherapy, Radiation therapy
Developmental/Structural	Cryptorchidism/Orchidopexy, Varicocele
Hormonal	Kallmann syndrome, hypogonadotropic hypogonadism, hyperprolactinemia/prolactinoma

2. Treatment of Non-Obstructive Azoospermia

Effective management of infertility in men with NOA requires testicular sperm retrieval as well as ART in the form of ICSI. Since sperm retrieval involves finding one of

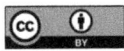

the very limited sites of sperm production within a highly dysfunctional testis of a man with NOA, it is not surprising that the approach used for sperm retrieval can substantially affect the chance of obtaining sperm for fertility.

A wide variety of approaches have been used for attempted sperm retrieval including fine needle aspiration of the testis (testicular sperm aspiration; TESA), random biopsies of testicular tissue to identify foci of sperm production (testicular sperm extraction; "conventional" TESE) as well as directed testicular surgical sperm retrieval using a microsurgical approach (microdissection testicular sperm extraction; microTESE or mTESE).

Each of these methods were compared using a meta-analysis of published literature [2]. Although a recent meta-analysis reported no difference in sperm retrieval rates when comparing conventional TESE to microTESE, it is important to note that this analysis did not require comparative studies so the heterogeneous nature of NOA patients treated at different sites invalidated any meaningful comparison of surgical techniques [3]. The superiority of microTESE is not surprising, as the surgery directs sampling of testicular tissue to the largest seminiferous tubules, which are those most likely to contain sperm [4]. From a laboratory perspective, the microTESE approach is ideal, as it limits the amount of tissue that must be examined by the andrologist to identify sperm to that which is richest in sperm production. Typical search times to find sperm in isolated, dispersed testicular tissue specimens is only 3 to 5 min at experienced centers. Of note, microTESE, although an invasive surgical procedure, has less effect on testicular function than other approaches for sperm retrieval [4].

3. Causes of Non-Obstructive Azoospermia

NOA occurs secondary to the disruption of spermatogenesis within the testicular parenchyma. This disruption of sperm production is a common phenotype with various underlying etiologies. Although understanding the underlying etiology of azoospermia may help in prognosis and counseling, the precise mechanisms by which spermatogenesis is disrupted in these disorders are not well understood. Men with NOA have varying ranges of spermatogenic failure, and even in 30–60% of those with severely dysfunctional histology (i.e., Sertoli Cell Only (SCO) or maturation arrest) small foci of spermatogenesis can be observed [5]. Furthermore, many other presumed idiopathic cases of NOA are likely to be caused by genetic abnormalities that are yet to be fully delineated.

3.1. Hormonal Imbalances

Men with hypogonadotropic hypogonadism (HH) suffer from a lack of gonadotropin stimulation, resulting in failure of the testis to produce testosterone or sperm. The defect can be congenital (e.g., Kallmann syndrome, Prader-Willi syndrome) or acquired (e.g., secondary to pituitary tumor or exogenous steroid administration). The resultant phenotype of these men is lack of development of secondary sexual characteristics (with prepubertal phenotype) and infertility. Importantly, because the phenotype is caused by a lack of gonadotropin, treatment of these men with exogenous gonadotropins (e.g., human chorionic gonadotropin (hCG) and recombinant follicle-stimulating hormone (FSH)) can result in the appropriate development of secondary sexual characteristics (i.e., pubic hair development, testis growth, development of muscle mass) and sperm [6]. Men with HH typically do not require ICSI to achieve pregnancy as treatment with exogenous gonadotropins is highly effective in inducing spermatogenesis adequate to allow return of sperm to the ejaculate, which is associated with an increase in endogenous testosterone production [6].

Hyperprolactinemia, or elevated serum prolactin levels, is a rare etiology for azoospermia but clinically relevant. Prolactin is produced by the posterior pituitary and elevated levels can result from a prolactin-secreting adenoma (or prolactinoma) [7]. One study examining prolactin levels in infertile men observed increased prolactin levels in men with asthenozoospermia, oligozoospermia, and azoospermia [8]. Since hyperprolactinemia is typically effectively treated with medical therapy, it is rarely a cause for persistent NOA requiring surgical intervention.

3.2. Klinefelter Syndrome

Klinefelter Syndrome (KS) is the most common sex chromosome aneuploidy in infertile men, with an estimated prevalence of approximately 10% in men with NOA [9]. This syndrome involves the addition of one or more extra X-chromosome(s), resulting most commonly in a 47,XXY karyotype [9–11]. KS is thought to occur secondary to chromosomal nondisjunction during meiosis [12,13]. Physical examination of KS men often reveals characteristic findings of tall stature, reduced testis size, reduced chest and facial hair, gynecomastia, eunuchoid appearance, wide hips, and narrow shoulders [13]. Small testis size is thought to occur due to fibrosis and hyalinization of the seminiferous tubules and is progressive through puberty and adult development [14,15]. Rare, small foci of spermatogenesis in the testes of KS men is hypothesized to be present due to the capability of XXY stem cells to undergo spermatogenesis, or more likely, mitotic errors within the XXY stem cell population resulting in diploid cells capable of completing the remaining spermatogenic process [16].

3.3. Y-Chromosome Microdeletions

One of the most common identifiable etiologies of NOA are microdeletions of the azoospermia factor (AZF) region of the Y chromosome, and up to 12% of men with NOA harbor AZF microdeletions [17]. There are three loci in the AZF region, which are designated AZFa, AZFb and AZFc, and each locus contains various genes responsible for different aspects of spermatogenesis [18–20]. Microdeletions within AZFc are the most common (up to 80%), whereas AZFa (up to 4%) and AZFb (up to 5%) are less common [21]. Polymerase chain reaction (PCR) is used to detect Y-chromosome microdeletions (YCMDs) as these chromosomal deletions are too small to detect by standard karyotype analysis. Current guidelines recommend testing for YCMD along with karyotype analysis in men with NOA or severe oligozoospermia (<5 million sperm/mL) [22]. Knowing the YCMD status in a man with severe infertility carries important prognostic information as the sperm retrieval rates (SRR) in men with complete AZFa and AZFb deletions is zero, whereas men with AZFc deletions can have SRR of approximately 50–60% [23].

3.4. Malignancy, Chemotherapy, and Radiation

Malignancy and associated treatments such as chemotherapy and radiation are important causes of azoospermia as approximately 50% of men will be affected by cancer in their lifetime [24]. Chemotherapy targets rapidly dividing cells and testicular germ cells which are mitotically and meiotically active and are highly sensitive to these systemic agents [25]. DNA alkylating agents, as well as platinum-containing chemotherapy agents (such as cisplatin), cross-link DNA and are particularly harmful to spermatogonial stem cells and may result in permanent azoospermia [26,27]. Other chemotherapy agents, such as anthracyclines, antimetabolites, and topoisomerase inhibitors, typically are less gonadotoxic and result only in transient decreases in sperm count because differentiating spermatogonia, and not stem cells, are primarily affected [26]. The CED, or cyclophosphamide-equivalent dose, may be used to determine estimated alkylating agent exposure [28]. One study of adult childhood cancer survivors found that when the CED was less than 4000 mg/m^2 men were normospermic, however there was substantial overlap in the CED values of normozoospermic, oligozoospermic, and azoospermic men [29]. Radiation therapy, on the other hand, may result in irreversible testicular damage secondary to the high radio-sensitivity of testicles [30]. Spermatogonial stem cells are highly sensitive to radiation and are adversely impacted even at low radiation doses (0.1 Gy), with permanent azoospermia typically occurring with doses of 16–20 Gy but reportedly occurring with radiation doses as low as 4 Gy [25,31]. Recovery of spermatogenesis after chemotherapy or radiation therapy depends on the chemotherapy agent used and cumulative chemotherapy or radiation dose [31].

Importantly, as the efficacy of cancer treatments has improved, the number of survivors has increased worldwide [24]. Therefore, strong recommendations from the American Urological Association (AUA), American Society of Clinical Oncology (ASCO), and American Society for Reproductive Medicine (ASRM) have been made to counsel and refer patients for discussion of fertility preservation prior to initiating cancer treatments [32–34]. Additionally, men undergoing chemotherapy or radiation therapy should avoid pregnancy for a minimum of twelve months after completing treatment because of potentially mutagenic effects of the treatments on germ cells [34,35]. Finally, in men with persistent azoospermia after gonadotoxic chemotherapy or radiation treatment, testicular sperm extraction may be performed to harvest sperm for ART [34].

3.5. Cryptorchidism

Cryptorchidism, or undescended testis, is a well-known risk factor for male infertility and a common genitourinary finding. This disorder affects 1–9% of all male neonates worldwide, with approximately 3% of boys remaining cryptorchid at one year of age [36,37]. Semen abnormalities are observed in up to 30% of men with a history of unilateral cryptorchidism and up to 80% of men with a history of bilateral cryptorchidism [38]. Recommended treatment is orchidopexy, or fixation of the testis within the scrotum, and typically is performed early in life (by 18 months of age) to prevent future testicular dysfunction [36,39,40]. The majority of men with a history of cryptorchidism, either unilateral or bilateral, are fertile, however some may develop azoospermia secondary to iatrogenic injury to the testis or testicular vasculature during orchidopexy, or baseline underlying severe spermatogenic dysfunction. For men with NOA secondary to cryptorchidism, testicular sperm extraction is generally favorable with success in the majority of these patients [41–46].

3.6. Varicocele

Varicoceles are a common cause of infertility, found in at least 5% of men with NOA, and the most common cause of secondary infertility [47,48]. Varicoceles are dilated veins (spermatic and pampiniform plexus veins) within the spermatic cord and may result in subsequent testicular dysfunction [49]. Different mechanisms of testicular dysfunction in men with varicoceles have been proposed, including testicular parenchymal hyperthermia, blood-testis barrier dysfunction, and testicular hypoxia [50]. The ultimate downstream effect is the generation of reactive oxygen species and damage to testicular cells [50–52]. Damage to Sertoli, Leydig, and germ cells can result in abnormal or decreased sperm production, as well as deficient testosterone production [49,53]. Although varicoceles clearly contribute to testicular dysfunction, a varicocele is unlikely to be the primary cause of NOA since only 5–10% of men with NOA and clinical varicocele will have enough sperm return to the ejaculate after varicocele repair to avoid testicular sperm extraction [54].

3.7. Other Causes of NOA

NOA may also be acquired for a wide variety of reasons including genitourinary infections, such as post-pubertal mumps orchitis, or various classes of medications. Common medication categories with documented negative impacts to fertility include exogenous testosterone or other androgen-modulating medications, psychiatric medications, and antihypertensive medications, which all have been documented to modulate the hormonal environment resulting in decreased or absent sperm production [55].

4. Optimization of Sperm Production Prior to Surgical Retrieval

Various abnormalities, including hormonal deficiencies and testicular dysfunction, may contribute to abnormal spermatogenesis and decreased or absent sperm production. The production of sperm requires adequate levels of (serum and intratesticular) testosterone, and the goal of optimization is to increase testosterone levels. Serum testosterone levels can be optimized prior to surgical sperm extraction by administration of hormone analogs and modulators, including gonadotropins, aromatase inhibitors (AI), and selective estrogen receptor modulators (SERM) (Table 2). Unfortunately, there is no high-level evidence to support use of medical therapy prior to sperm retrieval, despite many anecdotal applications of medical therapy prior to attempted sperm retrieval for NOA [22]. Certainly, it is conceptually appropriate to treat low testosterone levels in men with NOA. However, retrospective data from a large series of men with NOA suggest that the benefits of treatment are quite limited, with men receiving medical therapy to raise testosterone levels having SRR of 51% (151/307) compared with men not receiving medical therapy prior to surgical intervention who had SRR of 61% (25/41) ($p = 0.31$) [56].

Table 2. Medical therapy for hormonal optimization prior to sperm retrieval.

Class	Medication Name	Dose
AI	Anastrozole	1 mg/day
AI	Letrozole	2.5 mg/day
Gonadotropin	hCG	1500–3000 IU 2×/week
Gonadotropin	rhFSH	100–1500 IU 2–3×/week
SERM	Clomiphene Citrate	25–50 mg/day
SERM	Tamoxifen	20 mg/day

AI, aromatase inhibitor, SERM, selective estrogen receptor modulator; rhFSH, recombinant human follicle-stimulating hormone; hCG, human chorionic gonadotropin; IU, international unit.

Medical therapy used to optimize testosterone levels aims to increase testosterone production and decrease estradiol levels. Elevated estradiol levels, typically greater than 60 pg/mL, can suppress hypothalamic gonadotropin secretion and subsequently inhibit testosterone production [6]. Testosterone-to-estradiol (T:E) ratios are normally greater than 10, and fertile men have a mean T:E ratio of approximately 15 (14.5 ± 1.2) [57,58]. Men with infertility have lower T:E ratios, with NOA men typically in the range of 7 (6.9 ± 0.6) and men with KS approximately 5 (4.4 ± 0.5) [58–60]. Gonadotropins can stimulate testosterone production and spermatogenesis in men with low gonadotropin levels secondary to congenital or acquired disorders [60]. hCG may be used as an luteinizing hormone (LH) substitute alone or in combination with an FSH analog (recombinant human FSH (rhFSH) or human menopausal gonadotropin (hMG)) to stimulate testis growth, testosterone production, and spermatogenesis [60]. AIs, including anastrozole and letrozole, prevent the actions of aromatase, which is present in peripheral tissues, in converting testosterone to estrogen. AIs have been shown to be effective medical therapy to increase SRR in men with KS and in infertile, non-KS men with abnormal T:E ratios [61,62]. SERMs, such as clomiphene citrate and tamoxifen, provide benefits by inhibiting the negative feedback exerted on the hypothalamic-pituitary-testis (HPT) axis by estrogen. With decreased negative inhibition, higher levels of LH and FSH can be achieved, resulting in increased serum testosterone levels and improved sperm production. Several studies have demonstrated positive impacts on semen parameters in infertile men taking clomiphene citrate [63,64].

Repair of clinical varicoceles has been demonstrated to improve serum testosterone levels, as well as spermatogenesis in men with oligozoospermia [48]. After varicocele repair in men with NOA, the potential improvement of spermatogenesis may result in enhanced SRR, although there is no high-level evidence to support such intervention [54].

5. Intracytoplasmic Sperm Injection for NOA

Prior to the advent of ICSI, men with NOA had no means for conceiving biological children. ICSI was first introduced in 1992, and three years later, in 1995, sperm retrieved from an NOA patient was used successfully with ICSI [65,66]. Since the development of ICSI, numerous studies have been performed to examine factors that may predict or be associated with increased ICSI success.

5.1. Predictors of ICSI Outcomes

Limited pre-operative variables exist which predict success of SRR and ICSI. For predictors of SRR, patient age, serum hormone levels, and testicle size have been evaluated, however, conclusive evidence is lacking that any of these factors is predictive of successful sperm retrieval [67–69]. Testicular histopathology does provide some prognostic information for SRR, but it is not routinely recommended for diagnosis of NOA, as the diagnosis can be made clinically based on FSH > 7.6 and testis length < 4.5 cm in about 90% of men with this condition [22,68,70,71]. Similarly, no clinical or biochemical factors have been found to be predictive of ICSI outcomes [3]. Additionally, testis histology has not been shown to significantly influence clinical outcomes after ICSI [71]. There may, however, be an association of the number of sperm found at time of surgical retrieval with the number of clinical pregnancies [72]. Further work is needed to determine if any preoperative factors, in conjunction with female factors, can predict ICSI outcomes.

5.2. ICSI Outcomes in NOA Men

Understanding clinical outcomes after ICSI are important when counseling men with NOA and their partners prior to surgical sperm retrieval. A study derived from the National Assisted Reproductive Technology Surveillance System (NASS) found that men with infertility (including non-azoospermic and azoospermic men) had a clinical pregnancy rate (CPR) of 48% and live birth rate (LBR) of 40%, which was similar to rates in men with no infertility (CPR 44.9%, LBR 36.5%) [73]. A clear limitation of this study was that the various etiologies of male infertility were not specified or separately examined and thus, the CPR and LBR may not hold true for all etiologies of NOA. Although NOA men represent the most severe phenotype of those with male infertility, the majority of studies, similar to that previously described, have pooled men with NOA regardless of etiology which limits the overall generalizability of the data. A comprehensive summary of SRR, biochemical pregnancy rate (BCPR), CPR, and LBR from studies investigating ICSI outcomes between 1997 and 2020 in NOA men is presented in Table 3.

Table 3. Studies reporting intracytoplasmic sperm injection outcomes in men with non-obstructive azoospermia.

Study	Year	NOA Etiology	Sperm Retrieval	SRR (%)	(BCPR (%)) CPR (%)	LBR (%)	MR (%)
Fahmy et al. [74]	1997	NR	cTESE	NR	(16.6) 19.2	NR	NR
Friedler et al. [75]	1997	NR	TESA TESE	43.0	29.0	NR	NR
Ben-Yosef et al. [76]	1999	NR	TESE *	60.0	21.7–27	13.0–25.0	6.7–8.7
Palermo et al. [77]	1999	NR	mTESE	63.9	49.1	NR	12.5
Mercan et al. [78]	2000	NR	TESA TESE	64.4	29–46	NR	20.7–24.2
Chan et al. [79]	2001	Chemotherapy	cTESE mTESE	45.0	(44.5) 33.3	22.2	NR
Damani et al. [80]	2002	Chemotherapy	cTESE	65.2	60.0	53.0	NR
Friedler et al. [81]	2002	NR	cTESE	39.0–85.0	16.0–19.0	67.0–80.0	NR
Mátyás et al. [82]	2002	NR	cTESE	69.6	26.7	NR	NR
Bailly et al. [83]	2003	NR	cTESE	35.0	18.0	81.8	9.0

Table 3. Cont.

Study	Year	NOA Etiology	Sperm Retrieval	SRR (%)	(BCPR (%)) CPR (%)	LBR (%)	MR (%)
Mansour et al. [84]	2003	NR	cTESE	56.1	13.6–24.1	NR	NR
Meseguer et al. [85]	2003	Chemotherapy	cTESE	41.7	20.0	20.0	NR
Osmanagaoglu et al. [86]	2003	NR	TESE *	NR	NR	13.9	NR
Raman et al.—a [42]	2003	Cryptorchidism	cTESE mTESE	74.0	46.0	43.0	NR
Raman et al.—b [42]	2003	NR	cTESE mTESE	58.0	44.0	36.0	8.1
Vernaeve et al.—a [43]	2004	NOA (excluded cryptorchidism)	cTESE	33.3%	(20.7) 10.9	10.9	NR
Vernaeve et al.—b [43]	2004	Cryptorchidism	cTESE	51.9	(28.1) 17.2	17.2	NR
Aydos et al. [87]	2005	Cryptorchidism, idiopathic, nontestis cancer, RT, trauma, mumps, orchitis, chromosome anomaly	mTESE	57.0	36.0	NR	NR
Giorgetti et al. [88]	2005	NR	cTESE	46.0	35.3	25.0–29.0	NR
Mitchell et al. [89]	2005	NR	cTESE	N/A	8.7–26.7	17.4–33.3	NR
Wu et al. [90]	2005	NR	cTESE	76.7	33.3–62.5	33.3–41.7	0–20.8
Everaert et al. [91]	2006	NR	MESA mTESE	35.4	(13.2) 9.4	7.5	NR
Hibi et al. [92]	2007	Chemotherapy	mTESE	60.0	NR	40.0	NR
Mitchell et al. [93]	2007	NR	cTESE	N/A	26.0	13.3	NR
Kanto et al. [94]	2009	NR	mTESE	42.5	52.9	NR	NR
Ravizzini et al. [95]	2008	NR	mTESE	57.1	(50.0) 40.0	40.0	NR
Ishikawa et al. [96]	2009	NR	mTESE	N/A	(36.8) 30.9	26.5	NR
Wiser et al. [44]	2009	Cryptorchidism	cTESE	59.5	30.8–41.2	75.0–80.0	NR
Yarali et al.—a [97]	2009	non-KS	mTESE	44.0	(41.0) 33.0	26.0	NR
Yarali et al.—b [97]	2009	KS	mTESE	56.0	(61.0) 39.0	28.0	NR

Table 3. Cont.

Study	Year	NOA Etiology	Sperm Retrieval	SRR (%)	(BCPR (%)) CPR (%)	LBR (%)	MR (%)
Boitrelle et al. [98]	2011	Cryptorchidism, KS, YCMD, Y inversion, malignancy, idiopathic chemotherapy/RT	cTESE	53.2	42.7	37.0	7.9 5.3 €
Hauser et al. [99]	2011	NOA + cryptozoospermia	cTESE	N/A	(19.1–42.9) 12.8–42.9	12.8–42.9	NR
Hsiao et al. [100]	2011	Chemotherapy	mTESE	37.0	50.0	42.0	NR
Ashraf et al. [101]	2013	NR	mTESE	50.0	40.0	NR	NR
Choi et al.—a [102]	2013	NOA + AZFc YCMD	cTESE	21.0	NR	19.5	NR
Choi et al.—b [102]	2013	AZFc YCMD	cTESE	26.6	NR	24.3	NR
Karacan et al. [103]	2013	NR	mTESE	54.9	31.3	28.9	7.6
Arafa et al. [104]	2014	Familial and non-familial idiopathic NOA	mTESE	37.4	13.9	NR	NR
Esteves et al. [105]	2014	NR	mTESE	41.4	27.8	19.9	28.6
Karacan et al. [106]	2014	NR	mTESE	48.9	16.6–30.7	16.6–28.2	8.3
Aydin et al. [107]	2015	NR	mTESE	58.6	44.6	NR	NR
Tsai et al. [45]	2015	Cryptorchidism	TESE *	N/A	45.6	32.9	6.3
Vloeberghs et al. [108]	2015	NR	cTESE	40.5	(27.7–34) 21.7–26.7	20.6–25.3	NR
Ko et al. [109]	2016	NR	cTESE mTESE	44.9	(37.5) 30	25.0	NR
Alfano et al. [110]	2017	Idiopathic NOA	mTESE	48.9	21.7	13.0	NR
Arafa et al.—a [111]	2018	Idiopathic NOA + AZFc YCMD	TESE *	63.2	25.7	NR	NR
Arafa et al.—b [111]	2018	Idiopathic NOA	TESE *	65.8	26.6	NR	NR
Yu et al. [112]	2018	NR	mTESE	38.4	(34.3) 49.1	24.6	20.7

Table 3. Cont.

Study	Year	NOA Etiology	Sperm Retrieval	SRR (%)	(BCPR (%)) CPR (%)	LBR (%)	MR (%)
Chen et al. [41]	2019	Idiopathic, KS, YCMD, cryptorchidism, mumps orchitis, chemotherapy	mTESE	40.3	51.0–55.8	NR	NR
Yamaguchi et al.—a [113]	2020	NOA (excluded AZFc YCMD)	mTESE	74.0	28.9	NR	20.2
Yamaguchi et al.—b [113]	2020	AZFc YCMD	mTESE	20.4	24.7	NR	26.3

AZFRc, azoospermia factor region deletion in locus c; SRR, sperm retrieval rate; BCPR, biochemical pregnancy rate (elevated serum hCG); CPR, clinical pregnancy rate (heartbeat or gestational sac detectable by ultrasound); LBR, live birth rate; MR, miscarriage rate; NOA, non-obstructive azoospermia; NR, not reported; TESA, testicular sperm aspiration; cTESE, conventional TESE; mTESE, microdissection TESE; TESE *—type of TESE not specified; €, ectopic pregnancy rate; KS, Klinefelter syndrome; YCMD, Y-chromosome microdeletion; RT, radiation therapy; MESA, microsurgical epiddiymal sperm aspiration. "a" and "b" were used to denote different patient cohorts examined within one study.

A recent meta-analysis examining sperm retrieval as well as pregnancy and LBRs was performed [3]. This review compared SRR after conventional TESE (cTESE) with that after microTESE, and found that the per procedure SRR was 45–49%, and was not able to identify differences between conventional or microsurgical methods of sperm retrieval because the included studies did not include comparator trials [3]. Meta-regression analysis further demonstrated that SRR was independent of both age and hormonal parameters [3]. Testis volume greater than 12.5 mL was found to be associated with a greater than 60% chance of successful sperm retrieval with an accuracy of 86.2% [3]. The BCPR (diagnosed by positive serum hCG in the female partner) was 25–32% per ICSI cycle, and LBR was 20–28% [3]. It is important to note that the patient cohorts included in this meta-analysis were heterogenous with varying NOA etiologies, making the comparison of outcomes between cTESE and mTESE less valid. A previous meta-analysis which included fifteen comparative studies demonstrated a 17% higher likelihood of sperm retrieval success when performing mTESE compared to cTESE [2]. Additionally, it was noted that men who underwent mTESE had failed prior cTESE or TESA, which also may have underestimated the increase in sperm retrieval rate with mTESE [2]. Several, smaller studies have been performed examining NOA men based on underlying etiology, including KS, YCMD, malignancy, and cryptorchidism, and these will be discussed further.

5.2.1. Klinefelter Syndrome

A meta-analysis of 37 studies found a cumulative SRR of 44% (39–48%) per TESE procedure in KS patients, with no significant difference between cTESE and mTESE [114]. ICSI outcomes were available for 29 of the 37 studies in the meta-analysis, and reported a cumulative CPR, defined by ultrasound detection of a gestational sac or heartbeat, of 43% (36–50%), and LBR of 43% (34–53%) per ICSI cycle [114]. SRR, CPR, and LBR in this analysis were independent of patient age at time of retrieval as well as testis volume, and serum hormone parameters [114]. Additionally, no differences between use of fresh versus frozen sperm were observed [114]. Again, it is important to note that this meta-analysis examined studies where the patient cohorts were not entirely made up of KS patients. In one of the largest published studies on SRR in KS patients, we report a SRR of 66% (Table 4) [61]. In our experience with KS patients, the appearance of tubules within the testis is unique amongst men with NOA. Instead of typically having sperm production throughout an individual seminiferous tubule, KS patients tend to have focal enlargement of otherwise sclerotic tubules within the testes. This appearance requires an intensive search within these typically very atrophic testes to find the millimeter-sized segments of tubules that may contain sperm. In addition, the number of sperm retrieved tends to be so small that sperm are typically not able to be frozen for later use. Therefore, the numbers of sperm obtained may be only adequate to inject available oocytes during a programmed, fresh in vitro fertilization (IVF) cycle.

Table 4. Sperm retrieval rates in non-obstructive azoospermia by etiology.

NOA Etiology	Weill Cornell Medicine (P.N.S.)	Other Reports
Idiopathic	48.5% [46]	37.4–65.8% [104,111]
Klinefelter syndrome	61–66% [46,61]	44% [114]
YCMD (AZFc)	67–75% [17,46]	20.4–54.8% [102,113,115]
Chemotherapy	42% [46]	37–60% [79,92,100]
Cryptorchidism	62% [46]	52–85% [41–45]
Overall	48% [46]	45–49% [3]

P.N.S., Peter N. Schlegel, attending urologist at Weill Cornell Medicine.

5.2.2. Y-Chromosome Microdeletions

Little is known regarding ICSI and clinical outcomes in NOA men with YCMD given that many of these studies excluded men with YCMD or included men with YCMD in a larger cohort of azoospermic men (Tables 3 and 4). SRRs differ drastically depending on the site of microdeletion. Sperm can be surgically retrieved in up to 70% of men with AZFc deletions and a subset may have low concentrations of sperm in the ejaculate, whereas no reports of sperm retrieval in men with complete AZFa or AZFb deletions have been effectively documented [17,116]. One study examining ICSI outcomes using ejaculated sperm demonstrated no significant difference in pregnancy, live birth, and miscarriage rates in men with AZFc microdeletions compared to those with other sources of infertility and no evidence of YCMD [117]. Another study found that men with AZFc microdeletions had a significantly increased fertilization rate when ejaculated sperm was used compared to testicular sperm [118]. With ejaculated sperm, pregnancy rate was 47% compared to 14% with testicular sperm [118]. Unfortunately, no predictors of successful sperm retrieval have been identified in this cohort, and it is important to inform couples that any male offspring will harbor the same Y-chromosome mutations [118,119].

5.2.3. Chemotherapy-Associated NOA

In men treated with chemotherapy, SRR ranges from 37 to 60%, pregnancy rates 33–50%, and LBR 22–42% (Tables 3 and 4) [79,92,100]. Additional studies have been performed examining SRRs and ICSI outcomes, but men treated for malignancy (either with chemotherapy or radiation) are often pooled with men who have NOA due to other underlying etiologies. Therefore, the reported clinical outcomes may not be accurate for men with azoospermia solely secondary to chemotherapy or radiation treatment. One retrospective study of male cancer survivors found that following chemotherapy or radiation treatment, approximately 57% were azoospermic [120]. This percentage is higher than expected in a full cohort of men treated with chemotherapy, as it reflects a referral bias to an infertility center for selected cancer survivors. The CPR was 38.6% and the LBR was 30.5% after ICSI [120]. Overall, SRR and ICSI outcomes are generally favorable for men who have undergone treatment for malignancy. In testis cancer survivors, 3% (who received chemotherapy) and 6% (who received radiation therapy) remained azoospermic two years after therapy [121]. With increasingly aggressive chemotherapy treatment regimens, the rates of persistent azoospermia are higher [122]. However, fertility preservation prior to cancer treatment is still highly recommended as it is minimally invasive for men and can potentially portend less invasive treatments for the female partner [22].

5.2.4. Cryptorchidism

The mechanism underlying infertility in males with a history of cryptorchidism is not well understood. Men with bilateral cryptorchidism have a higher risk of infertility compared with those who have unilateral cryptorchidism [38,39,123]. Additionally, age at orchidopexy also affects sperm production and future fertility [40]. It is estimated that greater than 50% of men with a history of cryptorchidism will have varying degrees of spermatogenic failure and may require surgical sperm retrieval to conceive biological children [39,123].

Men who have had prior orchidopexy typically have substantial peri-testicular scar, no tunica vaginalis, and often have an abnormal lie or position of the testis with an anterior epididymis. Surgical treatment in these men also often reveals an atypical blood supply to the testis with variable patterns of vessels on the tunica albuginea. Within the testis, most tubules are typically sclerotic with distinctively different tubules containing isolated foci of spermatogenesis visible during microdissection. Studies examining ICSI outcomes solely in men with a history of cryptorchidism report SRR ranging from 52 to 85%, pregnancy rates ranging from 10–46%, LBR ranging from 33–100%, and miscarriage rates ranging from 6.3–8.1% (Tables 2 and 3) [41–45]. Patients with cryptorchidism have a wide range of fertility potential and more studies of these individuals is needed to determine the mechanisms underlying their infertility so that patients can be counseled with accurate prognostic information.

5.3. Sperm Effects on ICSI Outcomes

For men with severely impaired sperm production, embryo development appears to be adversely affected by the (testicular) source of sperm and level of sperm production with decreased development associated with higher FSH levels [124,125]. Men with NOA often have such low fertilization rates that a limited number of embryos exist on day 3. Therefore, transfer of day 3 embryos is routinely required, as further in vitro culture risks losing the embryos available for transfer on day 3. Of note, high-quality day 3 embryos have been suggested in some studies to be equivalent to day 5 blastocysts in terms of pregnancy and live birth rate [124]. However, existing data are limited with no interpretable data on embryo morphokinetic parameters, although some publications suggest that embryo development may be less efficient in me with lower sperm production [124,126]. Similarly, there are limited published data on blastocyst euploidy rates. Given the frequency of day 3 embryo transfer for couples where men have NOA, data obtained from the select group with blastocysts available for transfer may not reflect results that are generalizable for NOA patients as a whole.

Advances in the understanding of sperm biology have revealed important paternal effects on embryo development and quality. Poor semen parameters have been demonstrated to negatively affect blastocyst formation rates after IVF and ICSI [124,126–129]. Ejaculated sperm has been found to produce higher fertilization and pregnancy rates than testicular sperm [130]. Additionally, when compared to men with obstructive azoospermia undergoing ICSI, men with NOA undergoing ICSI have lower rates of fertilization, blastocyst formation, implantation, and pregnancy [124,126,131,132].

6. Improving ICSI Outcomes from the Male Perspective

Optimization of hormone levels in NOA men may improve SRR [71]. Increased numbers of sperm may allow selection of more optimal sperm to be used for ICSI. Currently, various methods exist for improving sperm selection, including viability assays, cell sorting methods and enhanced microscopic analysis for selection of sperm for ICSI, although manual selection of individual sperm is the most common approach used in men with NOA [133].

Conventional sperm selection methods including the swim-up method, migration density, and density gradients rely heavily on the motility of sperm, and cannot be used for sperm retrieved from the testis as certain maturation processes have not occurred in testicular sperm and these sperm are immotile. Magnetic activated cell sorting (MACS) is a method of sperm selection using annexin V-conjugated magnetic beads to isolate viable sperm. A systematic review analyzing five prospective, randomized trials evaluating MACS compared to standard sperm selection methods (including swim-up and density gradient methods) found significantly increased pregnancy rates resulted after MACS [134]. Intracytoplasmic morphologically selected sperm injection (IMSI) is the process of selecting sperm at x6,600 magnification to examine motile sperm organellar morphology [133]. A prospective, randomized study examining ICSI and IMSI in couples with severe male factor infertility reported higher CPR with IMSI (39.2% IMSI vs. 26.5% ICSI, $p = 0.004$) [135]. This study along with other studies, including one meta-analysis, also demonstrated a decreased miscarriage rate and improved implantation rates with IMSI compared with ICSI [133,135]. However, a recent Cochrane review of the efficacy of IMSI compared with traditional ICSI did not provide any conclusive evidence to suggest that IMSI is superior to ICSI in terms of clinical outcomes (CPR, LBR) [136].

Additional work on novel techniques is underway that will further optimize the sperm chosen for oocyte injection. One promising technique is microfluidic sorting of sperm, which allows for analysis of sperm count, motility, and morphology on a microscopic level, allowing for the identification and selection of sperm with the best qualities [137,138]. Studies examining microfluidics-sorted sperm have demonstrated improved ICSI and clinical outcomes compared to sperm selected by conventional methods [138,139]. However, further work is needed to fully develop this technology for mainstream use [140]. Given the limited numbers of sperm available for retrieval from men with NOA, it is more challenging to apply sperm selection techniques that could be used for sperm samples from men with oligozoospermia.

7. Conclusions

ICSI has permitted NOA men, who were previously unable, to conceive biological children. Studies have demonstrated varying rates of clinical (pregnancy and live birth rates) outcomes likely due to a heterogenous population of men with NOA included in these studies, and future studies would benefit from etiology-specific outcome reporting. Understanding clinical outcomes after ICSI is important for prognostic information and counseling of these NOA men and their partners prior to undergoing invasive surgical procedures. Further work is needed to delineate the molecular mechanisms and genetic defects that underlie this severe reproductive phenotype.

Author Contributions: Conceptualization P.N.S.; writing—C.K., N.P., and P.N.S.; review and editing—C.K., N.P., and P.N.S.; supervision P.N.S. All authors have read and agreed to the published version of the manuscript.

Funding: C.K. and N.P. are supported in part by the Frederick J. and Theresa Dow Wallace Fund of the New York Community Trust.

Data Availability Statement: Not applicable.

Conflicts of Interest: The authors have no conflict of interest to declare.

References

1. Leifke, E.; Nieschlag, E. Male infertility treatment in the light of evidence-based medicine. *Andrologia* **1996**, *28*, 23–30. [PubMed]
2. Bernie, A.M.; Mata, D.A.; Ramasamy, R.; Schlegel, P.N. Comparison of microdissection testicular sperm extraction, conventional testicular sperm extraction, and testicular sperm aspiration for nonobstructive azoospermia: A systematic review and meta-analysis. *Fertil. Steril.* **2015**, *104*, 1099–1103.e3. [CrossRef] [PubMed]
3. Corona, G.; Minhas, S.; Giwercman, A.; Bettocchi, C.; Dinkelman-Smit, M.; Dohle, G.; Fusco, F.; Kadioglou, A.; Kliesch, S.; Kopa, Z.; et al. Sperm recovery and ICSI outcomes in men with non-obstructive azoospermia: A systematic review and meta-analysis. *Hum. Reprod. Update* **2019**, *25*, 733–757. [CrossRef]
4. Schlegel, P.N. Testicular sperm extraction: Microdissection improves sperm yield with minimal tissue excision. *Hum. Reprod.* **1999**, *14*, 131–135. [CrossRef] [PubMed]
5. Esteves, S.C. Clinical management of infertile men with nonobstructive azoospermia. *Asian J. Androl.* **2015**, *17*, 459–470. [CrossRef]

6. Kumar, R. Medical management of non-obstructive azoospermia. *Clinics* **2013**, *68*, 75–79. [CrossRef]
7. Romijn, J.A. Hyperprolactinemia and prolactinoma. *Handb. Clin. Neurol.* **2014**, *124*, 185–195. [CrossRef]
8. Merino, G.; Carranza-Lira, S.; Martinez-Chéquer, J.C.; Barahona, E.; Morán, C.; Bermúdez, J.A. Hyperprolactinemia in men with asthenozoospermia, oligozoospermia, or azoospermia. *Arch. Androl.* **1997**, *38*, 201–206. [CrossRef]
9. Stahl, P.J.; Schlegel, P.N. Genetic evaluation of the azoospermic or severely oligozoospermic male. *Curr. Opin. Obstet. Gynecol.* **2012**, *24*, 221–228. [CrossRef]
10. Suganya, J.; Kujur, S.B.; Selvaraj, K.; Suruli, M.S.; Haripriya, G.; Samuel, C.R. Chromosomal Abnormalities in Infertile Men from Southern India. *J. Clin. Diagn. Res.* **2015**, *9*, GC05-10. [CrossRef]
11. Abramsky, L.; Chapple, J. 47,XXY (Klinefelter syndrome) and 47,XYY: Estimated rates of and indication for postnatal diagnosis with implications for prenatal counselling. *Prenat. Diagn.* **1997**, *17*, 363–368. [CrossRef]
12. Maduro, M.R.; Lamb, D.J. Understanding new genetics of male infertility. *J. Urol.* **2002**, *168*, 2197–2205. [CrossRef]
13. Bonomi, M.; Rochira, V.; Pasquali, D.; Balercia, G.; Jannini, E.A.; Ferlin, A.; Klinefelter Italia, N.G. Klinefelter syndrome (KS): Genetics, clinical phenotype and hypogonadism. *J. Endocrinol. Investig.* **2017**, *40*, 123–134. [CrossRef] [PubMed]
14. Lanfranco, F.; Kamischke, A.; Zitzmann, M.; Nieschlag, E. Klinefelter's syndrome. *Lancet* **2004**, *364*, 273–283. [CrossRef]
15. Aksglaede, L.; Wikstrom, A.M.; Rajpert-De Meyts, E.; Dunkel, L.; Skakkebaek, N.E.; Juul, A. Natural history of seminiferous tubule degeneration in Klinefelter syndrome. *Hum. Reprod. Update* **2006**, *12*, 39–48. [CrossRef]
16. Fainberg, J.; Hayden, R.P.; Schlegel, P.N. Fertility management of Klinefelter syndrome. *Expert Rev. Endocrinol. Metab* **2019**, *14*, 369–380. [CrossRef]
17. Hopps, C.V.; Mielnik, A.; Goldstein, M.; Palermo, G.D.; Rosenwaks, Z.; Schlegel, P.N. Detection of sperm in men with Y chromosome microdeletions of the AZFa, AZFb and AZFc regions. *Hum. Reprod.* **2003**, *18*, 1660–1665. [CrossRef]
18. Vogt, P.H.; Edelmann, A.; Kirsch, S.; Henegariu, O.; Hirschmann, P.; Kiesewetter, F.; Kohn, F.M.; Schill, W.B.; Farah, S.; Ramos, C.; et al. Human Y chromosome azoospermia factors (AZF) mapped to different subregions in Yq11. *Hum. Mol. Genet.* **1996**, *5*, 933–943. [CrossRef]
19. Vogt, P.H. AZF deletions and Y chromosomal haplogroups: History and update based on sequence. *Hum. Reprod. Update* **2005**, *11*, 319–336. [CrossRef]
20. Colaco, S.; Modi, D. Genetics of the human Y chromosome and its association with male infertility. *Reprod. Biol. Endocrinol.* **2018**, *16*, 14. [CrossRef]
21. Bansal, S.K.; Jaiswal, D.; Gupta, N.; Singh, K.; Dada, R.; Sankhwar, S.N.; Gupta, G.; Rajender, S. Gr/gr deletions on Y-chromosome correlate with male infertility: An original study, meta-analyses, and trial sequential analyses. *Sci. Rep.* **2016**, *6*, 19798. [CrossRef] [PubMed]
22. Schlegel, P.N.; Sigman, M.; Collura, B.; De Jonge, C.J.; Eisenberg, M.L.; Lamb, D.J.; Mulhall, J.P.; Niederberger, C.; Sandlow, J.I.; Sokol, R.Z.; et al. Diagnosis and Treatment of Infertility in Men: AUA/ASRM Guideline Part I. *J. Urol.* **2021**, *205*, 36–43. [CrossRef] [PubMed]
23. Georgiou, I.; Syrrou, M.; Pardalidis, N.; Karakitsios, K.; Mantzavinos, T.; Giotitsas, N.; Loutradis, D.; Dimitriadis, F.; Saito, M.; Miyagawa, I.; et al. Genetic and epigenetic risks of intracytoplasmic sperm injection method. *Asian J. Androl.* **2006**, *8*, 643–673. [CrossRef]
24. Osterberg, E.C.; Ramasamy, R.; Masson, P.; Brannigan, R.E. Current practices in fertility preservation in male cancer patients. *Urol. Ann.* **2014**, *6*, 13–17. [CrossRef] [PubMed]
25. Howell, S.J.; Radford, J.A.; Ryder, W.D.; Shalet, S.M. Testicular function after cytotoxic chemotherapy: Evidence of Leydig cell insufficiency. *J. Clin. Oncol.* **1999**, *17*, 1493–1498. [CrossRef] [PubMed]
26. Meistrich, M.L. Effects of chemotherapy and radiotherapy on spermatogenesis in humans. *Fertil. Steril.* **2013**, *100*, 1180–1186. [CrossRef] [PubMed]
27. Dasari, S.; Tchounwou, P.B. Cisplatin in cancer therapy: Molecular mechanisms of action. *Eur. J. Pharmacol* **2014**, *740*, 364–378. [CrossRef] [PubMed]
28. Green, D.M.; Nolan, V.G.; Goodman, P.J.; Whitton, J.A.; Srivastava, D.; Leisenring, W.M.; Neglia, J.P.; Sklar, C.A.; Kaste, S.C.; Hudson, M.M.; et al. The cyclophosphamide equivalent dose as an approach for quantifying alkylating agent exposure: A report from the Childhood Cancer Survivor Study. *Pediatr. Blood Cancer* **2014**, *61*, 53–67. [CrossRef]
29. Green, D.M.; Liu, W.; Kutteh, W.H.; Ke, R.W.; Shelton, K.C.; Sklar, C.A.; Chemaitilly, W.; Pui, C.H.; Klosky, J.L.; Spunt, S.L.; et al. Cumulative alkylating agent exposure and semen parameters in adult survivors of childhood cancer: A report from the St Jude Lifetime Cohort Study. *Lancet Oncol.* **2014**, *15*, 1215–1223. [CrossRef]
30. Okada, K.; Fujisawa, M. Recovery of Spermatogenesis Following Cancer Treatment with Cytotoxic Chemotherapy and Radiotherapy. *World J. Mens Health* **2019**, *37*, 166–174. [CrossRef]
31. Dohle, G.R. Male infertility in cancer patients: Review of the literature. *Int. J. Urol.* **2010**, *17*, 327–331. [CrossRef] [PubMed]
32. Loren, A.W.; Mangu, P.B.; Beck, L.N.; Brennan, L.; Magdalinski, A.J.; Partridge, A.H.; Quinn, G.; Wallace, W.H.; Oktay, K.; American Society of Clinical, O. Fertility preservation for patients with cancer: American Society of Clinical Oncology clinical practice guideline update. *J. Clin. Oncol.* **2013**, *31*, 2500–2510. [CrossRef] [PubMed]
33. Ethics Committee of the American Society for Reproductive Medicine. Fertility preservation and reproduction in patients facing gonadotoxic therapies: An Ethics Committee opinion. *Fertil. Steril.* **2018**, *110*, 380–386. [CrossRef] [PubMed]

34. Schlegel, P.N.; Sigman, M.; Collura, B.; De Jonge, C.J.; Eisenberg, M.L.; Lamb, D.J.; Mulhall, J.P.; Niederberger, C.; Sandlow, J.I.; Sokol, R.Z.; et al. Diagnosis and Treatment of Infertility in Men: AUA/ASRM Guideline PART II. *J. Urol.* **2021**, *205*, 44–51. [CrossRef] [PubMed]
35. Meistrich, M.L. Risks of genetic damage in offspring conceived using spermatozoa produced during chemotherapy or radiotherapy. *Andrology* **2020**, *8*, 545–558. [CrossRef] [PubMed]
36. Gurney, J.K.; McGlynn, K.A.; Stanley, J.; Merriman, T.; Signal, V.; Shaw, C.; Edwards, R.; Richiardi, L.; Hutson, J.; Sarfati, D. Risk factors for cryptorchidism. *Nat. Rev. Urol.* **2017**, *14*, 534–548. [CrossRef]
37. Cortes, D. Cryptorchidism–aspects of pathogenesis, histology and treatment. *Scand. J. Urol. Nephrol. Suppl.* **1998**, *196*, 1–54. [PubMed]
38. Hanson, B.M.; Eisenberg, M.L.; Hotaling, J.M. Male infertility: A biomarker of individual and familial cancer risk. *Fertil. Steril.* **2018**, *109*, 6–19. [CrossRef]
39. Cobellis, G.; Noviello, C.; Nino, F.; Romano, M.; Mariscoli, F.; Martino, A.; Parmeggiani, P.; Papparella, A. Spermatogenesis and cryptorchidism. *Front. Endocrinol.* **2014**, *5*, 63. [CrossRef]
40. Rodprasert, W.; Virtanen, H.E.; Mäkelä, J.A.; Toppari, J. Hypogonadism and Cryptorchidism. *Front. Endocrinol.* **2019**, *10*, 906. [CrossRef] [PubMed]
41. Chen, X.; Ma, Y.; Zou, S.; Wang, S.; Qiu, J.; Xiao, Q.; Zhou, L.; Ping, P. Comparison and outcomes of nonobstructive azoospermia patients with different etiology undergoing MicroTESE and ICSI treatments. *Transl. Androl. Urol.* **2019**, *8*, 366–373. [CrossRef] [PubMed]
42. Raman, J.D.; Schlegel, P.N. Testicular sperm extraction with intracytoplasmic sperm injection is successful for the treatment of nonobstructive azoospermia associated with cryptorchidism. *J. Urol.* **2003**, *170*, 1287–1290. [CrossRef] [PubMed]
43. Vernaeve, V.; Krikilion, A.; Verheyen, G.; Van Steirteghem, A.; Devroey, P.; Tournaye, H. Outcome of testicular sperm recovery and ICSI in patients with non-obstructive azoospermia with a history of orchidopexy. *Hum. Reprod.* **2004**, *19*, 2307–2312. [CrossRef] [PubMed]
44. Wiser, A.; Raviv, G.; Weissenberg, R.; Elizur, S.E.; Levron, J.; Machtinger, R.; Madgar, I. Does age at orchidopexy impact on the results of testicular sperm extraction? *Reprod. Biomed. Online* **2009**, *19*, 778–783. [CrossRef]
45. Tsai, Y.R.; Huang, F.J.; Lin, P.Y.; Kung, F.T.; Lin, Y.J.; Lan, K.C. Clinical outcomes and development of children born to couples with obstructive and nonobstructive azoospermia undergoing testicular sperm extraction-intracytoplasmic sperm injection: A comparative study. *Taiwan J. Obstet. Gynecol.* **2015**, *54*, 155–159. [CrossRef] [PubMed]
46. Dabaja, A.A.; Schlegel, P.N. Microdissection testicular sperm extraction: An update. *Asian J. Androl.* **2013**, *15*, 35–39. [CrossRef]
47. Gorelick, J.I.; Goldstein, M. Loss of fertility in men with varicocele. *Fertil. Steril.* **1993**, *59*, 613–616. [CrossRef]
48. Esteves, S.C.; Glina, S. Recovery of spermatogenesis after microsurgical subinguinal varicocele repair in azoospermic men based on testicular histology. *Int. Braz. J. Urol.* **2005**, *31*, 541–548. [CrossRef]
49. Sedaghatpour, D.; Berookhim, B.M. The Role of Varicocele in Male Factor Subfertility. *Curr. Urol. Rep.* **2017**, *18*, 73. [CrossRef]
50. Hassanin, A.M.; Ahmed, H.H.; Kaddah, A.N. A global view of the pathophysiology of varicocele. *Andrology* **2018**, *6*, 654–661. [CrossRef]
51. Shiraishi, K.; Naito, K. Effects of 4-hydroxy-2-nonenal, a marker of oxidative stress, on spermatogenesis and expression of p53 protein in male infertility. *J. Urol.* **2007**, *178*, 1012–1017, discussion 1017. [CrossRef] [PubMed]
52. Ogi, S.; Tanji, N.; Iseda, T.; Yokoyama, M. Expression of heat shock proteins in developing and degenerating rat testes. *Arch. Androl.* **1999**, *43*, 163–171. [CrossRef] [PubMed]
53. Tanrikut, C.; Goldstein, M.; Rosoff, J.S.; Lee, R.K.; Nelson, C.J.; Mulhall, J.P. Varicocele as a risk factor for androgen deficiency and effect of repair. *BJU Int.* **2011**, *108*, 1480–1484. [CrossRef] [PubMed]
54. Schlegel, P.N.; Kaufmann, J. Role of varicocelectomy in men with nonobstructive azoospermia. *Fertil. Steril.* **2004**, *81*, 1585–1588. [CrossRef] [PubMed]
55. Samplaski, M.K.; Nangia, A.K. Adverse effects of common medications on male fertility. *Nat. Rev. Urol.* **2015**, *12*, 401–413. [CrossRef]
56. Reifsnyder, J.E.; Ramasamy, R.; Husseini, J.; Schlegel, P.N. Role of optimizing testosterone before microdissection testicular sperm extraction in men with nonobstructive azoospermia. *J. Urol.* **2012**, *188*, 532–536. [CrossRef] [PubMed]
57. Schlegel, P.N. Aromatase inhibitors for male infertility. *Fertil. Steril.* **2012**, *98*, 1359–1362. [CrossRef]
58. Pavlovich, C.P.; King, P.; Goldstein, M.; Schlegel, P.N. Evidence of a treatable endocrinopathy in infertile men. *J. Urol.* **2001**, *165*, 837–841. [CrossRef]
59. Raman, J.D.; Schlegel, P.N. Aromatase inhibitors for male infertility. *J. Urol.* **2002**, *167*, 624–629. [CrossRef]
60. Ramasamy, R.; Stahl, P.J.; Schlegel, P.N. Medical therapy for spermatogenic failure. *Asian J. Androl.* **2012**, *14*, 57–60. [CrossRef]
61. Ramasamy, R.; Ricci, J.A.; Palermo, G.D.; Gosden, L.V.; Rosenwaks, Z.; Schlegel, P.N. Successful fertility treatment for Klinefelter's syndrome. *J. Urol.* **2009**, *182*, 1108–1113. [CrossRef] [PubMed]
62. Schiff, J.D.; Palermo, G.D.; Veeck, L.L.; Goldstein, M.; Rosenwaks, Z.; Schlegel, P.N. Success of testicular sperm extraction [corrected] and intracytoplasmic sperm injection in men with Klinefelter syndrome. *J. Clin. Endocrinol. Metab.* **2005**, *90*, 6263–6267. [CrossRef] [PubMed]
63. Moradi, M.; Moradi, A.; Alemi, M.; Ahmadnia, H.; Abdi, H.; Ahmadi, A.; Bazargan-Hejazi, S. Safety and efficacy of clomiphene citrate and L-carnitine in idiopathic male infertility: A comparative study. *Urol. J.* **2010**, *7*, 188–193. [PubMed]

64. Roth, L.W.; Ryan, A.R.; Meacham, R.B. Clomiphene citrate in the management of male infertility. *Semin. Reprod. Med.* **2013**, *31*, 245–250. [CrossRef] [PubMed]
65. Palermo, G.; Joris, H.; Devroey, P.; Van Steirteghem, A.C. Pregnancies after intracytoplasmic injection of single spermatozoon into an oocyte. *Lancet* **1992**, *340*, 17–18. [CrossRef]
66. Devroey, P.; Liu, J.; Nagy, Z.; Goossens, A.; Tournaye, H.; Camus, M.; Van Steirteghem, A.; Silber, S. Pregnancies after testicular sperm extraction and intracytoplasmic sperm injection in non-obstructive azoospermia. *Hum. Reprod.* **1995**, *10*, 1457–1460. [CrossRef]
67. Bernie, A.M.; Ramasamy, R.; Stember, D.S.; Stahl, P.J. Microsurgical epididymal sperm aspiration: Indications, techniques and outcomes. *Asian J. Androl.* **2013**, *15*, 40–43. [CrossRef]
68. Kavoussi, P.K.; West, B.T.; Chen, S.H.; Hunn, C.; Gilkey, M.S.; Machen, G.L.; Kavoussi, K.M.; Esqueda, A.; Wininger, J.D.; Kavoussi, S.K. A comprehensive assessment of predictors of fertility outcomes in men with non-obstructive azoospermia undergoing microdissection testicular sperm extraction. *Reprod. Biol. Endocrinol.* **2020**, *18*, 90. [CrossRef]
69. Pavan-Jukic, D.; Stubljar, D.; Jukic, T.; Starc, A. Predictive factors for sperm retrieval from males with azoospermia who are eligible for testicular sperm extraction (TESE). *Syst. Biol. Reprod. Med.* **2020**, *66*, 70–75. [CrossRef]
70. Dohle, G.R.; Elzanaty, S.; van Casteren, N.J. Testicular biopsy: Clinical practice and interpretation. *Asian J. Androl.* **2012**, *14*, 88–93. [CrossRef]
71. Guler, I.; Erdem, M.; Erdem, A.; Demirdağ, E.; Tunc, L.; Bozkurt, N.; Mutlu, M.F.; Oktem, M. Impact of testicular histopathology as a predictor of sperm retrieval and pregnancy outcome in patients with nonobstructive azoospermia: Correlation with clinical and hormonal factors. *Andrologia* **2016**, *48*, 765–773. [CrossRef]
72. Cavallini, G.; Cristina Magli, M.; Crippa, A.; Resta, S.; Vitali, G.; Pia Ferraretti, A.; Gianaroli, L. The number of spermatozoa collected with testicular sperm extraction is a novel predictor of intracytoplasmic sperm injection outcome in non-obstructive azoospermic patients. *Asian J. Androl.* **2011**, *13*, 312–316. [CrossRef]
73. Boulet, S.L.; Mehta, A.; Kissin, D.M.; Warner, L.; Kawwass, J.F.; Jamieson, D.J. Trends in use of and reproductive outcomes associated with intracytoplasmic sperm injection. *Jama* **2015**, *313*, 255–263. [CrossRef] [PubMed]
74. Fahmy, I.; Mansour, R.; Aboulghar, M.; Serour, G.; Kamal, A.; Tawab, N.A.; Ramzy, A.M.; Amin, Y. Intracytoplasmic sperm injection using surgically retrieved epididymal and testicular spermatozoa in cases of obstructive and non-obstructive azoospermia. *Int. J. Androl.* **1997**, *20*, 37–44. [CrossRef] [PubMed]
75. Friedler, S.; Raziel, A.; Strassburger, D.; Soffer, Y.; Komarovsky, D.; Ron-El, R. Testicular sperm retrieval by percutaneous fine needle sperm aspiration compared with testicular sperm extraction by open biopsy in men with non-obstructive azoospermia. *Hum. Reprod.* **1997**, *12*, 1488–1493. [CrossRef] [PubMed]
76. Ben-Yosef, D.; Yogev, L.; Hauser, R.; Yavetz, H.; Azem, F.; Yovel, I.; Lessing, J.B.; Amit, A. Testicular sperm retrieval and cryopreservation prior to initiating ovarian stimulation as the first line approach in patients with non-obstructive azoospermia. *Hum. Reprod.* **1999**, *14*, 1794–1801. [CrossRef]
77. Palermo, G.D.; Schlegel, P.N.; Hariprashad, J.J.; Ergün, B.; Mielnik, A.; Zaninovic, N.; Veeck, L.L.; Rosenwaks, Z. Fertilization and pregnancy outcome with intracytoplasmic sperm injection for azoospermic men. *Hum. Reprod.* **1999**, *14*, 741–748. [CrossRef]
78. Mercan, R.; Urman, B.; Alatas, C.; Aksoy, S.; Nuhoglu, A.; Isiklar, A.; Balaban, B. Outcome of testicular sperm retrieval procedures in non-obstructive azoospermia: Percutaneous aspiration versus open biopsy. *Hum. Reprod.* **2000**, *15*, 1548–1551. [CrossRef]
79. Chan, P.T.; Palermo, G.D.; Veeck, L.L.; Rosenwaks, Z.; Schlegel, P.N. Testicular sperm extraction combined with intracytoplasmic sperm injection in the treatment of men with persistent azoospermia postchemotherapy. *Cancer* **2001**, *92*, 1632–1637. [CrossRef]
80. Damani, M.N.; Master, V.; Meng, M.V.; Burgess, C.; Turek, P.; Oates, R.D. Postchemotherapy ejaculatory azoospermia: Fatherhood with sperm from testis tissue with intracytoplasmic sperm injection. *J. Clin. Oncol.* **2002**, *20*, 930–936. [CrossRef]
81. Friedler, S.; Raziel, A.; Schachter, M.; Strassburger, D.; Bern, O.; Ron-El, R. Outcome of first and repeated testicular sperm extraction and ICSI in patients with non-obstructive azoospermia. *Hum. Reprod.* **2002**, *17*, 2356–2361. [CrossRef] [PubMed]
82. Mátyás, S.; Rajczy, K.; Papp, G.; Bernard, A.; Korponai, E.; Kovács, T.; Krizsa, F.; Kulin, S.; Menyhárt, R.; Szmatona, G.; et al. Five years experiences with microinjection of testicular spermatozoa into oocytes in Hungary. *Andrologia* **2002**, *34*, 248–254. [CrossRef] [PubMed]
83. Bailly, M.; Guthauser, B.; Bergere, M.; Wainer, R.; Lombroso, R.; Ville, Y.; Selva, J. Effects of low concentrations of inhibin B on the outcomes of testicular sperm extraction and intracytoplasmic sperm injection. *Fertil. Steril.* **2003**, *79*, 905–908. [CrossRef]
84. Mansour, R.T.; Fahmy, I.M.; Taha, A.K.; Tawab, N.A.; Serour, G.I.; Aboulghar, M.A. Intracytoplasmic spermatid injection can result in the delivery of normal offspring. *J. Androl.* **2003**, *24*, 757–764. [CrossRef] [PubMed]
85. Meseguer, M.; Garrido, N.; Remohí, J.; Pellicer, A.; Simón, C.; Martínez-Jabaloyas, J.M.; Gil-Salom, M. Testicular sperm extraction (TESE) and ICSI in patients with permanent azoospermia after chemotherapy. *Hum. Reprod.* **2003**, *18*, 1281–1285. [CrossRef] [PubMed]
86. Osmanagaoglu, K.; Vernaeve, V.; Kolibianakis, E.; Tournaye, H.; Camus, M.; Van Steirteghem, A.; Devroey, P. Cumulative delivery rates after ICSI treatment cycles with freshly retrieved testicular sperm: A 7-year follow-up study. *Hum. Reprod.* **2003**, *18*, 1836–1840. [CrossRef] [PubMed]
87. Aydos, K.; Demirel, L.C.; Baltaci, V.; Unlü, C. Enzymatic digestion plus mechanical searching improves testicular sperm retrieval in non-obstructive azoospermia cases. *Eur. J. Obstet. Gynecol. Reprod. Biol.* **2005**, *120*, 80–86. [CrossRef]

88. Giorgetti, C.; Chinchole, J.M.; Hans, E.; Charles, O.; Franquebalme, J.P.; Glowaczower, E.; Salzmann, J.; Terriou, P.; Roulier, R. Crude cumulative delivery rate following ICSI using intentionally frozen-thawed testicular spermatozoa in 51 men with non-obstructive azoospermia. *Reprod. Biomed. Online* **2005**, *11*, 319–324. [CrossRef]
89. Mitchell, V.; Steger, K.; Marchetti, C.; Herbaut, J.C.; Devos, P.; Rigot, J.M. Cellular expression of protamine 1 and 2 transcripts in testicular spermatids from azoospermic men submitted to TESE-ICSI. *Mol. Hum. Reprod.* **2005**, *11*, 373–379. [CrossRef]
90. Wu, B.; Wong, D.; Lu, S.; Dickstein, S.; Silva, M.; Gelety, T.J. Optimal use of fresh and frozen-thawed testicular sperm for intracytoplasmic sperm injection in azoospermic patients. *J. Assist. Reprod. Genet.* **2005**, *22*, 389–394. [CrossRef]
91. Everaert, K.; De Croo, I.; Kerckhaert, W.; Dekuyper, P.; Dhont, M.; Van der Elst, J.; De Sutter, P.; Comhaire, F.; Mahmoud, A.; Lumen, N. Long term effects of micro-surgical testicular sperm extraction on androgen status in patients with non obstructive azoospermia. *BMC Urol.* **2006**, *6*, 9. [CrossRef]
92. Hibi, H.; Ohori, T.; Yamada, Y.; Honda, N.; Hashiba, Y.; Asada, Y. Testicular sperm extraction and ICSI in patients with post-chemotherapy non-obstructive azoospermia. *Arch. Androl.* **2007**, *53*, 63–65. [CrossRef]
93. Mitchell, V.; Lefebvre-Khalil, V.; Thomas, P.; Rigot, J.M.; Steger, K. Transition protein 1 mRNA expression is not related to pregnancy rate in azoospermic men undergoing TESE-ICSI. *Andrologia* **2007**, *39*, 124–127. [CrossRef] [PubMed]
94. Kanto, S.; Sugawara, J.; Masuda, H.; Sasano, H.; Arai, Y.; Kyono, K. Fresh motile testicular sperm retrieved from nonobstructive azoospermic patients has the same potential to achieve fertilization and pregnancy via ICSI as sperm retrieved from obstructive azoospermic patients. *Fertil. Steril.* **2008**, *90*, 2010.e5–2010.e7. [CrossRef] [PubMed]
95. Ravizzini, P.; Carizza, C.; Abdelmassih, V.; Abdelmassih, S.; Azevedo, M.; Abdelmassih, R. Microdissection testicular sperm extraction and IVF-ICSI outcome in nonobstructive azoospermia. *Andrologia* **2008**, *40*, 219–226. [CrossRef]
96. Ishikawa, T.; Shiotani, M.; Izumi, Y.; Hashimoto, H.; Kokeguchi, S.; Goto, S.; Fujisawa, M. Fertilization and pregnancy using cryopreserved testicular sperm for intracytoplasmic sperm injection with azoospermia. *Fertil. Steril.* **2009**, *92*, 174–179. [CrossRef]
97. Yarali, H.; Polat, M.; Bozdag, G.; Gunel, M.; Alpas, I.; Esinler, I.; Dogan, U.; Tiras, B. TESE-ICSI in patients with non-mosaic Klinefelter syndrome: A comparative study. *Reprod. Biomed. Online* **2009**, *18*, 756–760. [CrossRef]
98. Boitrelle, F.; Robin, G.; Marcelli, F.; Albert, M.; Leroy-Martin, B.; Dewailly, D.; Rigot, J.M.; Mitchell, V. A predictive score for testicular sperm extraction quality and surgical ICSI outcome in non-obstructive azoospermia: A retrospective study. *Hum. Reprod.* **2011**, *26*, 3215–3221. [CrossRef]
99. Hauser, R.; Bibi, G.; Yogev, L.; Carmon, A.; Azem, F.; Botchan, A.; Yavetz, H.; Klieman, S.E.; Lehavi, O.; Amit, A.; et al. Virtual azoospermia and cryptozoospermia–fresh/frozen testicular or ejaculate sperm for better IVF outcome? *J. Androl.* **2011**, *32*, 484–490. [CrossRef]
100. Hsiao, W.; Stahl, P.J.; Osterberg, E.C.; Nejat, E.; Palermo, G.D.; Rosenwaks, Z.; Schlegel, P.N. Successful treatment of postchemotherapy azoospermia with microsurgical testicular sperm extraction: The Weill Cornell experience. *J. Clin. Oncol.* **2011**, *29*, 1607–1611. [CrossRef]
101. Ashraf, M.C.; Singh, S.; Raj, D.; Ramakrishnan, S.; Esteves, S.C. Micro-dissection testicular sperm extraction as an alternative for sperm acquisition in the most difficult cases of Azoospermia: Technique and preliminary results in India. *J. Hum. Reprod. Sci.* **2013**, *6*, 111–123. [CrossRef] [PubMed]
102. Choi, D.K.; Gong, I.H.; Hwang, J.H.; Oh, J.J.; Hong, J.Y. Detection of Y Chromosome Microdeletion is Valuable in the Treatment of Patients With Nonobstructive Azoospermia and Oligoasthenoteratozoospermia: Sperm Retrieval Rate and Birth Rate. *Korean J. Urol.* **2013**, *54*, 111–116. [CrossRef]
103. Karacan, M.; Alwaeely, F.; Erkan, S.; Çebi, Z.; Berberoğlugil, M.; Batukan, M.; Uluğ, M.; Arvas, A.; Çamlıbel, T. Outcome of intracytoplasmic sperm injection cycles with fresh testicular spermatozoa obtained on the day of or the day before oocyte collection and with cryopreserved testicular sperm in patients with azoospermia. *Fertil. Steril.* **2013**, *100*, 975–980. [CrossRef] [PubMed]
104. Arafa, M.M.; ElBardisi, H.T.; AlSaid, S.S.; Majzoub, A.; AlMalki, A.H.; ElRobi, I.; AlAnsari, A.A. Outcome of microsurgical testicular sperm extraction in familial idiopathic nonobstructive azoospermia. *Andrologia* **2015**, *47*, 1062–1067. [CrossRef] [PubMed]
105. Esteves, S.C.; Prudencio, C.; Seol, B.; Verza, S.; Knoedler, C.; Agarwal, A. Comparison of sperm retrieval and reproductive outcome in azoospermic men with testicular failure and obstructive azoospermia treated for infertility. *Asian J. Androl.* **2014**, *16*, 602–606. [CrossRef]
106. Karacan, M.; Ulug, M.; Arvas, A.; Cebi, Z.; Erkan, S.; Camlıbel, T. Live birth rate with repeat microdissection TESE and intracytoplasmic sperm injection after a conventional testicular biopsy in men with nonobstructive azoospermia. *Eur. J. Obstet. Gynecol. Reprod. Biol.* **2014**, *183*, 174–177. [CrossRef] [PubMed]
107. Aydin, T.; Sofikerim, M.; Yucel, B.; Karadag, M.; Tokat, F. Effects of testicular histopathology on sperm retrieval rates and ICSI results in non-obstructive azoospermia. *J. Obstet. Gynaecol.* **2015**, *35*, 829–831. [CrossRef] [PubMed]
108. Vloeberghs, V.; Verheyen, G.; Haentjens, P.; Goossens, A.; Polyzos, N.P.; Tournaye, H. How successful is TESE-ICSI in couples with non-obstructive azoospermia? *Hum. Reprod.* **2015**, *30*, 1790–1796. [CrossRef] [PubMed]
109. Ko, J.K.; Chai, J.; Lee, V.C.; Li, R.H.; Lau, E.; Ho, K.L.; Tam, P.C.; Yeung, W.S.; Ho, P.C.; Ng, E.H. Sperm retrieval rate and pregnancy rate in infertile couples undergoing in-vitro fertilisation and testicular sperm extraction for non-obstructive azoospermia in Hong Kong. *Hong Kong Med. J.* **2016**, *22*, 556–562. [CrossRef] [PubMed]

110. Alfano, M.; Ventimiglia, E.; Locatelli, I.; Capogrosso, P.; Cazzaniga, W.; Pederzoli, F.; Frego, N.; Matloob, R.; Saccà, A.; Pagliardini, L.; et al. Anti-Mullerian Hormone-to-Testosterone Ratio is Predictive of Positive Sperm Retrieval in Men with Idiopathic Non-Obstructive Azoospermia. *Sci. Rep.* **2017**, *7*, 17638. [CrossRef]
111. Arafa, M.M.; Majzoub, A.; AlSaid, S.S.; El Ansari, W.; Al Ansari, A.; Elbardisi, Y.; Elbardisi, H.T. Chromosomal abnormalities in infertile men with azoospermia and severe oligozoospermia in Qatar and their association with sperm retrieval intracytoplasmic sperm injection outcomes. *Arab. J. Urol.* **2018**, *16*, 132–139. [CrossRef] [PubMed]
112. Yu, Y.; Xi, Q.; Pan, Y.; Jiang, Y.; Zhang, H.; Li, L.; Liu, R. Pregnancy and Neonatal Outcomes in Azoospermic Men After Intracytoplasmic Sperm Injection Using Testicular Sperm and Donor Sperm. *Med. Sci. Monit* **2018**, *24*, 6968–6974. [CrossRef] [PubMed]
113. Yamaguchi, K.; Ishikawa, T.; Mizuta, S.; Takeuchi, T.; Matsubayashi, H.; Kokeguchi, S.; Habara, T.; Ichioka, K.; Ohashi, M.; Okamoto, S.; et al. Clinical outcomes of microdissection testicular sperm extraction and intracytoplasmic sperm injection in Japanese men with Y chromosome microdeletions. *Reprod. Med. Biol.* **2020**, *19*, 158–163. [CrossRef] [PubMed]
114. Corona, G.; Pizzocaro, A.; Lanfranco, F.; Garolla, A.; Pelliccione, F.; Vignozzi, L.; Ferlin, A.; Foresta, C.; Jannini, E.A.; Maggi, M.; et al. Sperm recovery and ICSI outcomes in Klinefelter syndrome: A systematic review and meta-analysis. *Hum. Reprod. Update* **2017**, *23*, 265–275. [CrossRef]
115. Park, S.H.; Lee, H.S.; Choe, J.H.; Lee, J.S.; Seo, J.T. Success rate of microsurgical multiple testicular sperm extraction and sperm presence in the ejaculate in korean men with y chromosome microdeletions. *Korean J. Urol.* **2013**, *54*, 536–540. [CrossRef] [PubMed]
116. Stahl, P.J.; Masson, P.; Mielnik, A.; Marean, M.B.; Schlegel, P.N.; Paduch, D.A. A decade of experience emphasizes that testing for Y microdeletions is essential in American men with azoospermia and severe oligozoospermia. *Fertil. Steril.* **2010**, *94*, 1753–1756. [CrossRef]
117. Liu, X.H.; Qiao, J.; Li, R.; Yan, L.Y.; Chen, L.X. Y chromosome AZFc microdeletion may not affect the outcomes of ICSI for infertile males with fresh ejaculated sperm. *J. Assist. Reprod. Genet.* **2013**, *30*, 813–819. [CrossRef]
118. Oates, R.D.; Silber, S.; Brown, L.G.; Page, D.C. Clinical characterization of 42 oligospermic or azoospermic men with microdeletion of the AZFc region of the Y chromosome, and of 18 children conceived via ICSI. *Hum. Reprod.* **2002**, *17*, 2813–2824. [CrossRef]
119. De Vries, J.W.; Repping, S.; Oates, R.; Carson, R.; Leschot, N.J.; van der Veen, F. Absence of deleted in azoospermia (DAZ) genes in spermatozoa of infertile men with somatic DAZ deletions. *Fertil. Steril.* **2001**, *75*, 476–479. [CrossRef]
120. Schmidt, K.L.; Larsen, E.; Bangsbøll, S.; Meinertz, H.; Carlsen, E.; Andersen, A.N. Assisted reproduction in male cancer survivors: Fertility treatment and outcome in 67 couples. *Hum. Reprod.* **2004**, *19*, 2806–2810. [CrossRef]
121. Gandini, L.; Sgrò, P.; Lombardo, F.; Paoli, D.; Culasso, F.; Toselli, L.; Tsamatropoulos, P.; Lenzi, A. Effect of chemo- or radiotherapy on sperm parameters of testicular cancer patients. *Hum. Reprod.* **2006**, *21*, 2882–2889. [CrossRef] [PubMed]
122. Van der Kaaij, M.A.; van Echten-Arends, J.; Simons, A.H.; Kluin-Nelemans, H.C. Fertility preservation after chemotherapy for Hodgkin lymphoma. *Hematol. Oncol.* **2010**, *28*, 168–179. [CrossRef] [PubMed]
123. Cortes, D.; Thorup, J.M.; Visfeldt, J. Cryptorchidism: Aspects of fertility and neoplasms. A study including data of 1335 consecutive boys who underwent testicular biopsy simultaneously with surgery for cryptorchidism. *Horm. Res.* **2001**, *55*, 21–27. [CrossRef]
124. Zorn, B.; Virant-Klun, I.; Drobni, S.; Sinkovec, J.; Meden-Vrtovec, H. Male and female factors that influence ICSI outcome in azoospermia or aspermia. *Reprod. Biomed. Online* **2009**, *18*, 168–176. [CrossRef]
125. Desai, N.; Gill, P.; Tadros, N.N.; Goldberg, J.M.; Sabanegh, E.; Falcone, T. Azoospermia and embryo morphokinetics: Testicular sperm-derived embryos exhibit delays in early cell cycle events and increased arrest prior to compaction. *J. Assist. Reprod. Genet.* **2018**, *35*, 1339–1348. [CrossRef]
126. Loutradi, K.E.; Tarlatzis, B.C.; Goulis, D.G.; Zepiridis, L.; Pagou, T.; Chatziioannou, E.; Grimbizis, G.F.; Papadimas, I.; Bontis, I. The effects of sperm quality on embryo development after intracytoplasmic sperm injection. *J. Assist. Reprod. Genet.* **2006**, *23*, 69–74. [CrossRef]
127. Janny, L.; Menezo, Y.J. Evidence for a strong paternal effect on human preimplantation embryo development and blastocyst formation. *Mol. Reprod. Dev.* **1994**, *38*, 36–42. [CrossRef]
128. Ron-el, R.; Nachum, H.; Herman, A.; Golan, A.; Caspi, E.; Soffer, Y. Delayed fertilization and poor embryonic development associated with impaired semen quality. *Fertil. Steril.* **1991**, *55*, 338–344. [CrossRef]
129. Shoukir, Y.; Chardonnens, D.; Campana, A.; Sakkas, D. Blastocyst development from supernumerary embryos after intracytoplasmic sperm injection: A paternal influence? *Hum. Reprod.* **1998**, *13*, 1632–1637. [CrossRef]
130. Göker, E.N.; Sendag, F.; Levi, R.; Sendag, H.; Tavmergen, E. Comparison of the ICSI outcome of ejaculated sperm with normal, abnormal parameters and testicular sperm. *Eur. J. Obstet. Gynecol. Reprod. Biol.* **2002**, *104*, 129–136. [CrossRef]
131. Vernaeve, V.; Tournaye, H.; Osmanagaoglu, K.; Verheyen, G.; Van Steirteghem, A.; Devroey, P. Intracytoplasmic sperm injection with testicular spermatozoa is less successful in men with nonobstructive azoospermia than in men with obstructive azoospermia. *Fertil. Steril.* **2003**, *79*, 529–533. [CrossRef]
132. Nicopoullos, J.D.; Gilling-Smith, C.; Almeida, P.A.; Ramsay, J.W. The results of 154 ICSI cycles using surgically retrieved sperm from azoospermic men. *Hum. Reprod.* **2004**, *19*, 579–585. [CrossRef] [PubMed]
133. Sakkas, D. Novel technologies for selecting the best sperm for in vitro fertilization and intracytoplasmic sperm injection. *Fertil. Steril.* **2013**, *99*, 1023–1029. [CrossRef] [PubMed]

134. Gil, M.; Sar-Shalom, V.; Melendez Sivira, Y.; Carreras, R.; Checa, M.A. Sperm selection using magnetic activated cell sorting (MACS) in assisted reproduction: A systematic review and meta-analysis. *J. Assist. Reprod. Genet.* **2013**, *30*, 479–485. [CrossRef]
135. Antinori, M.; Licata, E.; Dani, G.; Cerusico, F.; Versaci, C.; d'Angelo, D.; Antinori, S. Intracytoplasmic morphologically selected sperm injection: A prospective randomized trial. *Reprod. Biomed. Online* **2008**, *16*, 835–841. [CrossRef]
136. Teixeira, D.M.; Hadyme Miyague, A.; Barbosa, M.A.; Navarro, P.A.; Raine-Fenning, N.; Nastri, C.O.; Martins, W.P. Regular (ICSI) versus ultra-high magnification (IMSI) sperm selection for assisted reproduction. *Cochrane Database Syst. Rev.* **2020**, *2*, Cd010167. [CrossRef]
137. Parrella, A.; Keating, D.; Cheung, S.; Xie, P.; Stewart, J.D.; Rosenwaks, Z.; Palermo, G.D. A treatment approach for couples with disrupted sperm DNA integrity and recurrent ART failure. *J. Assist. Reprod. Genet.* **2019**, *36*, 2057–2066. [CrossRef] [PubMed]
138. Xie, P.; Keating, D.; Parrella, A.; Cheung, S.; Rosenwaks, Z.; Goldstein, M.; Palermo, G.D. Sperm Genomic Integrity by TUNEL Varies throughout the Male Genital Tract. *J. Urol.* **2020**, *203*, 802–808. [CrossRef]
139. Quinn, M.M.; Jalalian, L.; Ribeiro, S.; Ona, K.; Demirci, U.; Cedars, M.I.; Rosen, M.P. Microfluidic sorting selects sperm for clinical use with reduced DNA damage compared to density gradient centrifugation with swim-up in split semen samples. *Human. Reprod.* **2018**, *33*, 1388–1393. [CrossRef]
140. Samuel, R.; Feng, H.; Jafek, A.; Despain, D.; Jenkins, T.; Gale, B. Microfluidic-based sperm sorting & analysis for treatment of male infertility. *Transl. Androl. Urol.* **2018**, *7*, S336–S347. [CrossRef]

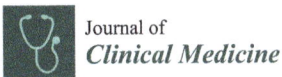

Review

Performing Microdissection Testicular Sperm Extraction: Surgical Pearls from a High-Volume Infertility Center

Giovanni M. Colpi [1,*] and Ettore Caroppo [2]

1. Andrology Unit, Procrea Institute, 6900 Lugano, Switzerland
2. Asl Bari, PTA "F Jaia", Andrology Outpatients Clinic, 70014 Conversano (Ba), Italy; ecaroppo@teseo.it
* Correspondence: gmcolpi@yahoo.com

Abstract: Microdissection testicular sperm extraction (mTESE) has been demonstrated to be the gold-standard surgical technique for retrieving testicular sperm in patients with non-obstructive azoospermia (NOA) as it enables the exploration of the whole testicular parenchyma at a high magnification, allowing the identification of the rare dilated seminipherous tubules that may contain sperm, usually surrounded by thinner or atrophic tubules. MTESE requires a skilled and experienced surgeon whose learning curve may greatly affect the sperm retrieval rate, as demonstrated in previous reports. The present review is intended to offer a precise and detailed description of the mTESE surgical procedure, accompanied by an extensive iconography, to provide urologists with valuable information to be translated into clinical practice. Advice about the pre-surgical and post-surgical management of patients is also offered.

Keywords: microTESE; sperm retrieval; non-obstructive azoospermia; male infertility

Citation: Colpi, G.M.; Caroppo, E. Performing Microdissection Testicular Sperm Extraction: Surgical Pearls from a High-Volume Infertility Center. *J. Clin. Med.* **2021**, *10*, 4296. https://doi.org/10.3390/jcm10194296

Academic Editor: Alberto Ferlin

Received: 21 July 2021
Accepted: 20 September 2021
Published: 22 September 2021

Publisher's Note: MDPI stays neutral with regard to jurisdictional claims in published maps and institutional affiliations.

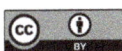

Copyright: © 2021 by the authors. Licensee MDPI, Basel, Switzerland. This article is an open access article distributed under the terms and conditions of the Creative Commons Attribution (CC BY) license (https://creativecommons.org/licenses/by/4.0/).

1. Introduction

Despite the lack of sperm in the ejaculate, patients with azoospermia due to spermatogenic dysfunction, the so-called non-obstructive azoospermia, may still be able to father children genetically on their own as residual, focal areas of spermatogenesis may be present in their testes. Due to the anatomical singularity of such a condition, often characterized by the heterogeneous distribution of histologically and functionally distinct seminiferous tubules (STs) [1], a randomly applied biopsy is able to retrieve sperm in about one third of the cases; on the other hand, by enabling the exploration of the whole testicular parenchyma, microdissection testicular sperm extraction (mTESE) is one point five times more successful than the conventional TESE (cTESE) [2] and is therefore considered the gold-standard surgical technique for patients with NOA. In addition, the exploration of the testicular parenchyma at a high magnification (24–36×) enables the retrieval of a significantly higher number of sperm to be used for intracytoplasmic sperm injection (ICSI) compared to that of cTESE.

The superiority of mTESE compared to other surgical techniques has been challenged by a more recent meta-analysis [3], whose results are, however, significantly affected by the heterogeneity of treated populations and reporting bias [4]. Esteves et al. re-evaluated the data of the meta-analysis on the basis of eligible controlled studies with histopathological data and found that the sperm retrieval rate (SRR) was 49% for mTESE vs. 35.8% for cTESE (RR 1.37 (1.14–1.65); $p = 0.0004$); for cases with Sertoli cell-only syndrome, SRR was 36.1% for mTESE vs. 13.3% for cTESE (RR 2.70 (1.72–4.24); $p < 0.0001$) [4].

Notably, when performing mTESE the skill and experience of the surgeon is key to a successful sperm retrieval. The sperm retrieval rate (SRR) of mTESE is strongly influenced by the surgeon's case volume: Ishikawa et al. [5] showed that the SRR increased after the first 100 mTESEs performed, and Dabaja and Schlegel [6] observed that the SRR further increased when the surgeon exceeded experience with more than 500 mTESE procedures. The surgical experience accumulated in the past twenty-three years by our leading urologist

(GMC) supports what is suggested by these authors: as displayed in Table 1, the mTESE sperm retrieval rates improved over time with the number of mTESE procedures.

Table 1. Comparison of the mTESE outcome performed by the same urologist (GMC) in two cohorts of patients with NOA.

	San Paolo Cohort	Procrea Cohort
Years	2004–2009	2015–2017
Number of patients	202	143
Overall sperm retrieval rate (SRR)	80/202 (39.6%)	79/143 (55.2%)
SRR per testis histology subcategories		
Sertoli cells only syndrome	28/125 (22.4%)	45/143 (31.5%)
Maturation arrest	6/16 (37.5%)	11/29 (37.9%)
Hypospermatogenesis	20/26 (76.9%)	27/28 (96.4%)
Focal Sertoli cells only syndrome	26/35 (74.2%)	9/9 (100%)
Hyalinosis	/	2/9 (22.2%)
Intraepithelial neoplasia	/	1/2 (50%)

San Paolo cohort: patients undergoing mTESE at San Paolo Hospital, Milan, Italy. Procrea Cohort: patients undergoing mTESE at Procrea Institute, Lugano, Switzerland.

The aim of the present narrative review is to share the surgical experience of an expert urologist by providing surgical tips and tricks in the management of patients with non-obstructive azoospermia.

2. Preoperative Patient Optimization

Spermatogenesis usually takes 74 days in humans. As physical (particularly occupational heat exposure) and lifestyle factors (recreational drug abuse, high fat diet, alcohol intake, etc.,) may compromise male reproductive health, it is advisable that men with NOA willing to undergo mTESE should be adequately counselled about those risks, which are more susceptible to undervaluation [7]. For men with known exposure, a three- to-six-month washout period may be advisable before proceeding with mTESE; those patients with previous surgical sperm retrieval should wait six months before undergoing a further surgical attempt.

Some patients with NOA may have a subclinical or clinical asymptomatic hypogonadism, in most cases due to primary testicular failure and in a few cases due to hypogonadotropic hypogonadism. As testosterone signaling is required for spermatogenesis to proceed beyond meiosis, it has been postulated that patients with hypogonadism should have their serum testosterone levels optimized before surgical sperm retrieval. Indeed, a pooled estimation of seven studies reporting the sperm retrieval rates in patients with subnormal vs. normal testosterone levels demonstrated that patients with normal testosterone levels had a significantly higher chance of successful sperm retrieval (SSR) compared to those with hypogonadism (OR 1.63, 95% CI 1.08–2.45, $p = 0.02$) [8]. The utility of the hormonal treatment of patients with NOA has been evaluated by a few studies, yet with conflicting results [8]. The recent AUA/ASRM guidelines on the diagnosis and management of male infertility recommend informing patients with NOA about the limited data supporting pharmacologic treatments prior to surgical intervention [9].

Performing scrotal ultrasound before surgery may provide valuable information for the surgeon. The testis volume should be evaluated by using the known formula of length × width × height × 0.52, while the ultrasonic texture may be evaluated according to Lenz et al. [10]. In addition, the testis ultrasound may reveal areas of fibrotic tissue, due to previous surgery or trauma, and the presence of testicular nodules, which may not be uncommon in men with NOA, given the significantly higher risk of testicular cancer in these patients compared to infertile men with less severe spermatogenic impairment (standardized incidence ratios—SIR 2.9, 95% CI 1.4–5.4), particularly in younger men

(SIR 3.7, 95% CI 1.7–7.0) [11]. The risk of testicular cancer may be even higher in patients with cryptorchidism [12].

Patients with NOA with clinical varicocele may undergo varicocele repair before surgical sperm retrieval as it may result in the detection of ejaculated sperm or in better sperm retrieval rates [13]. Such a beneficial effect may be more effective for patients with histological evidence of hypospermatogenesis than for patients with maturation arrest or Sertoli cell-only syndrome [14]. Postponing mTESE to let patients undergo varicocele repair may, however, be not advisable for couples with female factor fertility (e.g., female age > 38 years, poor ovarian reserve); as the potential benefits of varicocele repair are not obtained until at least 3–6 months after the repair, this would lead to unjustified delays in IVF treatments.

3. MTESE Procedure

The average duration of surgery, in our experience, is 87′ (range 60′–140′) for unilateral mTESE and 126′ (65–205′) for bilateral mTESE. MTESE is usually performed under general anesthesia; due to the inherent psychological stress, we try our best to avoid unneeded painful experiences for our patients by administering ketorolac 30 mg plus paracetamol 1 gr and pethidine 1 mg/kg one hour before awakening from anesthesia-induced unconsciousness. Ketorolac and paracetamol may be administered again eight hours later.

Generally, the larger testis is first chosen for the mTESE evaluation, apart from selected cases (the presence of testicular nodules or microlithiasis in the smaller testis at ultrasound or previous surgery on the larger testis). A 1.5–3 cm wide scrotal incision, performed in parallel to the skin vessels, ensures an almost invisible scar one month after surgery. Following the testis exposure, the tunica vaginalis is opened, then a 4–10× magnification allows the identification of a testicular surface area devoid of sub-albugineal vessels where an equatorial or para-equatorial incision can be safely made. In the case of a salvage mTESE after failed sperm retrieval attempts, the albugineal incision should be made far enough from the scars as the testicular tissue closer to the scars may be atrophic due to previous tissue excision and to vascular damage. Even testicular aspiration may inflict severe and irreversible damage to the testicular tissue and to the architecture of the tubules in the needle's path, as demonstrated by an animal study [15]; for this reason, performing a salvage mTESE after a failed multifocal TEFNA may be more challenging than after a cTESE.

Following albugineal incision, which may cover 180 to 270° of the testicular circumference (Figure 1), the two albugineal edges are held by two mosquito clamps, and the testicular parenchyma is observed at high magnification (×36) while the surgeon holds the testis firmly to allow a correct evaluation of the parenchyma under the operating microscope. The careful and thorough search for areas containing those STs that appear clearly dilated compared to the surroundings represents the most important step of mTESE as it has been demonstrated that dilated STs may contain sperm in 90% of cases [16]. Indeed, the testicular parenchyma of patients with NOA is commonly made of tiny tubules, containing only Sertoli cells, or with complete hyalinization, while dilated STs may lie solitary, surrounded by smaller size tubules or grouped in tiny heaps or, more rarely, occupy a small part of a lobule. Less frequently, STs may appear homogeneously dilated; this typically occurs in cases of early or late maturation arrest. Patients with NOA due to maturation arrest usually have normal FSH levels and testicular volume; in these cases, it may be advisable to make a less wide scrotal incision as the whole testicular parenchyma may be homogeneously made of dilated STs, and a larger incision would not improve the sperm retrieval outcome.

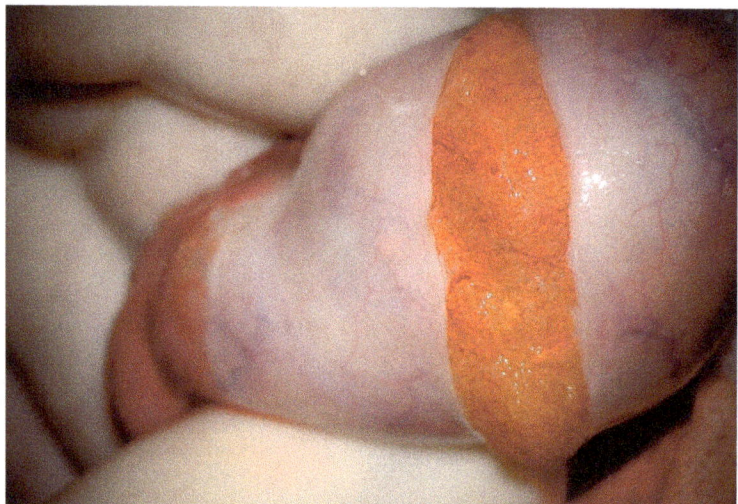

Figure 1. Wide incision of albuginea.

During the exploration at high magnification, the testicular parenchyma is gently detached (Figure 2) to individuate dilated tubules, avoiding any traction that may distort the STs caliber. Hemostasis with a bipolar microcoagulator should be avoided at this point (in some cases it may be applied only to the intra- or sub-albugineal vessels) and eventually limited to a gentle pressure on the testicular tissue for 4 min using gauze wet with Ringer solution. In this phase a small fragment of testicular tissue, representative of the overall appearance of the testicular parenchyma, is taken, fixed in Bouin's solution, and sent to the pathologist for histological examination. Testis histology is mandatory for classifying the predominant histological pattern and for excluding the presence of intraepithelial neoplasia [17], which is more common in patients with NOA compared to non-azoospermic infertile men [11]. In addition, a histopathological report may represent a cross-validation of the biological report: the presence of sperm in a previous histological section of a patient with sperm retrieval failure (e.g., Sertoli-only syndrome) may suggest the presence of focal areas of hypospermatogenesis that may justify a salvage mTESE.

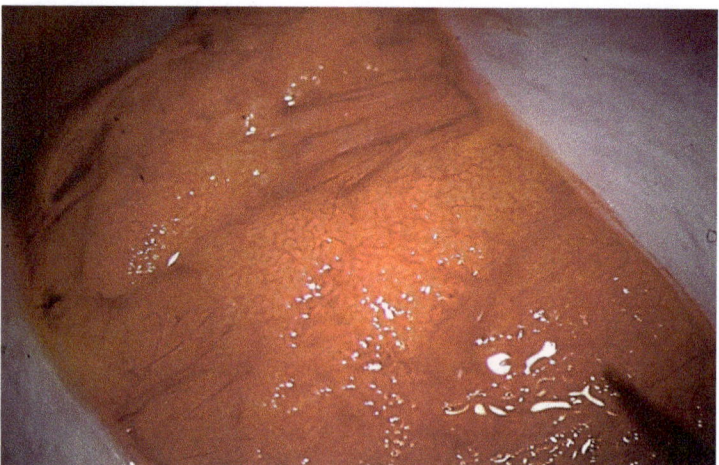

Figure 2. Testicular parenchyma at medium-high magnification.

The evaluation of the testicular parenchyma at high magnification (×36) enables the surgeon to discriminate between STs that, at a lower magnification, may appear of comparable size (Figure 3).

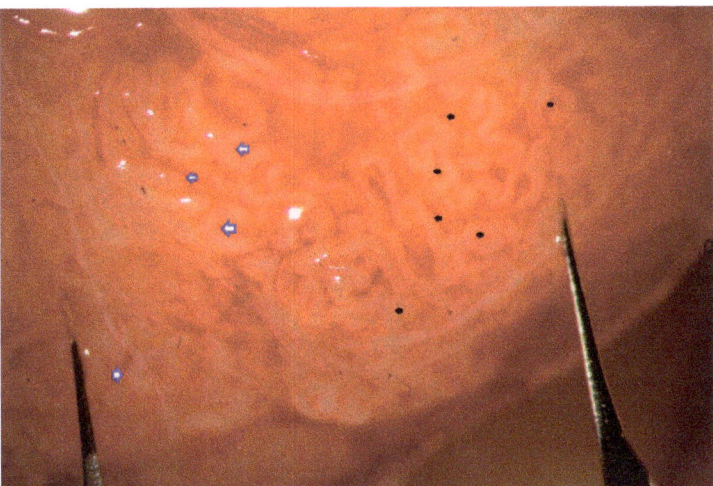

Figure 3. High magnification (×24- > ×36) allows the easy discrimination between seminiferous tubules of different sizes (those marked by blue arrows are very slightly larger than those marked by black arrows).

The STs of better caliber, which are often opaquer than the surroundings (Figure 4), are removed with Vannas micro-forceps, washed in human tubal fluid medium to remove the blood, and transferred to a sterile Petri dish containing Ham's F10 medium with serum substitute supplement; the embryologist then minces them extensively until they can be passed through a 24-gauge angiocatheter. Then, a 1 mL collagenase solution is added to the fragments, and the samples are incubated at 37° for two hours. The resulting cellular suspension is diluted with a medium and centrifuged twice at 800× g for ten minutes, then the pellet is observed under a phase contrast microscope. To save time, the procedure may be performed by two embryologists working in parallel. In a few minutes, the embryologist may give a response about the presence of sperm in the suspension; if sperm are found, the surgeon proceeds with the identification of STs of the same caliber, removes those grouped together with Vannas micro-forceps, and brings them to the embryologist for a rough estimate of the number and quality of sperm retrieved. When the number of sperm retrieved is adequate for the ICSI, the surgeon stops the research for dilated STs.

The number and quality of retrieved sperm, and their planned use in ICSI cycles (fresh or frozen), may affect the duration of surgery and the amount of tissue dissection. In the case of easily retrieved sperm, most of the testicular tissue is spared [18], which may represent an undoubted advantage in the case of a further salvage mTESE that could become necessary for further ICSI attempts. The search for sperm could be less extensive in the case of a fresh ICSI-mTESE as few viable sperm may be needed for the ICSI. For this reason, several authors prefer using freshly retrieved testicular sperm for the ICSI [19,20]; indeed, although no statistical difference has been demonstrated between the use of fresh versus cryopreserved-thawed testicular sperm with regard to fertilization and pregnancy rates in ICSI cycles [21], fresh ICSI-mTESE requires the yield of fewer sperm compared to the frozen ICSI-mTESE as only 33% of frozen-thawed testicular sperm will be viable for use with the ICSI [19]. Supernumerary testicular sperm should be frozen, obviously, for further use in the ICSI. Still, there are some drawbacks when using the fresh mTESE-ICSI, including the possibility of an otherwise unforeseeable sperm retrieval failure, with the consequent need for oocyte cryopreservation, as well as organizational issues. When the number of retrieved sperm is insufficient for the ICSI, the surgeon proceeds with a wider examination of the testicular parenchyma by a bivalve full opening (Figure 5). If needed, the deeper part of the testicular parenchyma is explored orthogonally to the para-equatorial section plan, avoiding as much as possible any possible vascular damage (Figure 6), and the tubules are examined both along the septa and by delicately detaching groups of them from the adjacent ones by Vannas micro-forceps. For large testes, if the initial incision does not adequately provide exposure to the entirety of the testicular parenchyma, a second parallel equatorial incision is performed. When no dilated STS are identified, any tubule whose caliber appears slightly larger than that of the surroundings is removed (the so-called slightly dilated tubules) [16]. If no sperm are found, then not-dilated tubules are excised according to a sort of mapping by removing tiny fragments of testicular tissue from the two separated surfaces at different depths from the albuginea to the hilum. In our experience, however, sperm are found in not-dilated tubules in only 7% of cases [16]. In the case of sperm retrieval failure, the contralateral testis is opened with the modality described above.

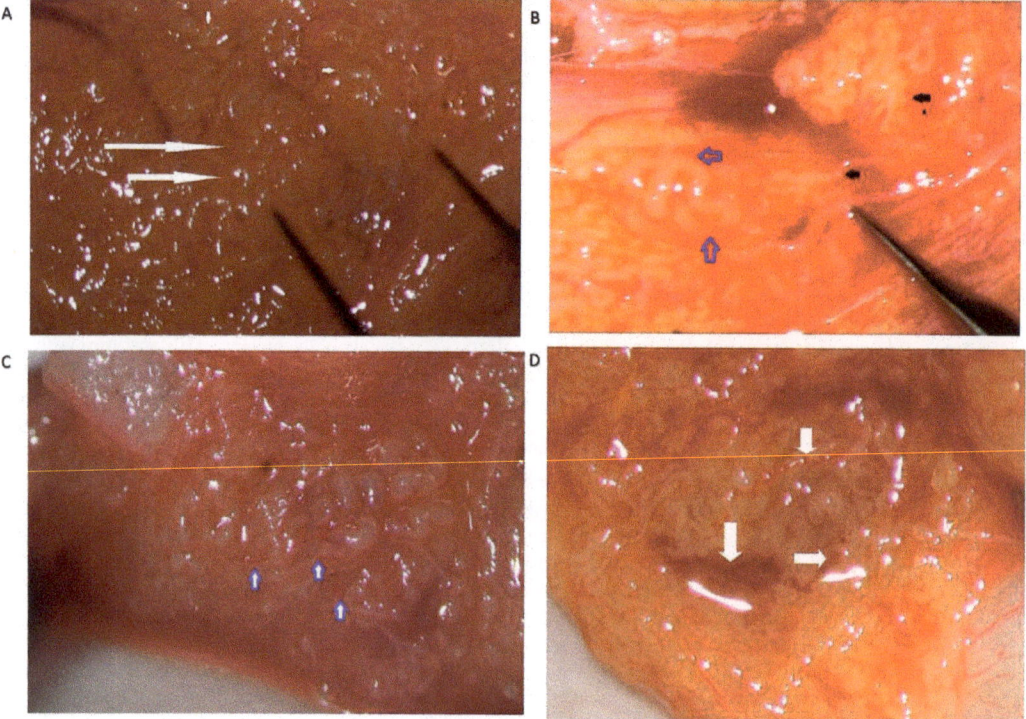

Figure 4. Dilated tubules. (**A**) Medium-sized group of dilated tubules (long arrows) among not-dilated tubules of different caliber. (**B**) Small group of dilated tubules (blue arrows) dispersed among non-dilated tubules (black arrows). (**C**) A small lobule of dilated tubules crossed and flanked by tiny blood vessels (arrows). (**D**) A group of large opaque tubules surrounded by blood vessels (arrows).

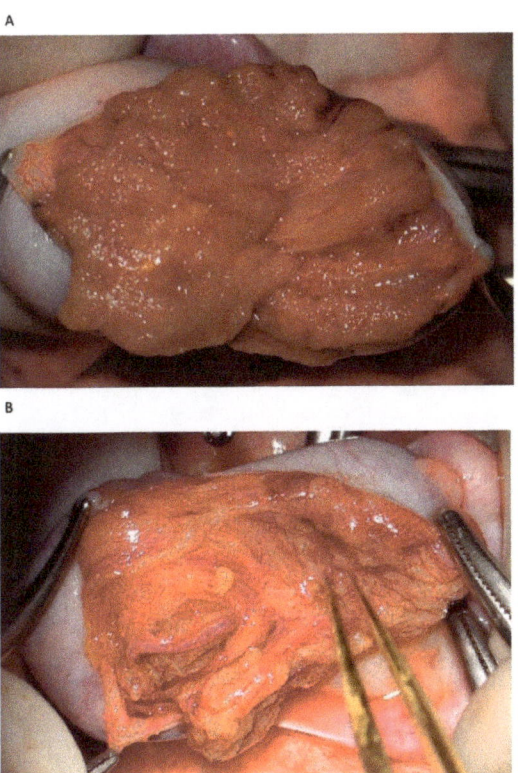

Figure 5. (**A**) Medium-degree bivalve testis opening; (**B**) large bivalve testis opening.

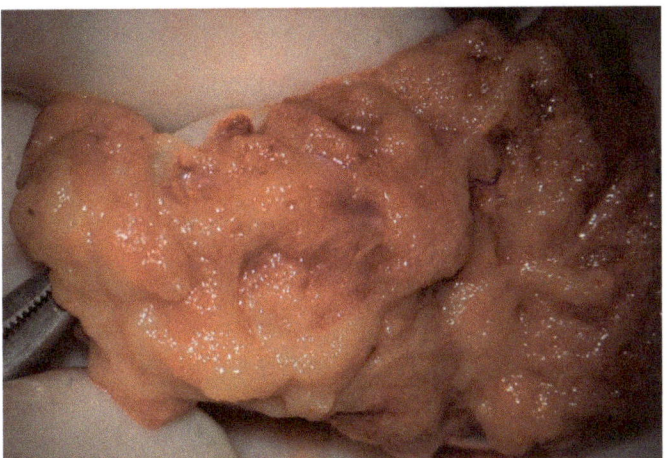

Figure 6. Extremely wide testis opening with exploration in the bi-polar direction and partial extrusion of lobules.

Our experience suggests that dilated STs containing sperm may be more easily found close to the small vessel, probably due to the better local blood perfusion, or to clustering Leydig cells ((Figure 4C,D and Figure 7). Sometimes groups of convoluted dilated STs are found (Figure 4) or occupy a small lobule that should be carefully detached and removed (Figure 7); in some cases only dilated segments of otherwise thin STs are found (Figure 8). The best tubules often display a slightly different color than the surrounding ones or may give the impression of being overdistended (Figure 9). The finding of large lobules made of dilated STs is an extremely rare event, at least in our experience (Figure 10).

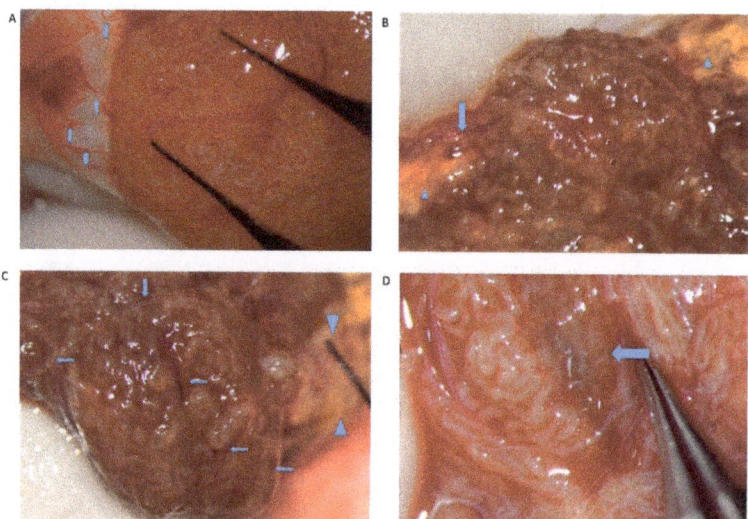

Figure 7. (**A**) Dilated tubules are found close to sub-albugineal vessels (arrows); (**B**) a lobule of dilated tubules supplied by a vessel (arrow), amidst two yellow areas full of Leydig cells (wedges); (**C**) an entire lobule of tubules with different calibers, but mainly dilated, well nourished by many vessels (arrows); in the background, out of focus, yellow tissue full of Leydig cells (between wedges); (**D**) a medium-sized group of dilated tubules close to blood vessels and a brown-yellowish Leydigian area (arrow).

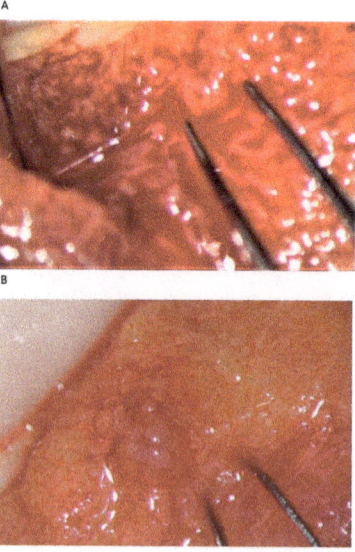

Figure 8. (**A**) An isolated dilated tubule; (**B**) a single dilated tubule surrounded by atrophic tubules.

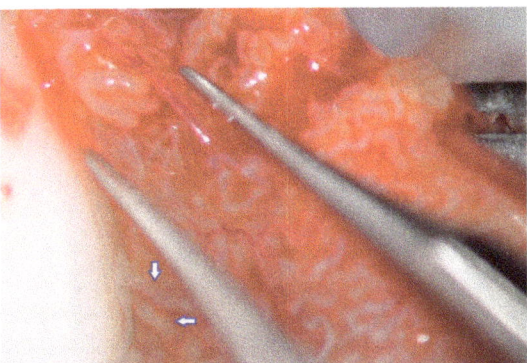

Figure 9. Sometimes dilated tubules appear bloated (between the forceps tips): see the contrast with the slightly less dilated tubules below (arrows).

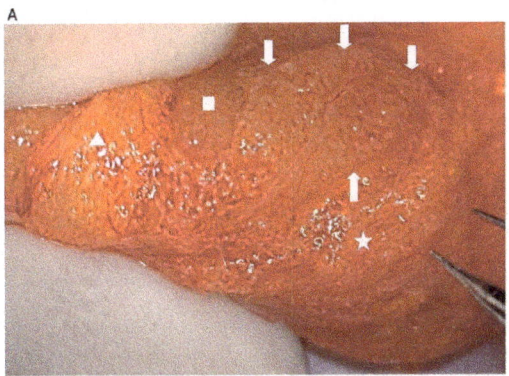

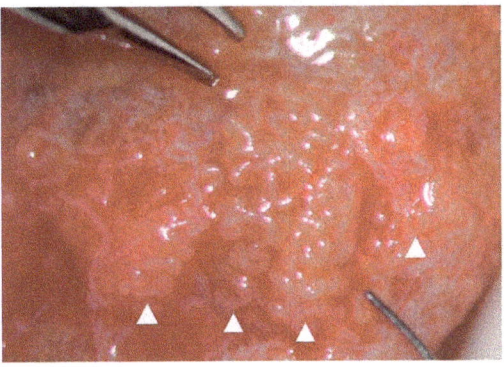

Figure 10. (**A**) Each lobule is made up of tubules of the same caliber, but the caliber decreases from lobule to lobule: dilated (delimited with arrows), less dilated (triangle), narrow (square), and atrophic (star); (**B**) four lobules of dilated tubules emerging from atrophic parenchyma.

At the end of the exploration of the testicular parenchyma at high magnification, the testicular tissue surface is irrigated for antisepsis with Ringer solution (with 80 mg gentamycin/100 mL). Hemostasis is performed when the blood pressure is normalized to avoid postoperative bleeding by gently pressing the testicular tissue for 4 min using gauze wet with the antiseptic solution and eventually (the least possible) using the microsurgical bipolar thermal device. The albuginea incision is closed with a continuous suture of Vicryl 5/0 with a taper-point needle in a running fashion (Figure 11), preferably involving only its external layer to avoid any additional damage to the sub-albugineal vessels. Vicryl is an absorbable suture that does not leave any detectable trace at the testis ultrasound when performed weeks later [22] (Figure 12). Other authors use a 5–0 non-absorbable monofilament suture, such as polydioxanone or a 6–0 nylon suture, to allow the clear identification of the site of incision if a repeat procedure is needed at a subsequent time [19]. The tunica vaginalis opening is repaired by a continuous Vicryl 4/0, after an instillation into the vaginalis cavity of 1 mL saline solution with 2 mg betamethasone, to prevent both pain and tunica vaginalis adhesions, as confirmed in the case of reoperation [23]. The dartos muscle layer and scrotal skin are closed by separate stitches with Vicryl 3/0 suture. MTESE is affected by a minimal blood loss (no more than 3 mL per testis).

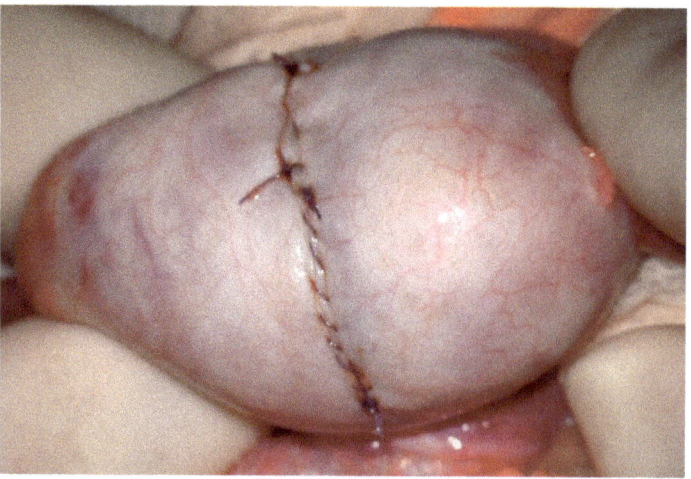

Figure 11. Closure of the albuginea after bivalve opening.

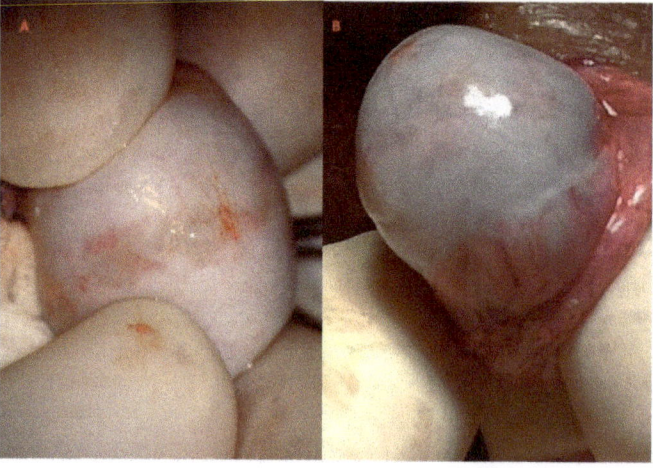

Figure 12. Salvage mTESE after (**A**) one previous failed mTESE (**B**) two previous mTESEs.

The mTESE procedure may proceed slightly differently in particular cases: (i) Incidental testicular lesions may be found in up to 2.9% of patients with NOA [24]. Such lesions are usually benign when their maximum diameter at ultrasound does not exceed 5 mm [25]. Following a preoperative testis ultrasound assessing the intraparenchymal coordinates of the nodule, incision of the albuginea is made to easily reach the nodule, which is completely removed together with a thin layer of intact parenchyma; a frozen section would guide the surgeon to proceed with mTESE in the case of benign lesions (e.g., leydigiomas), or to total orchiectomy, with a consequent search for sperm in the removed testis. (ii) Klinefelter patients may have very small, firm testes. The testicular parenchyma is usually darker, stiffer, and more fragile compared to that of patients with idiopathic NOA. Groups of hyperplastic Leydig cells are dispersed among hyalinized tubules, among which the rare dilated tubules may be found (Figure 13).

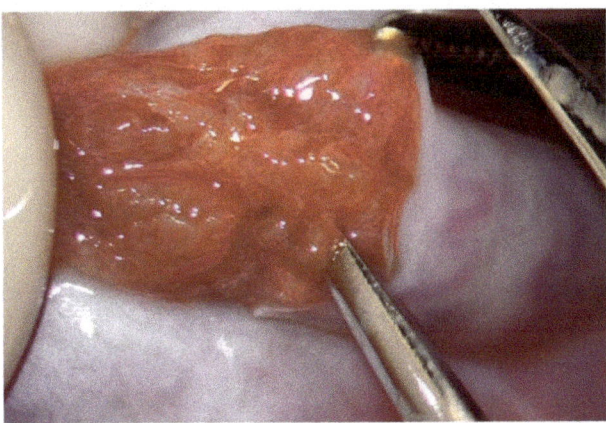

Figure 13. Testis in a patient with Klinefelter syndrome. (**A**) low magnification; (**B**) high magnification (×36): forceps tips indicate a tiny group of dilated tubules inside a brownish area rich with Leydig cells, with atrophic tubules in the background (one atrophic tubule is marked with a star).

4. Post-Operative Course

MTESE is a minimally invasive surgery when performed to preserve, as much as possible, the integrity of the testicular parenchyma: a testis ultrasound performed six months after mTESE does not usually reveal any visible scar [22]. Overnight hospitalization is always suggested, particularly for those patients living far away from the hospital. Patients should be examined for a scrotal hematoma prior to discharge. Other prescriptions include oral antibiotics (usually for a week); bed rest and an ice pack to the scrotum for the first 48 h; no scrotal supporters, to avoid testicular retraction in the upper scrotal position; and suture removal ten days after surgery. The post-operative course is usually painless, probably thanks to the betamethasone instillation in the vaginalis tunica and to the careful handling of the spermatic cord; in the case of pain, paracetamol is prescribed for a couple of days. The patient would be able to go back to work in three days, may resume normal sexual activity in ten days, and should wait for twenty days before resuming any intense physical activity.

Complications are extremely rare, particularly when a surgeon with great experience in microsurgery performs an mTESE. In our experience (GMC), intratesticular hematoma occurred once in 1300 procedures, due to hemostasis being performed during uncorrected hypotension after induction of general anesthesia; the testis was opened again, and no signs of testicular damage were seen at ultrasound two weeks and six months later. Complications are more frequently observed when a single or multiple biopsy cTESE is performed [26].

A testosterone follow up assay should be performed 9 and 18 months after surgery as a significant decrease in testosterone serum levels has been described at 3–6 months, with a return to 95% of the baseline testosterone levels at the end of 18 months [26]. Patients whose pre-surgical subnormal testosterone levels have been optimized prior to mTESE should receive testosterone replacement therapy if no further surgery for sperm retrieval is awaited.

Author Contributions: G.M.C. drafted the manuscript; E.C. drafted the English version and critically revised the manuscript. All authors have read and agreed to the published version of the manuscript.

Funding: The APC was funded by NextFertility Procrea, Lugano, Switzerland.

Institutional Review Board Statement: Not applicable.

Informed Consent Statement: Not applicable.

Data Availability Statement: Not applicable.

Conflicts of Interest: The authors declare no conflict of interest.

References

1. Silber, S.J.; Nagy, Z.; Devroey, P.; Tournaye, H.; Van Steirteghem, A.C. Distribution of spermatogenesis in the testicles of azoospermic men: The presence or absence of spermatids in the testes of men with germinal failure. *Hum. Reprod.* **1997**, *12*, 2422–2428. [CrossRef] [PubMed]
2. Bernie, A.M.; Mata, D.A.; RRamasamy, R.; Schlegel, P.N. Comparison of Microdissection Testicular Sperm Extraction, Conventional Testicular Sperm Extraction, and Testicular Sperm Aspiration for Nonobstructive Azoospermia: A Systematic Review and Meta-Analysis. *Fertil. Steril.* **2015**, *104*, 1099–1103. [CrossRef]
3. Corona, G.; Minhas, S.; Giwercman, A.; Bettocchi, C.; Dinkelman-Smit, M.; Dohle, G.; Fusco, F.; Kadioglou, A.; Kliesch, S.; Kopa, Z.; et al. Sperm recovery and ICSI outcomes in men with non-obstructive azoospermia: A systematic review and meta-analysis. *Hum. Reprod. Update* **2019**, *25*, 733–757. [CrossRef]
4. Esteves, S.C.; Ramasamy, R.; Colpi, G.M.; Carvalho, J.F.; Schlegel, P.N. Sperm retrieval rates by micro-TESE versus conventional TESE in men with non-obstructive azoospermia-the assumption of independence in effect sizes might lead to misleading conclusions. *Hum. Reprod. Update* **2020**, *26*, 603–605. [CrossRef] [PubMed]
5. Ishikawa, T.; Nose, R.; Yamaguchi, K.; Chiba, K.; Fujisawa, M. Learning curves of microdissection testicular sperm extraction for nonobstructive azoospermia. *Fertil. Steril.* **2010**, *94*, 1008–1011. [CrossRef] [PubMed]
6. Dabaja, A.A.; Schlegel, P.N. Microdissection testicular sperm extraction: An update. *Asian J. Androl.* **2013**, *15*, 35–39. [CrossRef]
7. Colpi, G.M.; Francavilla, S.; Haidl, G.; Link, K.; Behre, H.M.; Goulis, D.G.; Krausz, C.; Giwercman, A. European Academy of Andrology guideline: Management of oligo-astheno-teratozoospermia. *Andrology* **2018**, *6*, 513–524. [CrossRef] [PubMed]
8. Caroppo, E.; Colpi, G.M. Hormonal Treatment of Men with Nonobstructive Azoospermia: What Does the Evidence Suggest? *J. Clin. Med.* **2021**, *10*, 387. [CrossRef] [PubMed]
9. Schlegel, P.N.; Sigman, M.; Collura, B.; De Jonge, C.J.; Eisenberg, M.L.; Lamb, D.J.; Mulhall, J.P.; Niederberger, C.; Sandlow, J.I.; Sokol, R.Z.; et al. Diagnosis and treatment of infertility in men: AUA/ASRM guideline. Part II. *Fertil. Steril.* **2020**, *115*, 62–69. [CrossRef]

10. Lenz, S.; Thomsen, J.K.; Giwercman, A.; Hertel, N.T.; Hertz, J.; Skakkebaek, N.E. Ultrasonic texture and volume of testicles in infertile men. *Hum. Reprod.* **1994**, *9*, 878–881. [CrossRef] [PubMed]
11. Eisenberg, M.L.; Betts, P.; Herder, D.; Lamb, D.J.; Lipshultz, L.I. Increased risk of cancer among azoospermic men. *Fertil. Steril.* **2013**, *100*, 681–685. [CrossRef]
12. Pettersson, A.; Richiardi, L.; Nordenskjold, A.; Kaijser, M.; Akre, O. Age at surgery for undescended testis and risk of testicular cancer. *N. Engl. J. Med.* **2007**, *356*, 1835–1841. [CrossRef]
13. Esteves, S.C.; Miyaoka, R.; Roque, M.; Agarwal, A. Outcome of varicocele repair in men with nonobstructive azoospermia: Systematic review and meta-analysis. *Asian J. Androl.* **2016**, *18*, 246–253. [CrossRef]
14. Practice Committee of the American Society for Reproductive Medicine. Management of nonobstructive azoospermia: A committee opinion. *Fertil. Steril.* **2018**, *110*, 1239–1245. [CrossRef] [PubMed]
15. Shufaro, Y.; Prus, D.; Laufer, N.; Simon, A. Impact of repeated testicular fine needle aspirations (TEFNA) and testicular sperm extraction (TESE) on the microscopic morphology of the testis: An animal model. *Hum. Reprod.* **2002**, *17*, 1795–1799. [CrossRef]
16. Caroppo, E.; Colpi, E.M.; Gazzano, G.; Vaccalluzzo, L.; Piatti, E.; D'Amato, G.; Colpi, G.M. The seminiferous tubule caliber pattern as evaluated at high magnification during microdissection testicular sperm extraction predicts sperm retrieval in patients with non-obstructive azoospermia. *Andrology* **2019**, *7*, 8–14. [CrossRef] [PubMed]
17. Dohle, G.R.; Elzanaty, S.; van Casteren, N.J. Testicular biopsy: Clinical practice and interpretation. *Asian J. Androl.* **2012**, *14*, 88–93. [CrossRef]
18. Alrabeeah, K.; Doucet, R.; Boulet, E.; Phillips, S.; Al-Hathal, N.; Bissonnette, F.; Kadoch, I.J.; Zini, A. Can the rapid identification of mature spermatozoa during microdissection testicular sperm extraction guide operative planning? *Andrology* **2015**, *3*, 467–472. [CrossRef]
19. Flannigan, R.; Bach, P.V.; Schlegel, P.N. Microdissection testicular sperm extraction. *Transl. Androl. Urol.* **2017**, *6*, 745–752. [CrossRef] [PubMed]
20. Esteves, S.E. Clinical management of infertile men with nonobstructive azoospermia. *Asian J. Androl.* **2015**, *17*, 459–470. [CrossRef]
21. Ohlander, S.; Hotaling, J.; Kirshenbaum, E.; Niederberger, C.; Eisenberg, M.L. Impact of fresh versus cryopreserved testicular sperm upon intracytoplasmic sperm injection pregnancy outcomes in men with azoospermia due to spermatogenic dysfunction: A meta-analysis. *Fertil. Steril.* **2014**, *101*, 344–349. [CrossRef] [PubMed]
22. Colpi, G.M.; Piediferro, G.; Nerva, F.; Giacchetta, D.; Colpi, E.M.; Piatti, E. Sperm retrieval for intra-cytoplasmic sperm injection in non obstructive azoospermia. *Min. Urol. Nefrol.* **2005**, *57*, 99–107.
23. Colpi, G.M.; Piediferro, G.; Scroppo, F.I.; Colpi, E.M.; Sulpizio, P. Surgery for Male Infertility: Surgical Sperm Retrievals. In *Clinical Andrology*; Bjorndahl, L., Giwercman, A., Tournaye, T., Weidner, W., Eds.; Informa Healthcare: New York, NY, USA, 2010; pp. 148–162.
24. Carmignani, L.; Gadda, F.; Mancini, M.; Gazzano, G.; Nerva, F.; Rocco, F.; Colpi, G.M. Detection of testicular ultrasonographic lesions in severe male infertility. *J. Urol.* **2004**, *172*, 1045–1047. [CrossRef] [PubMed]
25. Eifler, J.B., Jr.; King, P.; Schlegel, P.N. Incidental testicular lesions found during infertility evaluation are usually benign and may be managed conservatively. *J. Urol.* **2008**, *180*, 261–264. [CrossRef]
26. Ramasamy, R.; Yagan, N.; Schlegel, P.N. Structural and functional changes to the testis after conventional versus microdissection testicular sperm extraction. *Urology* **2005**, *65*, 1190–1194. [CrossRef] [PubMed]

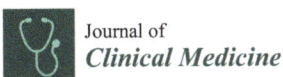

Review

Sperm Selection Procedures for Optimizing the Outcome of ICSI in Patients with NOA

Kaan Aydos [1,*] and Oya Sena Aydos [2]

1. Department of Urology, Reproductive Health Research Center, School of Medicine, University of Ankara, 06230 Ankara, Turkey
2. Department of Medical Biology, School of Medicine, University of Ankara, 06230 Ankara, Turkey; saydos@gmail.com
* Correspondence: drkaanaydos@gmail.com; Tel.: +90-533-748-8995

Abstract: Retrieving spermatozoa from the testicles has been a great hope for patients with non-obstructive azoospermia (NOA), but relevant methods have not yet been developed to the level necessary to provide resolutions for all cases of NOA. Although performing testicular sperm extraction under microscopic magnification has increased sperm retrieval rates, in vitro selection and processing of quality sperm plays an essential role in the success of in vitro fertilization. Moreover, sperm cryopreservation is widely used in assisted reproductive technologies, whether for therapeutic purposes or for future fertility preservation. In recent years, there have been new developments using advanced technologies to freeze and preserve even very small numbers of sperm for which conventional techniques are inadequate. The present review provides an up-to-date summary of current strategies for maximizing sperm recovery from surgically obtained testicular samples and, as an extension, optimization of in vitro sperm processing techniques in the management of NOA.

Keywords: testicular azoospermia; non-obstructive azoospermia; sperm selection; sperm; cryopreservation; in vitro maturation

---

1. Introduction

To date, although testicular spermatozoa from patients with non-obstructive azoospermia (NOA) have been used widely for intracytoplasmic sperm injection (ICSI), this method's effectiveness still has potential for further improvement. NOA is characterized by the absence of any spermatozoa, whether dead or alive, in the ejaculate due to reduced or nonexistent sperm production in the testicle [1]. Testicular fine needle aspiration (FNA or testicular sperm aspiration—TESA) is an effective and non-invasive method used to obtain sperm, especially from patients with obstructive azoospermia [2]. Although its simpler and less traumatic features have made FNA the preferred method, testicular sperm extraction (TESE) is the treatment of choice for patients with NOA, with a satisfactory number of successful spermatozoa retrieved in approximately half of the patients. In the conventional TESE procedure, the testis is exposed through a small incision in the tunica albuginea, and multiple biopsies are taken randomly [3]. However, microTESE carried out at high magnification under an operating microscope allows visualization of whitish, larger, and more opaque seminiferous tubules likely to contain mature germ cells [4]. Although not randomized, most studies have reported that the sperm recovery rate from microTESE is superior to that from conventional TESE [5–7]. In fact, a recent controlled, randomized study verified the efficacy of microTESE compared with that of TESE in retrieving spermatozoa from patients with NOA [8]. In addition to the surgical technique, however, in vitro extraction of sperm from surgically excised testicular tissue or tubules is also important for obtaining spermatozoa of sufficient quality and quantity for use in ICSI.

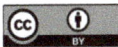

2. Processing and Selection of Surgically Retrieved Sperm for ICSI

2.1. Mechanical Processing of Testicular Tissue

The goal of TESE treatment in patients with NOA is to retrieve spermatozoa suitable for ICSI from the testicular tissue obtained by surgical intervention. Different methods have been described for processing TESE specimens in the laboratory. The most preferred tissue-processing procedure is mechanical treatment of testicular tissue pieces by shredding and mincing with fine needles, scissors, or glass slides [9–11]. In addition to the shredding, tubule pieces cut into short lengths can be squeezed into the medium with the help of a bent pipette [12,13]. The suspension can then be processed using either the swim-up or density gradient centrifugation method. In the former, following the sedimentation of tissue fragments, the most motile spermatozoa swim up the medium; in the density gradient method, during centrifugation, sperm cells are separated according to swimming rate while moving through discrete layers of density gradients [14,15]. Both methods have their advantages. Verheyen et al. compared rough shredding, fine mincing, vortexing, and crushing methods to evaluate the efficiency of obtaining a maximum number of sperm from testicular biopsy specimens, and fine mincing of testicular tissue followed by discontinuous Percoll centrifugation was found to be the most effective method of isolating a pure fraction of spermatozoa available for ICSI as well as cryopreservation [16]. However, the risk of cell loss through the discrete layers in Percoll gradient separation cannot be ignored. Therefore, if too few cells are present, it may be preferable to carefully mince the testicular tissue with fine forceps or microscissors and centrifuge the entire suspension immediately [10,17]. As another option, Haimov-Kochman et al. suggested that leaving tissue fragments from TESE in medium for 10 min and then centrifuging the supernatant could yield rapid sperm recovery without wasting time shredding the tissue [18]. Interestingly, when the supernatant was spermatozoa-negative, no spermatozoa were present in the tissue either. Therefore, this method makes it possible to quickly predict the success of TESE. Nevertheless, when it comes to choosing the optimal method, in addition to the structural features of the testicular tissue, personal experience and laboratory facilities should also be taken into consideration.

2.2. Use of Erythrocyte-Lysing Buffer (ELB)

One of the most frequently encountered problems during the search for spermatozoa in fragmented TESE specimens is abundant erythrocyte infiltration. Attempting to identify rare spermatozoa among dense erythrocyte clusters is time consuming and associated with a reduced recovery rate. The use of erythrocyte lysing buffer (ELB) for the elimination of red blood cells present in the mechanically shredded testicular tissues of patients with NOA was first described by Verheyen et al. [19]. Resuspending the testicular sperm pellet in ELB (155 mM NH_4Cl, 10 mM $KHCO_3$, and 2 mM EDTA; pH 7.2) yielded recovery of additional motile spermatozoa in a shorter time. Treatment of TESE samples with ELB shortens the processing time and increases the success of cell retrieval without decreasing the fertilization potential of the embryo [17]. However, treatment of sperm suspensions with ELB has also been shown to impair sperm quality [20]. When spermatozoa were incubated in ELB for 10 min, their motility and viability decreased and DNA fragmentation increased. This effect of ELB on sperm may be due to the fact that the same mechanism of disruption in ammonium equilibrium responsible for the lysis in erythrocytes is also present in the sperm. In addition, osmotic stress caused by the chemical structure of this buffer may damage the plasma membrane and alter sperm metabolism [21]. Conversely, Soygur et al. showed that ELB itself and the cellular stress caused by erythrocyte lysis did not have detrimental effects on the survival of ejaculated sperm [22]. According to their protocol, however, ELB incubation was only allowed for 5–10 s, so there may not have been enough time for damage to occur. Despite the fact that the potential influence of this buffer on sperm parameters remains uncertain, at present, ELB medium is widely used during testicular germ cell extraction to clean the cellular suspension from erythrocytes that interfere with visualization [23,24].

2.3. Enzymatic Digestion

In TESE, the goal of mechanically shredding tissues is to free the germ cells that are trapped in seminiferous tubules or adhered to the tissue. However, digestion of tissues using enzymes can be expected to facilitate the release of gametes by loosening the cellular contacts in the tubular wall. In fact, collagenase has been shown to provide sufficient dissolution in the tissue without decreasing cell viability [25] (Table 1). This was also confirmed by Salzbrunn et al. for cryopreserved testicular tissue, and enzymatic preparation of tissues using collagenase type AI provided high yields of vital spermatids and spermatozoa [26]. Subsequently, Fischer et al. reported the first pregnancy using spermatozoa extracted using the same method in ICSI [27]. However, when compared to type AI, collagenase type IV has been shown to be more effective in isolation and recovery of viable spermatozoa and round spermatids from testicular samples [28]. Type IV collagenase is preferred for the processing of testicular tissue, since type IV collagen is specifically localized in the basement membrane of the seminiferous tubules and within the extracellular matrix (ECM) layers [29]. On the other hand, collagenase type IV is produced by Sertoli cells (SCs), and its target (collagen IV) has been shown to affect the dynamics of SC-tight junctions, which mediates translocation of preleptotene and leptotene spermatocytes residing at the basal compartment of the seminiferous epithelium into the adluminal compartment for further development [30]. However, the exact mechanisms regulating the events of spermiation and sperm release have not yet been clearly elucidated. A disintegrin and metalloproteinase with thrombospondin motifs (ADAMTSs), which belong to the M12 metallopeptidase family, are responsible for the migration of differentiated germ cells through the seminiferous tubule wall by organizing the degradation and reformation of the ECM [31]. In fact, we recently demonstrated that ADAMTS1 and ADAMTS5 protein levels expressed in Sertoli cells were decreased approximately 2-fold in cases of NOA [32]. The effect of enzymatic digestion on the success of sperm retrieval in cases where these proteases are defective is a subject of further research. For these reasons, the use of type IV collagen has been widely preferred to increase sperm recovery rates, because of both its disrupting effect on the integrity of the tubule basement membrane and its ability to break the connections of germ cells with Sertoli cells [33]. During the process, clotting caused by free DNA released from dead cells can be prevented by the addition of DNAase enzyme [28].

Since enzymatic digestion of testicular tissue allows obtainment of an isolated germ cell suspension free of tissue artifacts, its efficiency is higher compared to rough mechanical separation, which causes contamination with large amounts of damaged cells, free nuclei, and residual tissue fragments in the cell suspension. Indeed, spermatozoa retrieval rates (SRRs) between 7% and 33% were reported following enzymatic processing of tissue suspension in TESE cases in which no spermatozoa could be obtained by mechanical mincing [33–36]. The differences between the SRRs reported in the studies may be due to the experience of the embryologists, the histopathological status of the testicular tissues, and variations in the number of cases. In particular, the time spent and effort expended during the mechanical shredding of seminiferous tubules have significant effects on the chance of sperm detection in the laboratory. The crucial role of laboratory handling, especially in the management of compromised testicular specimens, has been discussed previously [37]. Similarly, Modarresi et al. reported serum follicle-stimulating hormone (FSH) and luteinizing hormone levels as factors that may affect SRRs after enzymatic digestion treatment [33]. On the other hand, collagenase treatment has been shown to increase the cytokine population in the testis by stimulating an immune response, but its effects on spermatozoa remain unclear [38]. In general, processing with enzymatic digestion from testes in which very few spermatozoa are predicted to be present should be considered an effective practice.

Table 1. Clinical results of enzymatically tissue processing methods for sperm recovery by TESE.

Compound	Control	Results	Refs.
DNase plus collagenase type IV	Mechanical searching	Increased SRR 9% of cases where no spermatozoa were found after mechanical searching.	[33]
DNase plus collagenase type IV	Mechanical searching	Increased SRR 26% of cases where no spermatozoa were found after mechanical searching	[34]
DNase plus collagenase type IV	Mechanical searching	Increased SRR 33% of cases where no spermatozoa were found after mechanical searching	[35]
DNase plus collagenase type IV	Mechanical searching	Increased SRR 7% of cases where no spermatozoa were found after mechanical searching	[36]
Collagenase type IV and collagenase type IA	Untreated samples	Vitality in control, collagenase IV and IA; 74.7%, 84.9% and 79.5%, respectively, motility; 86%, 86% and 71%, respectively ($p > 0.05$). Recovered spermatozoa by collagenase IV and IA; 0.34×10^6 and 0.22×10^6, respectively $p = 0.017$	[28]

2.4. Motility Enhancers

The success of ICSI in patients with NOA is closely related to the recovery of motile spermatozoa during TESE. Indeed, fertilization success decreases significantly when immotile spermatozoa are injected into oocytes [39,40]. However, in most patients with NOA, only a small number of spermatozoa with very poor motility or complete immotility can be obtained from minced testicular tissue. Less than 3% sperm motility was reported following the initial processing of biopsy samples [41]. However, the primary goal in the treatment of NOA is to extract spermatozoa with sufficient motility from tissue fragments during TESE for use in ICSI. It has been suggested that viable sperm ratios increase after in vitro culture of testicular cell suspension with various motility enhancers [15] (Table 2). Among the many tested compounds for stimulating sperm motility in vitro, phosphodiesterase (PDE) inhibitors have been the most promising. The most common chemical component used as a motility enhancer in the laboratory is pentoxifylline. Pentoxifylline is a PDE inhibitor of the methylxanthine group shown to induce sperm motility [42]. In human sperm, adenylyl cyclase catalyzes the formation of cyclic adenosine monophosphate (cAMP) from adenosine triphosphate. The role of cAMP in the regulation of sperm motility has been defined [43]. Previous studies have suggested that cAMP is the primary signal for the onset of progressive motility under proper conditions [44]. Compounds such as pentoxifylline, caffeine, and theophylline are known to inhibit cyclic nucleotide phosphodiesterase, which breaks down cAMP to 5'-AMP [45,46]. However, it is not certain that theophylline and caffeine directly stimulate sperm motility by increasing the cAMP compound; they may also act on other enzymes in addition to PDE [43]. Caffeine was shown to increase cytochrome oxidase activity, an important compound of the electron transport chain in mitochondria, by stimulating the cAMP and protein kinase A pathway [47]. Experimental studies revealed that the addition of caffeine to semen samples increased sperm motility and stimulated capacitation and spontaneous acrosome reaction [48,49]. It was also shown that incubation of post-freezing human spermatozoa with caffeine for 15 min increased progressive motility through mitochondrial energy metabolism [50]. However, teratogenic consequences of high-dose caffeine and its derivatives have been established in animal models [51]. It has been suggested that by washing away the motility enhancers, the putative toxic effects on embryo development will disappear; however, it has also been shown that the removal of these compounds by centrifugation may lead to total motility loss [52]. Although the results in current literature are encouraging, the toxic effects of caffeine on embryo development and the potential prevention of these effects require further investigation.

In a comparative study, Mangoli et al. demonstrated that using pentoxifylline in the selection of viable spermatozoa from a testicular non-motile spermatozoa population significantly increased the success of fertilization (62% vs. 41%) and pregnancy (32% vs. 16%) more than the hypo-osmotic swelling test [53]. Pentoxifylline was found to increase the pregnancy success rate of IVF with its stimulating effect on acrosome reaction [54]. Similarly, Kovacic et al. reported that if immotile sperm in TESE tissue were cultured with pentoxifylline for 20 min, 97% of them started to move; hence, vital spermatozoa could be distinguished more easily, the procedure was shortened, and the fertilization rates and numbers of embryos increased [55]. The use of pentoxifylline to stimulate sperm motility in fresh or frozen/thawed suspensions has also been reported in other studies [56–58]. Since the cAMP level in spermatozoa with normal motility is sufficiently high to activate the subsequent cascades, PDE inhibitors have the most pronounced effect on sperm with poor motility [59]. This explains why pentoxifylline is rather successful on poorly motile sperms recovered with TESE. Above all, artificial oocyte activation was indicated as the main determining factor for ICSI success, regardless of the restoration of testicular sperm motility after pentoxifylline treatment [58]. Therefore, when evaluating the clinical results of in vitro sperm processing methods, the female factor should also be taken into consideration in certain aspects.

Theophylline, with its similar molecular structure to pentoxifylline, has also been shown to increase sperm motility and fertilizing capacity in in vitro studies [52,60,61]. Ebner et al. reported that when frozen/thawed testicular sperm samples from TESE were treated with theophylline, sperm motility improved in most cases, and the clinical pregnancy rate increased from 23% to 53% [45]. The positive effect of theophylline on sperm motility has also been demonstrated in other studies [62,63]. Although there is concern that motility-enhancing chemicals may have toxic effects on embryo development [64], no evidence of anomalies in offspring has been shown for either theophylline or pentoxifylline [63,65].

Spermatozoa contain various forms of PDEs with different regulatory interactions. Results from in vitro studies with PDE5, which represents a small functional fraction of spermatozoa, are contradictory. Glenn et al. reported that Sildenafil citrate, a widely used PDE5 inhibitor, produced a sustained improvement in sperm motility, but this was accompanied by a significant increase in acrosome-reacted sperm count [66]. Others have reported PDE5 inhibitors to yield similar improvements in motility; however, these studies did not confirm that sildenafil and tadalafil (another PDE5 inhibitor) triggered the acrosome reaction [67,68]. Overall, concentration and exposure time of PDE5 inhibitors have been indicated as the main decisive factors for sperm motility [66,69]. Nevertheless, the early acrosome reaction before reaching the oocyte renders sperm unable to fertilize; this constitutes the main concern. Furthermore, paucity of PDE in spermatozoa, as demonstrated in proteomic studies, may also have led to inconsistent results in in vitro studies [70]. In addition, the scarcity of studies on aberrant PDE expression and the role of biochemical pathways with different molecular interactions prevent further conclusions [71].

Table 2. Clinical results of motility enhancers for sperm recovery by TESE.

Compound	Control	Results	Refs.
Pentoxifylline	Hypoosmotic test	Increased fertilization rate (62% vs. 41% $p < 0.05$) Increased pregnancy rate (32% vs. 16% $p < 0.05$)	[53]
Pentoxifylline	Untreated immotile sperm	Initiated motility in 95.7% of the samples. Increased fertilization rate (66% vs. 50.9%; $p < 0.005$) Increased mean number of embryos per cycle (4.7 vs. 2.7 $p < 0.01$).	[55]
Pentoxifylline	In-group	Induced additional motility in 33.3% and 69.3% of cases where fresh and frozen samples were used, respectively.	[57]
Pentoxifylline	Untreated immotile sperm	Initiated motility in 70.8% of the samples.	[42]
Theophylline	Untreated motile or immotile sperm	Improved motility in 98.5% of the cases. Increased fertilization (79.9% vs. 63.3% $p < 0.001$) and pregnancy (53.9% vs. 23.8% $p < 0.05$) rates.	[45]

2.5. Short-Term Culture vs. Simultaneous ICSI

The impact of enhancers on sperm motility in TESE samples may also be related to in vitro incubation conditions. In fact, when the effects of culture time and ambient temperature on sperm motility in testicular tissue samples were evaluated, 24 h incubation at room temperature was found to be ideal for optimal sperm motion [72] (Table 3). Balaban et al. showed that incubating testicular tissue samples in recombinant FSH-supplemented medium for 24 h increased the motility of the spermatozoa and, thus, the success of ICSI [73]. Similarly, Wu et al. evaluated the laboratory and clinical results of fresh and post-freezing culturing of tissue samples taken by TESE from a group of patients with NOA [41]. According to their results, after 24 h of in vitro culture at 37 °C, the number of motile sperm increased remarkably, and sperm reached a maximum motility rate at 72 h. Similar studies reported that sperm motility peaked upon extending the culture period to 48 h [74]. Likewise, post-freezing cultures of TESE samples showed results similar to those of fresh cultures. In contrast, the outcome of in vitro cultures of testicular spermatozoa from patients with NOA has not been confirmed by others to be predictable [11]. However, the main goal in the treatment of NOA is to obtain vital spermatozoa with sufficient motility during a TESE attempt. In this context, Karacan et al. who compared the outcome of 337 ICSI cycles using testicular sperm freshly obtained on the day of or the day before oocyte retrieval or after a freeze/thaw cycle, demonstrated that in the presence of motile spermatozoa, neither the timing of TESE nor the use of post-freezing sperm affected ICSI results [75]. On the other hand, since culturing of testicular sperm for up to 24 h was found to increase DNA fragmentation, it is recommended that retrieved sperms are used without delay [76]. Unfortunately, we do not have enough data to make a reliable comment on whether TESE samples should be taken one day in advance and kept in the laboratory or used fresh simultaneously with oocyte pick-up (OPU).

Table 3. Clinical results of short-term testicular tissue culturing.

Time of in Vitro Culture	Control	Results	Refs.
24 h	0 day	Improved motility from 13% to 76% (at 25 °C) and 67% (at 37 °C) ($p = 0.01$)	[72]
24 h supp recFSH	24 h simple medium	recFSH supplementation improved motility to 70.4% vs. 32.9%, fertilization 68.8% vs. 42.1%, implantation per embryo 20.1% vs. 13.2%, and clinical pregnancy 47.9% vs. 30% ($p < 0.005$)	[73]
24 h—72 h	0 day	After 24 h in culture, a marked increase of 5–8% in motile sperm was observed and a maximum motility rate appeared between 48 and 72 h of culture ($p < 0.05$)	[41]

2.6. Motile Sperm Identification with HOST

During the examination of testicular tissue under a microscope, the most important factor determining the vitality of the selected spermatozoa is movement of the tail. In recent years, researchers have used various techniques in attempts to develop an optimal selection method that can directly discriminate living spermatozoa, regardless of their motility, while visualized under a micromanipulator. If all spermatozoa are immotile, hypo-osmotic swelling test (HOST) is an option for choosing a viable one for ICSI. HOST, first described by Jeyendran et al., is a vitality test used to assess the functional integrity of the spermatozoa membrane [77]. Principally, viable but immotile spermatozoa incubated in hypo-osmotic solution are expected to have swollen tails due to osmotic challenge, as their membrane functions are healthy. In a semen sample, the percentage of viable spermatozoa selected with HOST is defined as the HOST score [78]. A randomized and controlled study showed that fertilization and pregnancy rates associated with ICSI increased significantly when viable sperm were selected from among immotile testicular spermatozoa using HOST [79]. Furthermore, the use of testicular spermatozoa with total absence of motility selected with HOST demonstrated pregnancy rates comparable to ejaculate [80]. Others also reported similar results [81–83]. Likewise, in cases where immotile sperm cannot be activated with known motility enhancers, HOST is a reliable and effective option for choosing viable spermatozoa for ICSI [84]. On the other hand, low HOST values of spermatozoa, an indicator of impaired membrane integrity, may be associated with increased DNA damage [85]. Therefore, HOST can be a valuable tool for the selection of viable and also DNA-intact spermatozoa [86].

In many couples with low HOST scores, pregnancy rates remain low, either in natural cycles or after conventional IVF [87]. However, even if the HOST score is low, acceptable implantation and pregnancy rates can be achieved with ICSI [88]. In these cases, decreased fecundation rates were explained as the toxic effect of a number of spermatozoa with a low HOST score attached to the zona pellucida [78]. Fertilization can be achieved by bypassing this effect, using a single sperm with ICSI. This proves the importance of choosing a viable spermatozoon using HOST for pregnancy success, regardless of the total HOST score of a whole sperm population. Besides, high occurrences of spontaneously developed tail swellings were reported to affect the accuracy of HOST in determining the viability of frozen-thawed spermatozoa, a drawback of HOST for processed sperm [89]. In addition, HOST is not recommended as a viability test. Since pregnancy could be achieved in the following ICSI trials while HOST demonstrated impaired membrane function, it is recommended to verify the HOST results with vitality tests [90]. Moreover, although HOST is practical, the procedure is time consuming and requires chemicals used in the process to be removed [84]. Loss of viability due to prolonged incubation, further dilution of an extremely small number of testicular sperm in HOST solution, and various methodological modification proposals are other troubles related with the test [91,92]. However, the ability to demonstrate in real time that immotile spermatozoa are not dead still makes HOST an indispensable part of ICSI practice.

2.7. Sperm Tail Flexibility Test to Check Sperm Viability

Another method of assessing the viability of immotile spermatozoa is the sperm tail flexibility test. Essentially, this test involves observing whether the sperm tail is moving by mechanical agitation with lateral touch of the microinjection pipette [93]. If the tail moves independently of the head, the immotile sperm is considered alive and can therefore be selected for ICSI. In contrast, a spermatozoon's tail remaining rigid in response to the same force indicates its non-viability. When sperm were selected based on this method, whether from frozen or fresh testicular tissue samples, the pregnancy and take-home baby percentages using immotile and motile sperm were found to be similar [94]. Mechanical assessment of the viability of immotile spermatozoa is a simple and cost-effective method that avoids the risk of chemical solutions and does not disrupt the structural integrity of the sperm [84]. The main disadvantages of this mechanical touching technique are the scarcity of data comparing its results with those of other techniques and, in particular, its dependence on the personal experience and skill of the practitioner.

2.8. Intracytoplasmic Morphologically Selected Sperm Injection (IMSI)

IMSI allows selection of spermatozoa with normal nuclear morphology under ultra-high magnification for use in ICSI [95]. Initially, IMSI was confirmed to significantly increase pregnancy rates, especially in cases with recurrent implantation failure following ICSI [96]. Considering that it increases the implantation and pregnancy rates by 50% and 60%, respectively, the use of IMSI in male factor infertility was encouraged [97]. Later, the effectiveness of IMSI was further emphasized in cases of severe compound sperm disorders [98]. However, a recent meta-analysis found low-quality evidence that IMSI increases the clinical chance of pregnancy; the analysis reported the probability of live birth to be 24% by regular ICSI and between 21% and 33% following IMSI coupled with ICSI [99]. Pregnancy with testicular sperm selected by IMSI has also been reported [100]. In cases with high sperm DNA fragmentation, however, spermatozoa from the testicles doubled the live birth rates compared to ejaculated spermatozoa selected with IMSI (49.8% vs. 28.7%) [101]. The relatively high pregnancy percentages in TESE/TESA cases can be explained by the avoidance of testicular sperm from oxidative DNA damage during epididymal transit. Nevertheless, before making a firm conclusion about the role of IMSI in male factor infertility, further studies are needed to confirm whether the magnified morphological structure of a spermatozoon is an indicator of its functionality.

2.9. Laser-Assisted Sperm Selection

Laser-assisted (LA) sperm selection has been suggested as a novel technique to check the viability of immotile spermatozoa. To assess viability with a laser, a direct shot is made to the tip of the sperm tail for approximately 2 ms, using 200 µJ of energy. Curling of the tail following the laser shot indicates that the sperm is viable and can therefore be selected for ICSI [102]. In 2004, for the first time, Aktan et al. reported the selection of viable testicular sperm using a laser system [103]. The viability percentages of the selected immotile spermatozoa were similar to those of HOST. However, compared with randomly selected spermatozoa, the authors reported that fertilization and take-home baby rates of laser-selected spermatozoa increased from 20% to 45% and 5% to 19%, respectively. Subsequently, pregnancy with viable but immotile sperm selected using the LA technique in ICSI was reported [104]. A healthy birth was also achieved with laser-selected immotile but living frozen/thawed spermatozoa [105]. Furthermore, live births were reported with LA selection of pentoxifylline-resistant immotile sperm in cases of Kartagener's Syndrome [106]. Thus, viable sperm selection using LA technology, which is simpler and faster than HOST and does not require the use of chemical agents, now allows immotile sperm to be cryostored in order to preserve fertility. Apart from the instrument cost and the need for experienced personnel, LA sperm selection is considered a promising method for the future [84].

2.10. Birefringence-Based Sperm Selection

Another new strategy proposed to distinguish healthy and viable sperm for use in ICSI is the birefringence-based selection technique. Birefringence is defined as the splitting of a light wave into two unequally reflected waves by an optically anisotropic medium. The orderly longitudinal orientation of the nucleoprotein filaments in the protoplasmic texture of the nucleus and acrosomal complex gives mature sperm a characteristic intrinsic birefringent appearance. By evaluating the birefringence of sperm heads with the use of polarized light microscopy, mature and viable sperm can be selected. When compared with spermatozoa selected with HOST, significantly higher pregnancy rates were found in TESE-ICSI cases in which birefringent-headed spermatozoa were used (11% vs. 45%) [107]. Similarly, Gianoroli et al. reported that implantation and pregnancy rates from ICSI cycles were significantly higher when testicular sperm selection was performed using the birefringent method compared to couples using conventionally selected sperm [108]. Although available results from birefringent-selected sperm appear to indicate a better option than conventional methods or HOST, currently, there are not enough existing studies to validate this [109]. Cost and equipment supply in clinical practice are other issues that require resolution.

2.11. Microfluidics-Assisted Sperm Sorting

Besides the aforementioned methods, one alternative to functional spermatozoa separation techniques from semen samples has been the use of microfluidics [110]. For this purpose, special devices have been designed in which seminal fluid and media flow simultaneously through a microscopic channel without a physical barrier between them [111]. Due to the unique characteristics of microfluidics, the motile sperm in the sample swim into the parallel-flowing media. A comparative study showed that microfluidic sorting of semen allows highly motile sperm selection with minimal DNA fragmentation compared to standard processing methods [112]. Unfortunately, few studies have examined the use of microfluidic systems for sperm selection in testicular cell suspensions. Recently, a new microfluidic system has been developed to facilitate rapid and efficient sperm isolation from TESE samples [113]. This system processes testicular tissue extract in two successive modules. The first module is a spiral microchannel that separates sperm from red blood cells and cellular debris through microfluidics using inertial forces. In the second module, excess media is removed by means of a hollow fiber membrane designed for mammalian cell isolation, thus enriching the suspension. This system yielded an 8-fold increase in sperm identification time due to the low output volume of the cell suspension and the almost complete elimination of non-sperm bio-particles. However, it remains to be explained whether there is sperm loss in microfluidic processing, especially in samples containing very rare spermatozoa. Loss of immotile but viable sperm can also be a disadvantage of this procedure. The promising initial results have yet to be confirmed by further studies in terms of clinical practice.

2.12. Raman Spectroscopy-Assisted Sperm Retrieval

Raman spectroscopy (RS) has been used as a feasible and reliable method for the identification of seminiferous tubules with spermatogenesis in testicular tissues from humans and rats [114–116]. RS is a laser-scattering technique that provides information about the internal structure of molecules through chemical fingerprints [117]. Although the available data indicate that RS may be useful in real-time intra-operative distinguishing of seminiferous tubules containing full spermatogenesis during microTESE, a special probe designed for this purpose has not yet been developed. In addition, further studies are needed to investigate the extent of laser-induced testicular tissue damage, confirm genetic safety, and optimize the technical parameters of this system. However, whether microscopy-assisted or combined with microfluidics, RS may be a promising diagnostic tool capable of detecting the molecular characteristics of sperm [118,119].

2.13. Fluorescence-Activated Cell Sorting (FACS)

FACS is based on the isolation of living spermatozoa labeled with fluorophore-conjugated antibodies from seminal fluid when irritated by a laser [120]. In a pilot study, testicular spermatozoa could be isolated using this technique in cases of NOA where sperm recovery could not be achieved in previous TESE attempts [121]. However, alterations in cell viability due to fluorophores and antibodies, the cost of the system, high cell loss, and its time-consuming nature are potential limiting factors for the use of FACS in testicular cell selection for ICSI [122].

Comparison of different methods for viable sperm recovery by TESE is shown in Table 4.

Table 4. Clinical outcomes of different methods for viable sperm recovery by TESE. NS: no significant.

Method	Comparison	Results	Refs.
HOST	Sperm morphology	Significantly higher fertilization 43.6% vs. 28.2%, pregnancy 27.3% vs. 5.7% and ongoing pregnancy 20.5% vs. 2.9%.	[79]
	Testicular vs. ejaculated spermatozoa	Fertilization 30.1% vs. 42.7% (NS), pregnancy 16.7% vs. 13.3% (NS) and delivery/ongoing pregnancy 8.3% vs. 6.7% (NS), respectively.	[80]
Sperm tail flexibility test	Motile vs. immotile sperm selected by the test	In frozen-thawed samples; fertilization 74.3% vs. 65.7%, and pregnancies three vs. two, respectively (NS). In fresh samples; fertilization 64.4% vs. 73.4%, and pregnancies nine vs. three, respectively (NS).	[94]
Laser-assisted sperm selection	Random sperm selection	Higher fertilization 45.4% vs. 20.4% $p < 0.0001$, cleavage 64.4% vs. 30.6% $p < 0.0001$, and take-home-baby rate 9.0% vs. 5.9%.	[103]
Sperm birefringence	Normal motility/morphology	Improved grade I/II embryo 71.2% vs. 63.4% and pregnancy 46.6% vs. 33.3%, respectively.	[107]
	Routine sperm selection	Improved pregnancy 58% vs. 18% $p = 0.053$, implantation 42.1% vs. 12.5% $p = 0.049$ and ongoing pregnancy 58% vs. 9% $p = 0.018$, respectively.	[108]
Microfluidics-assisted sperm sorting	Standard sample processing	Improved sperm yield 13.5 sperm per min vs. 1.52 sperm per min.	[113]
Fluorescence-activated cell sorting	Standard sample processing	Improved sperm recovery 50% vs. 38%, respectively.	[121]

2.14. Other Emerging Technologies for Predicting Spermatogenesis in the Testes

In addition to the testicular sperm extraction methods mentioned above, various other techniques have been attempted; they are expected to identify spermatogenesis foci precisely and rapidly but are not yet used in routine clinical practice. Multiphoton microscopy (MPM), based on low-energy infrared laser technology, is a technique that uses radiated energy as intracellular autofluorescence. A study in rats using an MPM laser showed that seminiferous tubules with or without sperm could be distinguished in real time depending on the differences in fluorescence [123]. The same group later found an 86% concordance between human testicular biopsy results and MPM diagnoses [124]. In another study, ex vivo testicular tissues from rats were imaged with full-field optical coherence tomography, which uses white light interference microscopy; thus, spermatogenesis within the seminiferous tubules could be identified without the use of contrast or a fixative [125]. Although these novel technologies represent a promising tool for predicting outcomes in cases of NOA, sperm functionality results have yet to be verified.

Although other techniques (e.g., annexin V magnetic-activated cell sorting, hyaluronic acid binding, Zeta method, and mechanisms based in sperm guidance) have also been used in the selection of ejaculated spermatozoa, their efficiency and safety for testicular sperm have not yet been investigated [126].

3. Cryopreservation of Surgically Retrieved Sperm for ICSI

Sperm can be retrieved with TESE in approximately 35–52% of men with NOA [127]; however, in cases where pregnancy cannot be achieved, repeated TESE in subsequent cycles does not ensure sperm retrieval in every case of NOA with the same success. Under such circumstances, sperm cryopreservation has made an important contribution to the medical and social rehabilitation of couples by protecting their fertility. Establishing that the length of the storage time in liquid nitrogen does not affect the quality of spermatozoa (or, consequently, the fertilization potential) has allowed the widespread practice of sperm cryopreservation [128].

3.1. Fresh vs. Frozen/Thawed TESE

Even though ICSI is traditionally performed using fresh sperm, ready-to-use spermatozoa may not always be available when the oocyte is picked up from the partner, especially if it requires harvesting from the testis. In this context, performing TESE one day before oocyte retrieval or using cryopreserved testicular sperm provides several advantages. First, since sperm can be frozen at any time, there is no need for synchronized OPU planning. Thus, scheduling ICSI cycles and freezing testicular sperm eliminates the risks of ovulation induction and the unnecessary cost of canceled cycles [75]. When TESE is not repeated, the extra expense of a new surgical intervention is also avoided. Moreover, in repeated ICSI cycles, the use of frozen residual spermatozoa from fresh TESE cycles prevents re-surgical trauma of the testicle. Cryopreservation of tissue samples taken with TESE also saves time for further treatment of women who are not eligible for implantation that day. For example, changes in endometrial receptivity have been demonstrated as a contributing factor in recurrent implantation failures [129]. Postponing the embryo transfer may give the woman an opportunity to prepare for the best time for implantation. Likewise, injury to the endometrium may also increase the success of implantation in subsequent cycles [130,131]. Other benefits of sperm cryopreservation are the availability of spermatozoa when ovarian stimulation begins and the opportunity to perform a programmed embryo biopsy to eliminate those with anomalies from ICSI [56], ensuring sperm storage before vasectomy, and making use of sperm banking and sperm donation [132,133]. However, simultaneous TESE on the day of OPU has the advantages of preventing sperm loss after thawing and avoiding sperm damage or loss of quality due to cryopreservation, as explained later [134]. Additionally, if sperm is retrieved successfully, the need for a second course of treatment is eliminated, as OPU and subsequent ICSI will be completed on the same day.

Nevertheless, in many studies, the use of cryopreserved testicular spermatozoa in ICSI has yielded results comparable to or better than those of fresh cycles [135–137]. When compared to those with fresh spermatozoa, the cumulative miscarriage rate was significantly lower [4% vs. 14.7%) and the cumulative live birth rate was significantly higher (34.7% vs. 16%) for ICSI cycles with frozen/thawed spermatozoa obtained during the previous fresh TESE [57]. Likewise, a recent meta-analysis showed that fertilization and pregnancy rates were similar when using fresh vs. frozen sperm from testicles, even in men with poor spermatogenesis [138]. In contrast, higher miscarriage rates and lower live birth rates were observed in patients who underwent ICSI cycles with cryopreserved spermatozoa vs. fresh spermatozoa from microTESE [139]. Similarly, in men with Klinefelter's syndrome, the use of fresh testicular sperm provided higher pregnancy rates than frozen sperm (60% vs. 25%) [140]. These differences may be due to male-related parameters, such as FSH concentration, testicular volumes, and degree of spermatogenesis defect, in addition to the number of testicular samplings, sperm preparation techniques, method of sperm selection, woman's preparation protocol, and experience of the assisted reproductive technology (ART) center [141]. Additionally, the retrospective designs of most studies, relatively small numbers of participants, and scarcely provided confounding factors limit the ability to achieve a definitive conclusion about fresh vs. frozen/thawed TESE. Overall, recent technological and methodological advances in sperm cryopreservation with minimal damage have allowed this option to be used safely and effectively in many ART attempts.

3.2. Whole Tissue or Isolated Spermatozoa

Experimental studies comparing the cryopreservation of germ cells after isolation or within testicular tissue showed that the latter provides a higher rate of cell survival and the tissue structure remains unchanged [142,143]. As a common use, cryostorage of testicular tissue as fragments after gentle mincing was found to be more effective for maintaining viability after thawing than cell suspension [144]. However, in humans, there is no consensus regarding the storage of post-TESE germ cells as whole tissue or cell solution. Although spermatozoa frozen in seminal fluid are more resistant to the freezing process than washed sperm [145], the progressive motility of the samples, whether with or without seminal plasma, did not change in sperm bank donations after long-term cryostorage [128]. Besides, in cases of NOA where the sperm number is very limited within testicular specimens, it is preferable to freeze the whole tissue samples intact, as minimal processing of the tissue may allow the sperm to better maintain their surveillance and motility after thawing [146,147]. According to a comparative study, there were no significant differences between ICSI cycles with fresh or testicular spermatozoa cryopreserved in whole tissue in terms of clinical pregnancy rates (26% and 27%, respectively) and delivery or ongoing pregnancy rates (21% and 9%, respectively) [148]. However, clinical results similar to those with fresh sperm were also obtained in cases in which a few isolated testicular spermatozoa were frozen in glycerol-containing cryopreservation medium [149]. Cryopreservation of isolated testicular spermatozoa in straws is a widely used method all over the world [19,148,150,151]. Regarding such storage, it has been suggested that fully filling a small-volume straw would provide better protection than filling a larger straw up halfway, as the negative effect of the partial volume is associated with free radicals and intratubular pressure as well as biological effects [128].

Storing testicular tissue samples from which spermatozoa can be retrieved provides the opportunity not only for use in subsequent ICSI cycles but also to perform both tissue and cell therapy for in vitro maturation of immature germ cells. Thus, cryostored tissue samples can be used for future testicular grafting or organ culture procedures as well as for testicular transplantation or in vitro maturation with germ cells isolated from the tissue. At the same time, the niche microenvironment formed by Sertoli, Leydig, peritubular, and somatic cells in the preserved testicular tissue allows germ cells to maintain their viability and function after thawing [152,153]. On the other hand, cryopreservation of homogenized isolated spermatogenic cell fractions has been shown to preserve cell viability more than whole testicular extracts [154]. This can be explained by the detrimental role of toxins in the tissue suspension, which are secreted by non-germ cells. However, according to the available data, it may be more efficient to store a small number of low-quality spermatozoa while preserving tissue support. Conversely, for spermatozoa retrieved in sufficient numbers and with excellent motility, cryostorage may be preferred after isolation. Nevertheless, the choice between cryopreservation with isolated cells or using whole tissue should be made based upon personal experience and the facilities of the institution. However, in cases where extremely few spermatozoa have been dealt with, sufficient data has not yet been collected to make a definite decision on which method is more effective. The experience gained from the use of novel technological resources in laboratory procedures will be the deciding factor for this issue.

3.3. Cryopreservation Methods

Cell survival after cryopreservation depends on how minimally intracellular ice crystals are formed. By using cryoprotectants and adjusting the freezing/warming rate, it is possible to reduce the amount of intracellular water and, eventually, ice formation. Different cryopreservation methods have been developed with different freezing rates, cryoprotectant concentrations, and temperature reductions. Conventional freezing is a manual storage technique using liquid nitrogen and can be done using fast or slow freezing methods or with a programmable freezer [155]. Vitrification is an ultra-fast method developed as an alternative to rapid freezing in nitrogen vapor [156]. Unlike the gradual cooling in the conventional freezing method, during vitrification, the sample is submerged directly and quickly in liquid nitrogen at −196 °C without being exposed to its vapor. A comparative study demonstrated that progressive sperm motility and vitality were higher after conventional rapid freezing than after vitrification, whereas vitrification was more successful if normal morphology was the criterion [157]. Despite the widespread preference of the conventional technique in ART clinics, vitrification is recommended as a fast, practical, and low-cost method [158,159]. Rapid freezing also prevents damage due to intracellular ice crystallization during cooling [160]. According to a recent meta-analysis on cryopreservation of spermatozoa, vitrification is superior to conventional freezing in terms of total and progressive motility, but the post-thawing DNA fragmentation index and morphology are similar for both methods. Although the most commonly used method for cryopreservation of samples from TESE is conventional rapid freezing in liquid nitrogen vapor [161], vitrification has also been encouraged, especially in the freezing of rare spermatozoa. Due to the absence of permeable cryoprotectants and the sudden exposure to cold, vitrification has become advantageous in the storage of surgically retrieved spermatozoa concentrated in very small volumes [162]. Limited numbers of studies with NOA cases have reported healthy pregnancies in ICSI cycles using testicular spermatozoa frozen by vitrification [151,163,164]. For this purpose, specially designed tools have been developed that can allow freezing of a small number of spermatozoa [165]. Spis et al. compared the results of TESE spermatozoa cryopreserved by conventional freezing with those frozen using cryoprotectant and cryoprotectant-free vitrification methods [163]. They vitrified spermatozoa in 50-µL plastic capillaries in culture medium with 0.25 M sucrose. After a capillary was placed in a straw, it was plunged into liquid nitrogen and cooled at 600 °C/min. When thawed, the motility of small volumes of vitrified spermatozoa was found to be significantly higher than that of spermatozoa frozen using the conventional method (8.0% vs. 0.6%). The vitrification-in-straws method has also yielded highly efficient results in the cryopreservation of human testicular diploid germ cells in terms of recovery and viability [166]. However, the efficiency of vitrification varies depending on protocol and sperm quality. The roles of slow-programmable freezing [167], ultra-rapid freezing [168], solid-surface vitrification [169], and cryoprotectant-free freezing [170] on the molecular and structural effects of cooling have been further investigated in other studies.

3.4. Choosing the Proper Cryoprotectant

Another important factor that can determine sperm retrieval efficiency and quality in cryopreservation is the protectant used. In addition to permeable cryoprotectants such as glycerol, dimethyl sulfoxide (DMSO), dimethyl acetaldehyde, propylene glycol, ethylene glycol, and 1,2-propanediol, which are routinely used in cryopreservation, non-permeable agents—glucose, sucrose, egg yolk citrate, albumin, polyethylene glycol, and trehalose—have also been validated for use [171,172]. Pregnancy has been achieved for decades with frozen/thawed testicular spermatozoa using glycerol as a cryoprotectant [173,174]. Although experimental studies have shown the protective effect of glycerol on sperm structure to be better than that of dimethyl sulfoxide (DMSO) [175], Keros et al. recommended DMSO as an ideal penetrating agent if permeable protectants are to be used in cryopreservation of testicular specimens [176]. Additionally, compared to glycerol DMSO was found to be the most effective protectant in cryostorage of immature testicular samples [144]. In fact, immature testis tissue was demonstrated to be more susceptible to cryoprotectant toxicity with cell-specific sensitivity. However, when human testicular tissue was stored separately in DMSO, 1,2-propanediol, ethylene glycol, or glycerol using the slow freezing method, 52% to 58% of the cells remained alive, indicating that the selection of cryoprotectant did not affect viability after thawing [177]. However, the use of testicular samples with normal spermatogenesis and the lack of recovered cell numbers limit the interpretation of these results. Furthermore, different results have also been reported with regard to the cryoprotectant selection depending on the patient's age, the agents being compared, and the procedure used [144].

Since permeable protectants easily pass through the cell membrane, they form an osmotic gradient that draws water out of the cell, thereby preventing the formation of intracellular ice crystals [162]. However, these reactions can have toxic effects on the sperm plasma membrane due to lipid peroxidation as well as the stress created during processing [178]. In contrast, non-permeable cryoprotectants cannot pass through the cell membrane due to their high molecular weight, and extracellular solute accumulation allows the intracellular water to be discharged; thus, dehydration occurs in the cell. Medrano et al. reported the first birth of a healthy infant following ICSI using the permeable cryoprotectant-free sperm vitrification protocol [179]. Furthermore, the use of non-penetrating cryoprotectants at low concentrations has also pioneered the design of minimal-sized carriers to reduce fluctuations in cell volume, thus initiating a new era in the storage of small volume sperm obtained from TESE material. Subsequently, Spis et al. reported better sperm quality in epididymis and TESE spermatozoa when they used the cryoprotectant-free vitrification method compared to the conventional method using permeable cryoprotectants, and ICSI with cryoprotectant-free vitrified spermatozoa resulted in delivery of healthy babies [151]. Similarly, sperm droplets frozen on cryoloops showed that the motility of vitrified spermatozoa in the absence of cryoprotectant was not different from that of conventional freezing with protectants and did not affect DNA integrity [180]. In current practice, low chemical toxicity and limited osmotic shock have made non-penetrating cryoprotectants a feasible option for testicular sperm storage. As an alternative, combining two different protectants can reduce the marked toxic effects of cryoprotectants [180,181]. For this purpose, loading a small number of spermatozoa on a cryoloop in a 50:50 mixture of test yolk buffer with glycerol and modified human tubal fluid medium supplemented with 6% Plasmanate was shown to preserve sperm viability and function [182]. Various protectant mixtures have been investigated to reduce the concentration of compounds in order to ensure their maximum efficiency without reaching toxic levels [165].

3.5. Cryopreservation of Very Few Spermatozoa

In some TESE cases, despite all efforts, only an extremely small number of sperms can be extracted. Such situations pose a serious problem—namely, the loss of the few sperms after freezing/thawing processes [41,135]. There is an ongoing effort to develop optimized freezing protocols and effective technologies that will shorten the post-thaw search time and minimize sperm loss. However, current technologies have given patients with NOA the opportunity to retain their fertility by implementing cryopreservation of even a single sperm [165]. Freezing in microstraws was proposed as an option for the cryostorage of few spermatozoa. After thawing, microstraw samples reached a significantly higher rate of sperm motility than the traditional straw samples [183]. As microstraws are thinner and a very small volume of medium is loaded, this method allows faster freezing. Likewise, Desai et al. isolated motile spermatozoa individually with an ICSI needle, loaded them into a capillary tube, and then carefully inserted the tube into the outer straw [184]. Samples were frozen using the conventional method by plunging into liquid nitrogen. The post-thaw recovery rate ranged from 33% to 100%, and pregnancy was successful. In experimental studies, sperm vitrification in straws was demonstrated to preserve motility better than the spheres method where permeable cryoprotectants were not used [185].

In extreme cases, storage in empty zona, non-biological carriers, or vitrification devices has also been suggested for freezing and storing lone or very few sperm cells. A novel option for preserving only a few spermatozoa is to reduce the volume of cryoprotectant-added media and ensure efficient identification after thawing. For this purpose, the insertion of spermatozoa into encapsulated porous capsules has been suggested to allow easy visualization and manipulation during cryopreservation processes. It was shown that oocyte zona pellucida (ZP) can be used as a vehicle following removal of cellular material. Subsequently, empty ZPs prepared from humans and mice were used as frozen vectors in experimental studies [165,186,187]. Walmsley et al. reported the first live human birth associated with this procedure using testicular sperm [188]. Although an animal ZP is a biological carrier, it has not been widely used due to its low availability and bioethical issues as well as procedural problems (e.g., the risks of residual host DNA fragments and foreign DNA transfer and impaired sperm quality due to an artificially induced acrosome reaction) [186]. As a solution to the constraints of human oocyte use, algae Volvox globator spheres offered a promising approach to the cryopreservation of a single motile sperm, but the possibility of foreign DNA transfer was questionable [189]. With the encouragement of these studies, fabricated non-biological carriers, such as alginic acid capsules [190], agarose capsules [191], and hyaluronan-phenolic hydroxyl microcapsules [192], have also been developed as empty capsules for single-sperm freezing. However, empty capsules are not widely used due to the complexity of their fabrication and problems associated with their storage.

Although non-biological spheres give hope for future use due to their low toxicity, lack of ethical problems, and acceptable post-thawing motile sperm retrieval and survival results, the lack of existing clinical outcomes makes it difficult to reach a definitive conclusion. Recently, non-labor, non-biological, bioethically acceptable, and inexpensive commercialized alternative devices have been designed for the cryopreservation of a small number of spermatozoa. The Cryotop device developed for this purpose is formed by inserting a fine polypropylene strip on which sperm droplets are placed into a cover straw [193]. Recently, Ohno et al. evaluated the efficiency of cryopreservation of three or fewer spermatozoa loaded on the Cryotop using a modified permeable cryoprotectant-free vitrification method [194]. Clinical pregnancies resulting from vitrified spermatozoa from the ejaculate, fresh spermatozoa from the ejaculate, and vitrified spermatozoa from the testis were found at similar rates (25%, 24%, and 16%, respectively). Only the sperm survival rate and the oocyte fertilization rate were found to be significantly lower in attempts using vitrified spermatozoa from the testis compared with vitrified spermatozoa from the ejaculate. The researchers concluded that this technique was particularly effective for the cryopreservation of samples with fewer than 10 testicular spermatozoa. Cryoloops represent another efficient and non-labor-intensive method for the cryopreservation of individual spermatozoa [195]. With the aid of micromanipulator equipment, selected spermatozoa loaded onto an open cryoloop are enclosed in a vial and stored in liquid nitrogen. After loading 5–10 spermatozoa into each loop, total recovery and post-thaw survival rates were reported as 68% and 70%, respectively [182]. Individual testicular spermatozoa cryopreserved on cryoloops have also been shown to successfully fertilize oocytes [196]. Although open systems allow rapid cooling, direct exposure of semen to liquid nitrogen poses a potential risk of contamination [159]. Another closed system developed for sperm cryopreservation is the Cell Sleeper. Initially, the recovery and viability rates of individually vitrified spermatozoa using the Cell Sleeper were reported as 100% and 72%, respectively [194]. In this method, individual spermatozoa are transferred into freezing medium on an inner tray with a micromanipulator needle. Once the tray is placed in a vial, the cap is screwed on and it is immersed in liquid nitrogen. In a case of NOA, the authors reported that when ICSI was performed with spermatozoa frozen using the Cell Sleeper, five out of six oocytes were fertilized, resulting in the birth of a healthy baby [193]. Likewise, various carrier devices based on the same principle, such as Cryolock [197], Cryoleaf [198], Cryopiece [199], and SpermVD [163], have also been designed and applied in vitrification.

During the thawing of the vitrified samples, the warm-up speed should be high so that the frozen water inside spermatozoa can switch to the liquid phase without crystallization. The optimal thawing temperature to maintain membrane integrity and sperm function is still the subject of investigation. Depending on the methodological differences used in vitrification, temperatures ranging from 37 °C to 44 °C have been attempted [157,200,201]. However, there are limited cohort studies evaluating the sperm retrieval, fertilization, and pregnancy rates of these methods in IVF following cryopreservation. Moreover, the need for skilled personnel in handling the devices and the prolonged time of the laboratory processes have restricted the routine use of manufactured carriers. Although the fact that these novel devices can store a single spermatozoon has met an important need with respect to the management of patients with NOA, further research confirming their feasibility and efficiency is needed to adapt these systems for clinical practice.

3.6. Drawbacks of Sperm Cryopreservation

To some extent, cooling, thawing, and exposure to cryoprotectants may cause destructive changes to sperm function and structure [135]. Most importantly, in cases of NOA, post-thawing viability may be reduced significantly, since sperms obtained by TESE have reduced resistance to mechanical, thermal, and osmotic stress due to structural or functional defects [202]. For this reason, if very few spermatozoa were found in the initial search, the possibility of their disappearance after thawing (and, consequently, cancellation of the ICSI cycle) may be encountered. Up to a two-fold increase in the number of immotile sperm was found in frozen samples [137,203]. Sperm motility has also been shown to decrease from 50% in fresh semen to 7% in frozen/thawed samples [46]. Additionally, the broken neck abnormality observed after thawing is related to damaged centriole structure due to cryoinjury, causing fertilization failure in ICSI [19]. Quality impairment of frozen/thawed sperm is mostly attributed to DNA damage, which determines embryo quality and viability [204]. In fact, in cases of TESE, decreased concentration and reduced mitochondrial activity, as well as a significant increase in DNA fragmentation and reactive oxygen species (ROS) production, were reported in post-thawed sperms in comparison to freshly recovered samples [155]. Generation of ROS during sperm cryopreservation may damage many cellular components (e.g., membrane, cytoskeleton, DNA, and mitochondria), resulting in loss of function and genomic instability [205]. Thus, the decrease in sperm competence caused by excessive intracellular oxidative stress is accompanied by impaired fertilization and poor embryo development [206]. Although it is widely accepted that the freezing process causes remarkable changes in sperm parameters, the effects of various techniques may differ [207,208]. For example, in comparison to slow programmable freezing, rapid freezing has been found to be more advantageous in terms of post-thawing motility and cryosurvival [209]. With this knowledge, the advantages and disadvantages of each cryopreservation method should be evaluated on an individual basis.

When evaluating the drawbacks of cryopreservation, one should also take into account the functional capacity of sperm retrieved from the testicles, which are the products of defective spermatogenesis. Freezing of low-quality testicular specimens containing non-motile spermatozoa or spermatozoa with poor morphology has demonstrated a negative impact on embryo quality [210]. Moreover, Wu et al. showed that many sperms obtained from the testicles remained in the immature stage and the spermatozoa carried cytoplasmic droplets in the neck and mid-piece [41]. In fact, when compared with ejaculated sperm, miscarriage rates were found to be higher in cases of ICSI using testicular sperm. Chromosomal aneuploidy is more likely to be encountered in testicular sperm from patients with NOA [211,212]. Moreover, cryopreservation of testicular cells or tissues poses the risk of the presence of residual cancer cells during the transplantation of autologous cells in patients scheduled for oncotherapy, which may trigger the disease [153]. However, the absence of such a risk, at least in experimental studies, has been demonstrated by the lack of increase in cancer incidence or survival reduction after testicular transplantation of propagated spermatogonial stem cells (SSCs) [213]. Furthermore, the contamination risk of frozen sperm samples has not yet been completely resolved. The source of contamination may be the sample itself or the infected frozen carrier, liquid nitrogen, or storage tank. As single-sperm cryopreservation is performed with a more controlled technique, particularly in closed systems, a potentially reduced risk of contamination is expected [165].

Notably, in recent decades, some environmental, occupational, and lifestyle-related risk factors have accompanied the declining trend in semen quality through certain genetic and metabolic pathways whose exact causes have not been fully elucidated [214]. Therefore, when interpreting IVF results of fresh vs. frozen sperm, the quality of the sperm chosen for injection into the oocyte and the presence of DNA damage should be considered as the deciding factors. These parameters may also have potential impacts on the consistency of the results. Indeed, unlike in the aforementioned studies, Semião-Francisco et al. reported that the pregnancy and miscarriage rates of sperm taken from the testicles, whether in obstructive or NOA cases, did not differ significantly [215]. Likewise, pregnancy rates remained similar whether frozen or fresh TESE samples were used (32.1% and 35.7%, respectively; $p = 0.62$) and did not show a significant correlation with the use of motile or immotile sperm (46.3% and 66.7%, respectively; $p = 0.59$) [216]. Regarding the inconsistencies between results, a methodological analysis evaluating the success of TESE results in men with NOA emphasized the current lack of knowledge, especially regarding the quantity and quality of sperm retrieved [217]. Recently, OMICS technologies such as genomics, transcriptomics, proteomics, and metabolomics, in combination with advanced bioinformatics technology (e.g., Illumina RNA sequencing, high-throughput next-generation sequencing, multiplexed enzyme-linked immunosorbent assays), have provided an extensive opportunity for research on how cryopreservation affects sperm structure and function [218]. Nevertheless, no matter how few sperm can be retrieved, it has been suggested that cryopreservation should be considered as a feasible method in every surgical sperm retrieval case [148]. Beyond all, carefully and accurately recording data and respecting ethical considerations and legal regulations are also essential steps to maintaining trust.

3.7. Minimizing the Harmful Effects of Cryopreservation

When it comes to dealing with cellular damage due to cryopreservation, recent nanotechnological trends are promising [219]. Due to their unique physical and chemical nature as well as their low toxicity, nanoparticles can increase the absorption and bioavailability of protective ingredients by spermatozoa. Supplementation of the tris-based SHOTOR™ extender with zinc and selenium nanoparticles was shown to enhance sperm progressive motility, vitality, and membrane integrity after cryopreservation by reducing apoptosis and lipid peroxidation [220]. Similarly, in testes, the use of nanoparticles containing necrosis-inhibitory factors greatly improved tissue integrity and survival of germ cells [221]. Artificial or natural nanovesicles, such as liposomes and exosomes, are also promising measures for protecting sperm from the harmful consequences of freezing and thawing [222]. After exosomes are secreted from the cell, they are taken in by the target cells and transfer their protein and RNA contents to those cells. In experimental studies, seminal plasma and mesenchymal stem cell-derived exosomes have been shown to improve the quality of frozen/thawed spermatozoa [223,224]. A liposome is an artificially manufactured, exosome-like, spherical nanovesicle with a lipid bilayer that can transfer cryoprotectant contents to a spermatozoon by fusing with the sperm plasma membrane [225]. In animal studies, liposomes were shown to increase sperm motility and viability, strengthen the membrane structure, and improve fertility [226]. Likewise, testicular experimental studies involving gene technology have shown that knockout serum replacement (KSR) supplement, a chemically defined medium, provides a cryoprotective effect comparable to that of conventional sera but more consistent in quality [227]. The beneficial effects of using antioxidants in seminal plasma (but not yet in testicular tissue) on sperm parameters and

ROS production during the freeze/thaw process were widely discussed in a systematic review and meta-analysis by Bahmyari et al. [228]. The addition of exogenous antioxidants into the freezing medium may ameliorate sperm damage by reducing the oxidative stress caused by cryopreservation. For frozen semen, resveratrol, lycopene, vitamin E, and quercetin are the most commonly used agents to protect sperm from ROS damage [229,230]. However, further studies are needed to evaluate how nanoparticles and additives affect clinical practice outcomes and embryo development when used for small numbers of poor-quality testicular spermatozoa.

4. Processing Immature Germ Cells

Despite extensive searching, mature spermatozoa can be obtained with TESE in only approximately 40% to 60% of cases of NOA for use in ICSI [231,232]. In the remaining cases, round spermatids were attempted as a last resort, although until recently, the results were not satisfactory enough to encourage routine practice [233]. However, in 2015, Tanaka et al. reported 14 healthy babies born with round spermatid injection (ROSI) in oocytes previously activated by electric current; 3 years later, from the 2-year follow-up results of 90 ROSI babies, it was determined that round spermatids enabled patients with NOA to have their own genetic offspring [23,234]. Subsequently, Papuccu et al. reported their results of 472 couples who underwent 904 cycles using elongating (Sb2) spermatids for the ROSI technique and achieved a 9.6% ongoing pregnancy rate [235]. Since transformation of immature germ cells into spermatozoa with fully developed flagella has had limited success in in vitro experiments, culturing samples to achieve at least haploid round spermatids may have wider clinical application [236].

If testicular tissue samples from TESE do not contain spermatozoa, various approaches have been described for in vitro maturation of early stage germ cells. For in vitro maturation, either (1) testicular tissue is used in whole pieces while preserving its three-dimensional (3D) structure or (2) after isolation and purification, different cell types are exposed to culture conditions in which the spermatogenic process is recreated. In TESE-negative cases, it makes sense to try culturing small fragments of testicular tissue or intact pieces of tubules first. However, since the limited diffusion rates of the tissue do not allow tissue viability to be maintained over a long period, it is challenging to culture the tissue as a whole. After long-standing efforts, in 2011, Sato et al. reported healthy offspring from haploid cells developed from testicular fragments cultured on agarose gel in modified Minimum Essential Medium (α-MEM) supplemented with knockout serum replacement [237]. Others have also shown culturing of frozen/thawed testicular tissue on agarose gel to restore spermatogenesis up to haploid spermatids, leading to offspring [238]. Furthermore, from seminiferous tubule segments cultured in chitosan hydrogel bioreactors, the development of spermatids and spermatozoa were achieved on days 34 and 55, respectively [239]. In another organotypic culture system described for human immature testicular tissue, germ cells were shown to differentiate up to round spermatids within 16 days [240]. However, the inability of organ culture systems to restore spermatogenesis in cryopreserved human testicular specimens has also been reported [241]. These contradictions in results may be due to the fact that culture methods are not yet fully optimized or that the nature of subcellular defects is different [242]. Later, developed microfluidic technology further improved organotypic culture systems, allowing ex vivo sustainability of the structure and viability of germ cells in testicular tissue for producing mature sperm [243]. As an option for in vitro maturation of isolated germ cells, 2D culture systems have been developed to support enzymatically digested testicular cell suspensions. In 2D cultures, isolated SSCs are maintained either on feeder cells or on mixed cell populations co-cultured with somatic cells [244]. Different feeders, including SIM mouse embryo-derived thioguanine and ouabain resistant (STO), mouse embryonic fibroblast, bovine Sertoli cells and laminin-coated plate were used to support spermatogenesis [245]. Apart from feeders, different culture systems, such as human amnion mesenchymal stem cells [246], in vitro reprogramming of fibroblasts to human induced Sertoli-like cells [247], and isolated cell culture with growth factor supplementation [248], have been defined to support in vitro spermatogenesis. Nevertheless, 2D culture systems provided in vitro restoration of spermatogenesis and supported the development of haploid spermatids with fertilization potential [249]. Experiences gained from previous studies ultimately led to the development of artificially constructed 3D structures [250]. By creating structures that mimic the composition of the main testicular components, 3D cultures allow immature germ cells to be reconstructed similarly to their original tissue architecture, thereby allowing further maturation [251–254]. Although this system has the ability to direct the differentiation of germ cells, microenvironmental conditions favorable for complete maturation must also be achieved.

In addition to attempting complex and intricate methods for in vitro maturation of immature germ cells from testicular tissue, there is a need for simple methods that can be used more easily in clinical practice. When Aslam et al. compared suspensions of mixed cell populations and isolated homogeneous populations of spermatogenic cells prepared from testicular tissue, they showed that most of the isolated round spermatids developed tails and remained intact and viable for 72 h in modified Eagle's minimum essential medium with no hormonal supplementation [154]. However, since they used a mixture of obstructive and non-obstructive tissue samples, the contribution of in vitro culturing to the development of flagella in immature germ cells in cases of NOA is not clear. Similarly, it has been shown that human round spermatids can mature up to spermatozoa when cocultured on Vero cell monolayers [255]. Other researchers have also verified the maturation of primary spermatocytes into haploid spermatids through in vitro coculture with Vero cells [256]. Subsequently, round spermatids generated from human SSCs were shown to fertilize mouse oocytes [248]. However, even without a co-culture, in vitro hormonal supplementation has been demonstrated to be capable of providing sufficient support to mature premeiotic germ cells [257]. Thus, culturing testicular samples from patients with NOA in medium containing recombinant FSH and testosterone for 48 h transformed FISH-proven primary spermatocytes into mature round spermatids, after which injection into the oocyte resulted in healthy offspring [258]. It has been shown that hormones added to in vitro culture medium in cases of NOA not only accelerate spermiogenesis but also improve apoptosis-related cell damage in enhancing the reproductive performance of germ cells [259]. Contrary to most studies indicating that FSH and testosterone added to testicular culture media play a role in the development of different stages of in vitro spermatogenesis, it has also been suggested that their supplementation does not induce meiotic and post-meiotic cells and therefore cannot differentiate premeiotic germ cells [260]. Differences in germ cell development in in vitro maturation studies may be due to insufficient support of established culture conditions. The maintenance of healthy spermatogenesis from SSCs can only be achieved with the support of a complicated and precise "niche" microenvironment [261]. Sertoli cells establish the most important component of the "niche," and by producing growth factors and cytokines, they regulate proper self-renewing and differentiation of SSCs, transition to meiosis, and, finally, differentiation of round spermatids into spermatozoa [262].

Under proper culture conditions, reaggregation of Sertoli cells forms organized monolayer structures. Therefore, in most of the in vitro maturation studies performed on testicular tissue samples, a co-culture with Sertoli cells has been used effectively to provide structural and nutritional support for differentiation of germ cells [263–265]. In the co-culture of round spermatids and Sertoli cells, it has been shown that supplementation with recombinant FSH and testosterone contributes significantly to the differentiation of round spermatids into elongating spermatids [266]. However, other studies have also reported that no matter how much FSH stimulation in organotypic cultures of immature testicular tissue increases the percentage of premeiotic cells, it does not allow for further maturation [242]. Some similar studies have also confirmed that FSH supplementation in cultures does not support post-meiotic maturation [267]. Actually, the underlying mechanism for the contradictions in the reports may be the impaired ability of testes to respond to the endogenous hormonal milieu due to compromised androgen receptor and FSH receptor (FSHR) signaling pathways [268]. In fact, when compared to obstructive azoospermia, the FSHR expression level in isolated and purified Sertoli cell cultures was found to be 2.7 times lower in the NOA group; hence, it has been claimed that there may be an altered Sertoli cell response to in vitro FSH stimulation [269]. Alternatively, without the need for hormone supplementation, spermatogenesis from testicular SSCs to fertility-competent sperm formation could be induced in organ cultures using different techniques [270,271]. Considering this fact, before choosing a method to be used in co-culture studies with Sertoli cells, it is important to investigate the hormone/receptor interaction along with the response to FSH and testosterone.

To date, a number of studies have been conducted on the development of many different culture systems, with varying levels of success. Furthermore, with their innovations in in vitro germ cell maturation, advanced technology products created in the field of regenerative medicine using cell/tissue culture, biomaterials, and bioactive products have become promising treatment alternatives for patients with NOA [272,273]. However, before suggesting potential clinical uses of haploid male gametes exposed to in vitro manipulations, further analyses of fecundity, epigenetic consequences, and safety are essential.

5. Conclusions

The primary outcome associated with the efficiency of ARTs is successful, healthy live births. In addition to allowing only a small amount of sperm retrieval, cases of NOA require a more demanding process in the treatment of infertility due to the fact that the available sperm are also products of impaired spermatogenesis. The whole process begins with collection of the highest-quality surgical specimens possible. Following microTESE, with its verified efficacy, researchers have attempted sophisticated techniques such as Raman spectroscopy, multiphoton microscopy, and full field optical coherence tomography to identify testicular tubules with spermatogenesis. As further developments, laser-assisted sperm selection and microfluidic systems appear to be promising for extracting viable spermatozoa from surgically removed testicular samples. Moreover, there is an ongoing effort to develop optimized freezing protocols and effective technologies that will allow patients with NOA to retain their fertility by implementing cryopreservation of even a single sperm. However, the initial promising results of all of these developments must be confirmed by large studies in the context of clinical practice. The use of nanoparticles for in vitro maturation of germ cells is also another promising innovation, as it will allow previously unsuccessful patients with NOA to have children using their own biological material. Undoubtedly, the clinical consequences of all of these manipulations that could result from potential changes in the offspring's genomes must be followed very carefully.

Author Contributions: K.A.: Conceptualization, investigation, methodology, software, data curation, writing—original draft preparation, writing—review and editing, validation; O.S.A.: Conceptualization, investigation, resources, visualization, supervision, project administration. All authors have read and agreed to the published version of the manuscript.

Funding: This research received no external funding.

Institutional Review Board Statement: Not applicable.

Informed Consent Statement: Not applicable.

Data Availability Statement: The data presented in this study are openly available in PubMed, PubMed Central (PMC) https://pubmed.ncbi.nlm.nih.gov/.

Conflicts of Interest: The authors declare no conflict of interest.

References

1. Deruyver, Y.; Vanderschueren, D.; Van der Aa, F. Outcome of microdissection TESE compared with conventional TESE in non-obstructive azoospermia: A systematic review. *Andrology* **2014**, *2*, 20–24. [CrossRef]
2. Meng, M.V.; Cha, I.; Ljung, B.M.; Turek, P.J. Testicular fine-needle aspiration in infertile men: Correlation of cytologic pattern with biopsy histology. *Am. J. Surg. Pathol.* **2001**, *25*, 71–79. [CrossRef]
3. Ubaldi, F.; Nagy, Z.; Liu, J.; Tournaye, H.; Camus, M.; Smitz, J.; Liebaers, I.; Devroey, P.; Van Steirteghem, A. A survey of four years of experience with intracytoplasmic sperm injection. *Acta Eur. Fertil.* **1995**, *26*, 7–11.
4. Schlegel, P.N. Testicular sperm extraction: Microdissection improves sperm yield with minimal tissue excision. *Hum. Reprod.* **1999**, *14*, 131–135. [CrossRef] [PubMed]
5. Amer, M.; Ateyah, A.; Hany, R.; Zohdy, W. Prospective comparative study between microsurgical and conventional testicular sperm extraction in non-obstructive azoospermia: Follow-up by serial ultrasound examinations. *Hum. Reprod.* **2000**, *15*, 653–656. [CrossRef]
6. Okada, H.; Dobashi, M.; Yamazaki, T.; Hara, I.; Fujisawa, M.; Arakawa, S.; Kamidono, S. Conventional versus microdissection testicular sperm extraction for nonobstructive azoospermia. *J. Urol.* **2002**, *168*, 1063–1067. [CrossRef]
7. Westlander, G. Utility of micro-TESE in the most severe cases of non-obstructive azoospermia. *Ups J. Med. Sci.* **2020**, *125*, 99–103. [CrossRef]
8. Colpi, G.M.; Colpi, E.M.; Piediferro, G.; Giacchetta, D.; Gazzano, G.; Castiglioni, F.M.; Magli, M.C.; Gianaroli, L. Microsurgical TESE versus conventional TESE for ICSI in non-obstructive azoospermia: A randomized controlled study. *Reprod. Biomed. Online* **2009**, *18*, 315–319. [CrossRef]
9. Silber, S.J.; Van Steirteghem, A.C.; Liu, J.; Nagy, Z.; Tournaye, H.; Devroey, P. High fertilization and pregnancy rate after intracytoplasmic sperm injection with spermatozoa obtained from testicle biopsy. *Hum. Reprod.* **1995**, *10*, 148–152. [CrossRef]
10. Edirisinghe, W.R.; Junk, S.M.; Matson, P.L.; Yovich, J.L. Changes in motility patterns during in-vitro culture of fresh and frozen/thawed testicular and epididymal spermatozoa: Implications for planning treatment by intracytoplasmic sperm injection. *Hum. Reprod.* **1996**, *11*, 2474–2476. [CrossRef]
11. Liu, J.; Tsai, Y.L.; Katz, E.; Compton, G.; Garcia, J.E.; Baramki, T.A. Outcome of in-vitro culture of fresh and frozen-thawed human testicular spermatozoa. *Hum. Reprod.* **1997**, *12*, 1667–1672. [CrossRef]
12. Allan, J.A.; Cotman, A.S. A new method for freezing testicular biopsy sperm: Three pregnancies with sperm extracted from cryopreserved sections of seminiferous tubule. *Fertil. Steril.* **1997**, *68*, 741–744. [CrossRef]
13. Popal, W.; Nagy, Z.P. Laboratory processing and intracytoplasmic sperm injection using epididymal and testicular spermatozoa: What can be done to improve outcomes? *Clinics (Sao Paulo)* **2013**, *68* (Suppl. 1), 125–130. [CrossRef]
14. Pousette, A.; Akerlöf, E.; Rosenborg, L.; Fredricsson, B. Increase in progressive motility and improved morphology of human spermatozoa following their migration through Percoll gradients. *Int. J. Androl.* **1986**, *9*, 1–13. [CrossRef]
15. Verheyen, G.; Popovic-Todorovic, B.; Tournaye, H. Processing and selection of surgically-retrieved sperm for ICSI: A review. *Basic Clin. Androl.* **2017**, *27*, 6. [CrossRef]
16. Verheyen, G.; De Croo, I.; Tournaye, H.; Pletincx, I.; Devroey, P.; van Steirteghem, A.C. Comparison of four mechanical methods to retrieve spermatozoa from testicular tissue. *Hum. Reprod.* **1995**, *10*, 2956–2959. [CrossRef]
17. Crabbé, E.; Verheyen, G.; Tournaye, H.; Van Steirteghem, A. Freezing of testicular tissue as a minced suspension preserves sperm quality better than whole-biopsy freezing when glycerol is used as cryoprotectant. *Int. J. Androl.* **1999**, *22*, 43–48. [CrossRef]
18. Haimov-Kochman, R.; Imbar, T.; Lossos, F.; Nefesh, I.; Zentner, B.S.; Moz, Y.; Prus, D.; Bdolah, Y.; Hurwitz, A. Technical modification of testicular sperm extraction expedites testicular sperm retrieval. *Fertil. Steril.* **2009**, *91*, 281–284. [CrossRef]
19. Verheyen, G.; Nagy, Z.; Joris, H.; De Croo, I.; Tournaye, H.; Van Steirteghem, A. Quality of frozen-thawed testicular sperm and its preclinical use for intracytoplasmic sperm injection into in vitro-matured germinal-vesicle stage oocytes. *Fertil. Steril.* **1997**, *67*, 74–80. [CrossRef]
20. Yazdinejad, F.; Heydari, L.; Motamed Zadeh, L.; Seifati, S.M.; Agha-Rahimi, A. Application of erythrocyte lysing buffer (ELB) has detrimental effects on human sperm quality parameters, DNA fragmentation and chromatin structure. *Andrologia* **2020**, *52*, e13702. [CrossRef]
21. Ball, B.A. Oxidative stress, osmotic stress and apoptosis: Impacts on sperm function and preservation in the horse. *Anim. Reprod. Sci.* **2008**, *107*, 257–267. [CrossRef] [PubMed]
22. Soygur, B.; Celik, S.; Celik-Ozenci, C.; Sati, L. Effect of erythrocyte-sperm separation medium on nuclear, acrosomal, and membrane maturity parameters in human sperm. *J. Assist. Reprod. Genet.* **2018**, *35*, 491–501. [CrossRef] [PubMed]
23. Tanaka, A.; Nagayoshi, M.; Takemoto, Y.; Tanaka, I.; Kusunoki, H.; Watanabe, S.; Kuroda, K.; Takeda, S.; Ito, M.; Yanagimachi, R. Fourteen babies born after round spermatid injection into human oocytes. *Proc. Natl. Acad. Sci. USA* **2015**, *112*, 14629–14634. [CrossRef] [PubMed]
24. Goswami, G.; Singh, S.; Devi, M.G. Successful fertilization and embryo development after spermatid injection: A hope for nonobstructive azoospermic patients. *J. Hum. Reprod. Sci.* **2015**, *8*, 175–177. [CrossRef] [PubMed]
25. Chemes, H.; Cigorraga, S.; Bergadá, C.; Schteingart, H.; Rey, R.; Pellizzari, E. Isolation of human Leydig cell mesenchymal precursors from patients with the androgen insensitivity syndrome: Testosterone production and response to human chorionic gonadotropin stimulation in culture. *Biol. Reprod.* **1992**, *46*, 793–801. [CrossRef] [PubMed]

26. Salzbrunn, A.; Benson, D.M.; Holstein, A.F.; Schulze, W. A new concept for the extraction of testicular spermatozoa as a tool for assisted fertilization (ICSI). *Hum. Reprod.* **1996**, *11*, 752–755. [CrossRef]
27. Fischer, R.; Baukloh, V.; Naether, O.G.; Schulze, W.; Salzbrunn, A.; Benson, D.M. Pregnancy after intracytoplasmic sperm injection of spermatozoa extracted from frozen-thawed testicular biopsy. *Hum. Reprod.* **1996**, *11*, 2197–2199. [CrossRef]
28. Crabbé, E.; Verheyen, G.; Tournaye, H.; Van Steirteghem, A. The use of enzymatic procedures to recover testicular germ cells. *Hum. Reprod.* **1997**, *12*, 1682–1687. [CrossRef]
29. Hadley, M.A.; Dym, M. Immunocytochemistry of extracellular matrix in the lamina propria of the rat testis: Electron microscopic localization. *Biol. Reprod.* **1987**, *37*, 1283–1289. [CrossRef]
30. Siu, M.K.; Lee, W.M.; Cheng, C.Y. The interplay of collagen IV, tumor necrosis factor-alpha, gelatinase B (matrix metalloprotease-9), and tissue inhibitor of metalloproteases-1 in the basal lamina regulates Sertoli cell-tight junction dynamics in the rat testis. *Endocrinology* **2003**, *144*, 371–387. [CrossRef]
31. Cheng, C.Y.; Mruk, D.D. Cell junction dynamics in the testis: Sertoli-germ cell interactions and male contraceptive development. *Physiol Rev.* **2002**, *82*, 825–874. [CrossRef]
32. Aydos, O.S.; Yukselten, Y.; Ozkavukcu, S.; Sunguroglu, A.; Aydos, K. ADAMTS1 and ADAMTS5 metalloproteases produced by Sertoli cells: A potential diagnostic marker in azoospermia. *Syst. Biol. Reprod. Med.* **2019**, *65*, 29–38. [CrossRef]
33. Modarresi, T.; Sabbaghian, M.; Shahverdi, A.; Hosseinifar, H.; Akhlaghi, A.A.; Gilani, M.A.S. Enzymatic digestion improves testicular sperm retrieval in non-obstructive azoospermic patients. *Iran. J. Reprod. Med.* **2013**, *11*, 447–452. [PubMed]
34. Crabbé, E.; Verheyen, G.; Silber, S.; Tournaye, H.; Van de Velde, H.; Goossens, A.; Van Steirteghem, A. Enzymatic digestion of testicular tissue may rescue the intracytoplasmic sperm injection cycle in some patients with non-obstructive azoospermia. *Hum. Reprod.* **1998**, *13*, 2791–2796. [CrossRef]
35. Aydos, K.; Demirel, L.C.; Baltaci, V.; Unlü, C. Enzymatic digestion plus mechanical searching improves testicular sperm retrieval in non-obstructive azoospermia cases. *Eur. J. Obstet Gynecol. Reprod. Biol.* **2005**, *120*, 80–86. [CrossRef]
36. Ramasamy, R.; Reifsnyder, J.E.; Bryson, C.; Zaninovic, N.; Liotta, D.; Cook, C.A.; Hariprashad, J.; Weiss, D.; Neri, Q.; Palermo, G.D.; et al. Role of tissue digestion and extensive sperm search after microdissection testicular sperm extraction. *Fertil. Steril.* **2011**, *96*, 299–302. [CrossRef] [PubMed]
37. Esteves, S.C.; Varghese, A.C. Laboratory handling of epididymal and testicular spermatozoa: What can be done to improve sperm injections outcome. *J. Hum. Reprod. Sci.* **2012**, *5*, 233–243. [CrossRef] [PubMed]
38. Bryniarski, K.; Szczepanik, M.; Ptak, M.; Ptak, W. The influence of collagenase treatment on the production of TNF-alpha, IL-6 and IL-10 by testicular macrophages. *J. Immunol. Methods* **2005**, *301*, 186–189. [CrossRef] [PubMed]
39. Liu, J.; Nagy, Z.; Joris, H.; Tournaye, H.; Smitz, J.; Camus, M.; Devroey, P.; Van Steirteghem, A. Analysis of 76 total fertilization failure cycles out of 2732 intracytoplasmic sperm injection cycles. *Hum. Reprod.* **1995**, *10*, 2630–2636. [PubMed]
40. Esfandiari, N.; Javed, M.H.; Gotlieb, L.; Casper, R.F. Complete failed fertilization after intracytoplasmic sperm injection–analysis of 10 years' data. *Int. J. Fertil. Womens Med.* **2005**, *50*, 187–192. [PubMed]
41. Wu, B.; Wong, D.; Lu, S.; Dickstein, S.; Silva, M.; Gelety, T.J. Optimal use of fresh and frozen-thawed testicular sperm for intracytoplasmic sperm injection in azoospermic patients. *J. Assist. Reprod. Genet.* **2005**, *22*, 389–394. [CrossRef] [PubMed]
42. Taşdemir, I.; Taşdemir, M.; Tavukçuoğlu, S. Effect of pentoxifylline on immotile testicular spermatozoa. *J. Assist. Reprod. Genet.* **1998**, *15*, 90–92. [CrossRef] [PubMed]
43. Tash, J.S.; Means, A.R. Cyclic adenosine 3′,5′ monophosphate, calcium and protein phosphorylation in flagellar motility. *Biol. Reprod.* **1983**, *28*, 75–104. [CrossRef] [PubMed]
44. Morisawa, M.; Okuno, M. Cyclic AMP induces maturation of trout sperm axoneme to initiate motility. *Nature* **1982**, *295*, 703–704. [CrossRef] [PubMed]
45. Ebner, T.; Tews, G.; Mayer, R.B.; Ziehr, S.; Arzt, W.; Costamoling, W.; Shebl, O. Pharmacological stimulation of sperm motility in frozen and thawed testicular sperm using the dimethylxanthine theophylline. *Fertil. Steril.* **2011**, *96*, 1331–1336. [CrossRef]
46. Pariz, J.R.; Ranéa, C.; Monteiro, R.A.C.; Evenson, D.P.; Drevet, J.R.; Hallak, J. Melatonin and Caffeine Supplementation Used, Respectively, as Protective and Stimulating Agents in the Cryopreservation of Human Sperm Improves Survival, Viability, and Motility after Thawing compared to Traditional TEST-Yolk Buffer. *Oxid. Med. Cell Longev.* **2019**, *2019*, 6472945. [CrossRef]
47. Verma, R.; Huang, Z.; Deutschman, C.S.; Levy, R.J. Caffeine restores myocardial cytochrome oxidase activity and improves cardiac function during sepsis. *Crit. Care Med.* **2009**, *37*, 1397–1402. [CrossRef]
48. Breininger, E.; Cetica, P.D.; Beconi, M.T. Capacitation inducers act through diverse intracellular mechanisms in cryopreserved bovine sperm. *Theriogenology* **2010**, *74*, 1036–1049. [CrossRef]
49. Marquez, B.; Suarez, S.S. Different signaling pathways in bovine sperm regulate capacitation and hyperactivation. *Biol. Reprod.* **2004**, *70*, 1626–1633. [CrossRef]
50. Pariz, J.R.; Hallak, J. Effects of caffeine supplementation in post-thaw human semen over different incubation periods. *Andrologia* **2016**, *48*, 961–966. [CrossRef]
51. York, R.G.; Randall, J.L.; Scott, W.J. Teratogenicity of paraxanthine (1,7-dimethylxanthine) in C57BL/6J. mice. *Teratology* **1986**, *34*, 279–282. [CrossRef]
52. Das, K.; Das, S.; Bhoumik, A.; Jaiswal, B.S.; Majumder, G.C.; Dungdung, S.R. In vitro initiated sperm forward motility in caput spermatozoa: Weak and transient. *Andrologia* **2012**, *44* (Suppl. 1), 807–812. [CrossRef]

53. Mangoli, V.; Mangoli, R.; Dandekar, S.; Suri, K.; Desai, S. Selection of viable spermatozoa from testicular biopsies: A comparative study between pentoxifylline and hypoosmotic swelling test. *Fertil. Steril.* **2011**, *95*, 631–634. [CrossRef] [PubMed]
54. Tasdemir, M.; Tasdemir, I.; Kodama, H.; Tanaka, T. Pentoxifylline-enhanced acrosome reaction correlates with fertilization in vitro. *Hum. Reprod.* **1993**, *8*, 2102–2107. [CrossRef] [PubMed]
55. Kovacic, B.; Vlaisavljevic, V.; Reljic, M. Clinical use of pentoxifylline for activation of immotile testicular sperm before ICSI in patients with azoospermia. *J. Androl.* **2006**, *27*, 45–52. [CrossRef] [PubMed]
56. Giorgetti, C.; Chinchole, J.M.; Hans, E.; Charles, O.; Franquebalme, J.P.; Glowaczower, E.; Salzmann, J.; Terriou, P.; Roulier, R. Crude cumulative delivery rate following ICSI using intentionally frozen-thawed testicular spermatozoa in 51 men with non-obstructive azoospermia. *Reprod. Biomed. Online* **2005**, *11*, 319–324. [CrossRef]
57. Aizer, A.; Dratviman-Storobinsky, O.; Noach-Hirsh, M.; Konopnicki, S.; Lazarovich, A.; Raviv, G.; Orvieto, R. Testicular sperm retrieval: What should we expect from the fresh and subsequent cryopreserved sperm injection? *Andrologia* **2021**, *53*, e13849. [CrossRef] [PubMed]
58. Kang, H.J.; Lee, S.H.; Park, Y.S.; Lim, C.K.; Ko, D.S.; Yang, K.M.; Park, D.W. Artificial oocyte activation in intracytoplasmic sperm injection cycles using testicular sperm in human in vitro fertilization. *Clin. Exp Reprod. Med.* **2015**, *42*, 45–50. [CrossRef]
59. Tardif, S.; Madamidola, O.A.; Brown, S.G.; Frame, L.; Lefièvre, L.; Wyatt, P.G.; Barratt, C.L.; Martins Da Silva, S.J. Clinically relevant enhancement of human sperm motility using compounds with reported phosphodiesterase inhibitor activity. *Hum. Reprod.* **2014**, *29*, 2123–2135. [CrossRef] [PubMed]
60. Chan, S.Y.; Tang, L.C.; Ma, H.K. Stimulation of the human spermatozoal fertilizing ability by dibutyryl 3′,5′-CAMP and theophylline in vitro. *Arch. Androl.* **1983**, *11*, 19–23. [CrossRef]
61. Loughlin, K.R.; Agarwal, A. Use of theophylline to enhance sperm function. *Arch. Androl.* **1992**, *28*, 99–103. [CrossRef]
62. Holubcová, Z.; Otevřel, P.; Koudelka, M.; Kloudová, S. Live birth achieved despite the absence of ejaculated spermatozoa and mature oocytes retrieved: A case report. *J. Assist. Reprod. Genet.* **2021**, *38*, 925–929. [CrossRef]
63. Ebner, T.; Shebl, O.; Mayer, R.B.; Moser, M.; Costamoling, W.; Oppelt, P. Healthy live birth using theophylline in a case of retrograde ejaculation and absolute asthenozoospermia. *Fertil. Steril.* **2014**, *101*, 340–343. [CrossRef] [PubMed]
64. Lacham-Kaplan, O.; Trounson, A. The effects of the sperm motility activators 2-deoxyadenosine and pentoxifylline used for sperm micro-injection on mouse and human embryo development. *Hum. Reprod.* **1993**, *8*, 945–952. [CrossRef]
65. Hattori, H.; Nakajo, Y.; Ito, C.; Toyama, Y.; Toshimori, K.; Kyono, K. Birth of a healthy infant after intracytoplasmic sperm injection using pentoxifylline-activated sperm from a patient with Kartagener's syndrome. *Fertil. Steril.* **2011**, *95*, 2431.e2439. [CrossRef] [PubMed]
66. Glenn, D.R.; McVicar, C.M.; McClure, N.; Lewis, S.E. Sildenafil citrate improves sperm motility but causes a premature acrosome reaction in vitro. *Fertil. Steril.* **2007**, *87*, 1064–1070. [CrossRef] [PubMed]
67. Lefièvre, L.; De Lamirande, E.; Gagnon, C. The cyclic GMP-specific phosphodiesterase inhibitor, sildenafil, stimulates human sperm motility and capacitation but not acrosome reaction. *J. Androl.* **2000**, *21*, 929–937. [PubMed]
68. Yang, Y.; Ma, Y.; Yang, H.; Jin, Y.; Hu, K.; Wang, H.X.; Wang, Y.X.; Huang, Y.R.; Chen, B. Effect of acute tadalafil on sperm motility and acrosome reaction: In vitro and in vivo studies. *Andrologia* **2014**, *46*, 417–422. [CrossRef]
69. Andrade, J.R.; Traboulsi, A.; Hussain, A.; Dubin, N.H. In vitro effects of sildenafil and phentolamine, drugs used for erectile dysfunction, on human sperm motility. *Am. J. Obstet Gynecol.* **2000**, *182*, 1093–1095. [CrossRef]
70. Wang, G.; Guo, Y.; Zhou, T.; Shi, X.; Yu, J.; Yang, Y.; Wu, Y.; Wang, J.; Liu, M.; Chen, X.; et al. In-depth proteomic analysis of the human sperm reveals complex protein compositions. *J. Proteom.* **2013**, *79*, 114–122. [CrossRef]
71. Dcunha, R.; Hussein, R.S.; Ananda, H.; Kumari, S.; Adiga, S.K.; Kannan, N.; Zhao, Y.; Kalthur, G. Current Insights and Latest Updates in Sperm Motility and Associated Applications in Assisted Reproduction. *Reprod. Sci.* **2020**. [CrossRef]
72. Hosseini, A.; Khalili, M.A. Improvement of motility after culture of testicular spermatozoa: The effects of incubation timing and temperature. *Transl. Androl. Urol.* **2017**, *6*, 271–276. [CrossRef] [PubMed]
73. Balaban, B.; Urman, B.; Sertac, A.; Alatas, C.; Aksoy, S.; Mercan, R.; Nuhoglu, A. In-vitro culture of spermatozoa induces motility and increases implantation and pregnancy rates after testicular sperm extraction and intracytoplasmic sperm injection. *Hum. Reprod.* **1999**, *14*, 2808–2811. [CrossRef] [PubMed]
74. Angelopoulos, T.; Adler, A.; Krey, L.; Licciardi, F.; Noyes, N.; McCullough, A. Enhancement or initiation of testicular sperm motility by in vitro culture of testicular tissue. *Fertil. Steril.* **1999**, *71*, 240–243. [CrossRef]
75. Karacan, M.; Alwaeely, F.; Erkan, S.; Çebi, Z.; Berberoğlugil, M.; Batukan, M.; Uluğ, M.; Arvas, A.; Çamlıbel, T. Outcome of intracytoplasmic sperm injection cycles with fresh testicular spermatozoa obtained on the day of or the day before oocyte collection and with cryopreserved testicular sperm in patients with azoospermia. *Fertil. Steril.* **2013**, *100*, 975–980. [CrossRef]
76. Dalzell, L.H.; McVicar, C.M.; McClure, N.; Lutton, D.; Lewis, S.E. Effects of short and long incubations on DNA fragmentation of testicular sperm. *Fertil. Steril.* **2004**, *82*, 1443–1445. [CrossRef]
77. Jeyendran, R.S.; Van der Ven, H.H.; Perez-Pelaez, M.; Crabo, B.G.; Zaneveld, L.J. Development of an assay to assess the functional integrity of the human sperm membrane and its relationship to other semen characteristics. *J. Reprod. Fertil.* **1984**, *70*, 219–228. [CrossRef]
78. Check, M.; Check, J.H.; Summers-Chase, D.; Swenson, K.; Yuan, W. An evaluation of the efficacy of in vitro fertilization with intracytoplasmic sperm injection for sperm with low hypoosmotic swelling test scores and poor morphology. *J. Assist. Reprod. Genet.* **2003**, *20*, 182–185. [CrossRef]

79. Sallam, H.N.; Farrag, A.; Agameya, A.F.; El-Garem, Y.; Ezzeldin, F. The use of the modified hypo-osmotic swelling test for the selection of immotile testicular spermatozoa in patients treated with ICSI: A randomized controlled study. *Hum. Reprod.* **2005**, *20*, 3435–3440. [CrossRef]
80. Sallam, H.; Farrag, A.; Agameya, A.; Ezzeldin, F.; Eid, A.; Sallam, A. The use of a modified hypo-osmotic swelling test for the selection of viable ejaculated and testicular immotile spermatozoa in ICSI. *Hum. Reprod.* **2001**, *16*, 272–276. [CrossRef]
81. Charehjooy, N.; Najafi, M.H.; Tavalaee, M.; Deemeh, M.R.; Azadi, L.; Shiravi, A.H.; Nasr-Esfahani, M.H. Selection of Sperm Based on Hypo-Osmotic Swelling May Improve ICSI Outcome: A Preliminary Prospective Clinical Trial. *Int. J. Fertil. Steril.* **2014**, *8*, 21–28. [PubMed]
82. Liu, J.; Tsai, Y.L.; Katz, E.; Compton, G.; Garcia, J.E.; Baramki, T.A. High fertilization rate obtained after intracytoplasmic sperm injection with 100% nonmotile spermatozoa selected by using a simple modified hypo-osmotic swelling test. *Fertil. Steril.* **1997**, *68*, 373–375. [CrossRef]
83. Goksan Pabuccu, E.; Sinem Caglar, G.; Dogus Demirkiran, O.; Pabuccu, R. Uncommon but devastating event: Total fertilisation failure following intracytoplasmic sperm injection. *Andrologia* **2016**, *48*, 164–170. [CrossRef]
84. Nordhoff, V. How to select immotile but viable spermatozoa on the day of intracytoplasmic sperm injection? An embryologist's view. *Andrology* **2015**, *3*, 156–162. [CrossRef]
85. Moskovtsev, S.I.; Willis, J.; Azad, A.; Mullen, J.B. Sperm DNA integrity: Correlation with sperm plasma membrane integrity in semen evaluated for male infertility. *Arch. Androl.* **2005**, *51*, 33–40. [CrossRef]
86. Stanger, J.D.; Vo, L.; Yovich, J.L.; Almahbobi, G. Hypo-osmotic swelling test identifies individual spermatozoa with minimal DNA fragmentation. *Reprod. Biomed. Online* **2010**, *21*, 474–484. [CrossRef] [PubMed]
87. Kiefer, D.; Check, J.H.; Katsoff, D. The value of motile density, strict morphology, and the hypoosmotic swelling test in in vitro fertilization-embryo transfer. *Arch. Androl.* **1996**, *37*, 57–60. [CrossRef] [PubMed]
88. Check, J.H.; Katsoff, D.; Check, M.L.; Choe, J.K.; Swenson, K. In vitro fertilization with intracytoplasmic sperm injection is an effective therapy for male factor infertility related to subnormal hypo-osmotic swelling test scores. *J. Androl.* **2001**, *22*, 261–265.
89. Hossain, A.; Osuamkpe, C.; Hossain, S.; Phelps, J.Y. Spontaneously developed tail swellings (SDTS) influence the accuracy of the hypo-osmotic swelling test (HOS-test) in determining membrane integrity and viability of human spermatozoa. *J. Assist. Reprod. Genet.* **2010**, *27*, 83–86. [CrossRef]
90. Bollendorf, A.; Check, J.H.; Kramer, D. The majority of males with subnormal hypoosmotic test scores have normal vitality. *Clin. Exp Obstet Gynecol.* **2012**, *39*, 25–26.
91. Barros, A.; Sousa, M.; Angelopoulos, T.; Tesarik, J. Efficient modification of intracytoplasmic sperm injection technique for cases with total lack of sperm movement. *Hum. Reprod.* **1997**, *12*, 1227–1229. [CrossRef]
92. Tsai, Y.L.; Liu, J.; Garcia, J.E.; Katz, E.; Compton, G.; Baramki, T.A. Establishment of an optimal hypo-osmotic swelling test by examining single spermatozoa in four different hypo-osmotic solutions. *Hum. Reprod.* **1997**, *12*, 1111–1113. [CrossRef]
93. Soares, J.B.; Glina, S.; Antunes, N.; Wonchockier, R.; Galuppo, A.G.; Mizrahi, F.E. Sperm tail flexibility test: A simple test for selecting viable spermatozoa for intracytoplasmic sperm injection from semen samples without motile spermatozoa. *Rev. Hosp. Clin. Fac Med. Sao Paulo* **2003**, *58*, 250–253. [CrossRef]
94. de Oliveira, N.M.; Vaca Sánchez, R.; Rodriguez Fiesta, S.; Lopez Salgado, T.; Rodríguez, R.; Bethencourt, J.C.; Blanes Zamora, R. Pregnancy with frozen-thawed and fresh testicular biopsy after motile and immotile sperm microinjection, using the mechanical touch technique to assess viability. *Hum. Reprod.* **2004**, *19*, 262–265. [CrossRef]
95. Kim, H.J.; Yoon, H.J.; Jang, J.M.; Oh, H.S.; Lee, Y.J.; Lee, W.D.; Yoon, S.H.; Lim, J.H. Comparison between intracytoplasmic sperm injection and intracytoplasmic morphologically selected sperm injection in oligo-astheno-teratozoospermia patients. *Clin. Exp Reprod. Med.* **2014**, *41*, 9–14. [CrossRef]
96. Boitrelle, F.; Guthauser, B.; Alter, L.; Bailly, M.; Bergere, M.; Wainer, R.; Vialard, F.; Albert, M.; Selva, J. High-magnification selection of spermatozoa prior to oocyte injection: Confirmed and potential indications. *Reprod. Biomed. Online* **2014**, *28*, 6–13. [CrossRef]
97. Setti, A.S.; Braga, D.P.; Figueira, R.C.; Iaconelli, A.; Borges, E. Intracytoplasmic morphologically selected sperm injection results in improved clinical outcomes in couples with previous ICSI failures or male factor infertility: A meta-analysis. *Eur. J. Obstet Gynecol. Reprod. Biol.* **2014**, *183*, 96–103. [CrossRef]
98. Schachter-Safrai, N.; Karavani, G.; Reuveni-Salzman, A.; Gil, M.; Ben-Meir, A. Which semen analysis correlates with favorable Intracytoplasmic morphologically selected sperm injection (IMSI) outcomes? *Eur. J. Obstet Gynecol. Reprod. Biol.* **2019**, *234*, 85–88. [CrossRef] [PubMed]
99. Teixeira, D.M.; Hadyme Miyague, A.; Barbosa, M.A.; Navarro, P.A.; Raine-Fenning, N.; Nastri, C.O.; Martins, W.P. Regular (ICSI) versus ultra-high magnification (IMSI) sperm selection for assisted reproduction. *Cochrane Database Syst Rev.* **2020**, *2*, CD010167. [CrossRef]
100. Văduva, C.C.; Constantinescu, C.; Radu, M.M.; Văduva, A.R.; Pănuş, T.; Ţenovici, M.; DiŢescu, D.; Albu, D.F. Pregnancy resulting from IMSI after testicular biopsy in a patient with obstructive azoospermia. *Rom. J. Morphol. Embryol.* **2016**, *57*, 879–883.
101. Bradley, C.K.; McArthur, S.J.; Gee, A.J.; Weiss, K.A.; Schmidt, U.; Toogood, L. Intervention improves assisted conception intracytoplasmic sperm injection outcomes for patients with high levels of sperm DNA fragmentation: A retrospective analysis. *Andrology* **2016**, *4*, 903–910. [CrossRef]

102. Chen, H.; Feng, G.; Zhang, B.; Zhou, H.; Wang, C.; Shu, J.; Gan, X.; Lin, R.; Huang, D.; Huang, Y. A new insight into male fertility preservation for patients with completely immotile spermatozoa. *Reprod. Biol. Endocrinol.* **2017**, *15*, 74. [CrossRef]
103. Aktan, T.M.; Montag, M.; Duman, S.; Gorkemli, H.; Rink, K.; Yurdakul, T. Use of a laser to detect viable but immotile spermatozoa. *Andrologia* **2004**, *36*, 366–369. [CrossRef]
104. Gerber, P.A.; Kruse, R.; Hirchenhain, J.; Krüssel, J.S.; Neumann, N.J. Pregnancy after laser-assisted selection of viable spermatozoa before intracytoplasmatic sperm injection in a couple with male primary cilia dyskinesia. *Fertil. Steril.* **2008**, *89*, 1826.e9–1826.e12. [CrossRef] [PubMed]
105. Chen, H.; Feng, G.; Zhang, B.; Zhou, H.; Shu, J.; Gan, X. A successful pregnancy using completely immotile but viable frozen-thawed spermatozoa selected by laser. *Clin. Exp. Reprod. Med.* **2017**, *44*, 52–55. [CrossRef] [PubMed]
106. Ozkavukcu, S.; Celik-Ozenci, C.; Konuk, E.; Atabekoglu, C. Live birth after Laser Assisted Viability Assessment (LAVA) to detect pentoxifylline resistant ejaculated immotile spermatozoa during ICSI in a couple with male Kartagener's syndrome. *Reprod. Biol. Endocrinol.* **2018**, *16*, 10. [CrossRef]
107. Ghosh, S.; Chattopadhyay, R.; Bose, G.; Ganesh, A.; Das, S.; Chakravarty, B.N. Selection of birefringent spermatozoa under Polscope: Effect on intracytoplasmic sperm injection outcome. *Andrologia* **2012**, *44* (Suppl. 1), 734–738. [CrossRef]
108. Gianaroli, L.; Magli, M.C.; Collodel, G.; Moretti, E.; Ferraretti, A.P.; Baccetti, B. Sperm head's birefringence: A new criterion for sperm selection. *Fertil. Steril.* **2008**, *90*, 104–112. [CrossRef] [PubMed]
109. McDowell, S.; Kroon, B.; Ford, E.; Hook, Y.; Glujovsky, D.; Yazdani, A. Advanced sperm selection techniques for assisted reproduction. *Cochrane Database Syst. Rev.* **2014**, CD010461. [CrossRef]
110. Huang, H.Y.; Wu, T.L.; Huang, H.R.; Li, C.J.; Fu, H.T.; Soong, Y.K.; Lee, M.Y.; Yao, D.J. Isolation of motile spermatozoa with a microfluidic chip having a surface-modified microchannel. *J. Lab. Autom.* **2014**, *19*, 91–99. [CrossRef]
111. Schuster, T.G.; Cho, B.; Keller, L.M.; Takayama, S.; Smith, G.D. Isolation of motile spermatozoa from semen samples using microfluidics. *Reprod. Biomed. Online* **2003**, *7*, 75–81. [CrossRef]
112. Quinn, M.M.; Jalalian, L.; Ribeiro, S.; Ona, K.; Demirci, U.; Cedars, M.I.; Rosen, M.P. Microfluidic sorting selects sperm for clinical use with reduced DNA damage compared to density gradient centrifugation with swim-up in split semen samples. *Hum. Reprod.* **2018**, *33*, 1388–1393. [CrossRef]
113. Samuel, R.; Son, J.; Jenkins, T.G.; Jafek, A.; Feng, H.; Gale, B.K.; Carrell, D.T.; Hotaling, J.M. Microfluidic System for Rapid Isolation of Sperm From Microdissection TESE Specimens. *Urology* **2020**, *140*, 70–76. [CrossRef]
114. Liu, Y.; Zhu, Y.; Di, L.; Osterberg, E.C.; Liu, F.; He, L.; Hu, H.; Huang, Y.; Li, P.S.; Li, Z. Raman spectroscopy as an ex vivo noninvasive approach to distinguish complete and incomplete spermatogenesis within human seminiferous tubules. *Fertil. Steril.* **2014**, *102*, 54–60.e52. [CrossRef]
115. Liu, Y.F.; Di, L.; Osterberg, E.C.; He, L.; Li, P.S.; Li, Z. Use of Raman spectroscopy to identify active spermatogenesis and Sertoli-cell-only tubules in mice. *Andrologia* **2016**, *48*, 1086–1091. [CrossRef]
116. Osterberg, E.C.; Laudano, M.A.; Ramasamy, R.; Sterling, J.; Robinson, B.D.; Goldstein, M.; Li, P.S.; Haka, A.S.; Schlegel, P.N. Identification of spermatogenesis in a rat sertoli-cell only model using Raman spectroscopy: A feasibility study. *J. Urol.* **2014**, *192*, 607–612. [CrossRef]
117. Mallidis, C.; Sanchez, V.; Wistuba, J.; Wuebbeling, F.; Burger, M.; Fallnich, C.; Schlatt, S. Raman microspectroscopy: Shining a new light on reproductive medicine. *Hum. Reprod. Update* **2014**, *20*, 403–414. [CrossRef]
118. Samuel, R.; Badamjav, O.; Murphy, K.E.; Patel, D.P.; Son, J.; Gale, B.K.; Carrell, D.T.; Hotaling, J.M. Microfluidics: The future of microdissection TESE? *Syst. Biol. Reprod. Med.* **2016**, *62*, 161–170. [CrossRef] [PubMed]
119. Jahmani, M.Y.; Hammadeh, M.E.; Al Smadi, M.A.; Baller, M.K. Label-Free Evaluation of Chromatin Condensation in Human Normal Morphology Sperm Using Raman Spectroscopy. *Reprod. Sci.* **2021**, 1–13. [CrossRef]
120. Haas, G.G.; D'Cruz, O.J.; DeBault, L.E. Assessment by fluorescence-activated cell sorting of whether sperm-associated immunoglobulin (Ig)G and IgA occur on the same sperm population. *Fertil. Steril.* **1990**, *54*, 127–132. [CrossRef]
121. Mittal, S.; Mielnik, A.; Bolyakov, A.; Schlegel, P.N.; Paduch, D. Pilot Study Results Using Fluorescence Activated Cell Sorting of Spermatozoa from Testis Tissue: A Novel Method for Sperm Isolation after TESE. *J. Urol.* **2017**, *197*, Pd68-01. [CrossRef]
122. Mangum, C.L.; Patel, D.P.; Jafek, A.R.; Samuel, R.; Jenkins, T.G.; Aston, K.I.; Gale, B.K.; Hotaling, J.M. Towards a better testicular sperm extraction: Novel sperm sorting technologies for non-motile sperm extracted by microdissection TESE. *Transl. Androl. Urol.* **2020**, *9*, S206–S214. [CrossRef]
123. Ramasamy, R.; Sterling, J.; Fisher, E.S.; Li, P.S.; Jain, M.; Robinson, B.D.; Shevchuck, M.; Huland, D.; Xu, C.; Mukherjee, S.; et al. Identification of spermatogenesis with multiphoton microscopy: An evaluation in a rodent model. *J. Urol.* **2011**, *186*, 2487–2492. [CrossRef]
124. Najari, B.B.; Ramasamy, R.; Sterling, J.; Aggarwal, A.; Sheth, S.; Li, P.S.; Dubin, J.M.; Goldenberg, S.; Jain, M.; Robinson, B.D.; et al. Pilot study of the correlation of multiphoton tomography of ex vivo human testis with histology. *J. Urol.* **2012**, *188*, 538–543. [CrossRef]
125. Ramasamy, R.; Sterling, J.; Manzoor, M.; Salamoon, B.; Jain, M.; Fisher, E.; Li, P.S.; Schlegel, P.N.; Mukherjee, S. Full field optical coherence tomography can identify spermatogenesis in a rodent sertoli-cell only model. *J. Pathol. Inform.* **2012**, *3*, 4. [CrossRef]
126. Oseguera-López, I.; Ruiz-Díaz, S.; Ramos-Ibeas, P.; Pérez-Cerezales, S. Novel Techniques of Sperm Selection for Improving IVF and ICSI Outcomes. *Front. Cell Dev. Biol.* **2019**, *7*, 298. [CrossRef]

127. Bernie, A.M.; Mata, D.A.; Ramasamy, R.; Schlegel, P.N. Comparison of microdissection testicular sperm extraction, conventional testicular sperm extraction, and testicular sperm aspiration for nonobstructive azoospermia: A systematic review and meta-analysis. *Fertil. Steril.* **2015**, *104*, 1099–1103.e3. [CrossRef]
128. Yogev, L.; Kleiman, S.E.; Shabtai, E.; Botchan, A.; Paz, G.; Hauser, R.; Lehavi, O.; Yavetz, H.; Gamzu, R. Long-term cryostorage of sperm in a human sperm bank does not damage progressive motility concentration. *Hum. Reprod.* **2010**, *25*, 1097–1103. [CrossRef] [PubMed]
129. Bashiri, A.; Halper, K.I.; Orvieto, R. Recurrent Implantation Failure-update overview on etiology, diagnosis, treatment and future directions. *Reprod. Biol. Endocrinol* **2018**, *16*, 121. [CrossRef] [PubMed]
130. Barash, A.; Dekel, N.; Fieldust, S.; Segal, I.; Schechtman, E.; Granot, I. Local injury to the endometrium doubles the incidence of successful pregnancies in patients undergoing in vitro fertilization. *Fertil. Steril.* **2003**, *79*, 1317–1322. [CrossRef]
131. Nastri, C.O.; Lensen, S.F.; Gibreel, A.; Raine-Fenning, N.; Ferriani, R.A.; Bhattacharya, S.; Martins, W.P. Endometrial injury in women undergoing assisted reproductive techniques. *Cochrane Database Syst. Rev.* **2015**, CD009517. [CrossRef]
132. Audrins, P.; Holden, C.A.; McLachlan, R.I.; Kovacs, G.T. Semen storage for special purposes at Monash IVF from 1977 to 1997. *Fertil. Steril.* **1999**, *72*, 179–181. [CrossRef]
133. Guan, H.T.; Wan, Z.; Zhang, L.; Meng, T.Q.; Xiong, C.L.; Li, C.L. Analysis of the Screening Results for 3,564 Student Sperm Donors in Hubei Province, China. *J. Reprod. Med.* **2015**, *60*, 409–414.
134. Talwar, P.; Singh, S. Chapter 7 Human Epididymal and Testicular Sperm Cryopreservation. *Methods Mol. Biol.* **2017**, *1568*, 85–104. [CrossRef] [PubMed]
135. Yu, Z.; Wei, Z.; Yang, J.; Wang, T.; Jiang, H.; Li, H.; Tang, Z.; Wang, S.; Liu, J. Comparison of intracytoplasmic sperm injection outcome with fresh versus frozen-thawed testicular sperm in men with nonobstructive azoospermia: A systematic review and meta-analysis. *J. Assist. Reprod. Genet.* **2018**, *35*, 1247–1257. [CrossRef] [PubMed]
136. Küpker, W.; Schlegel, P.N.; Al-Hasani, S.; Fornara, P.; Johannisson, R.; Sandmann, J.; Schill, T.; Bals-Pratsch, M.; Ludwig, M.; Diedrich, K. Use of frozen-thawed testicular sperm for intracytoplasmic sperm injection. *Fertil. Steril.* **2000**, *73*, 453–458. [CrossRef]
137. Kalsi, J.; Thum, M.Y.; Muneer, A.; Pryor, J.; Abdullah, H.; Minhas, S. Analysis of the outcome of intracytoplasmic sperm injection using fresh or frozen sperm. *BJU Int.* **2011**, *107*, 1124–1128. [CrossRef]
138. Ohlander, S.; Hotaling, J.; Kirshenbaum, E.; Niederberger, C.; Eisenberg, M.L. Impact of fresh versus cryopreserved testicular sperm upon intracytoplasmic sperm injection pregnancy outcomes in men with azoospermia due to spermatogenic dysfunction: A meta-analysis. *Fertil. Steril.* **2014**, *101*, 344–349. [CrossRef]
139. Zhang, Z.; Jing, J.; Luo, L.; Li, L.; Zhang, H.; Xi, Q.; Liu, R. ICSI outcomes of fresh or cryopreserved spermatozoa from micro-TESE in patients with nonobstructive azoospermia: CONSORT. *Medicine* **2021**, *100*, e25021. [CrossRef] [PubMed]
140. Madureira, C.; Cunha, M.; Sousa, M.; Neto, A.P.; Pinho, M.J.; Viana, P.; Gonçalves, A.; Silva, J.; Teixeira da Silva, J.; Oliveira, C.; et al. Treatment by testicular sperm extraction and intracytoplasmic sperm injection of 65 azoospermic patients with non-mosaic Klinefelter syndrome with birth of 17 healthy children. *Andrology* **2014**, *2*, 623–631. [CrossRef]
141. Park, Y.S.; Lee, S.H.; Lim, C.K.; Cho, J.W.; Yang, K.M.; Seo, J.T. Effect of testicular spermatozoa on embryo quality and pregnancy in patients with non-obstructive azoospermia. *Syst. Biol. Reprod. Med.* **2015**, *61*, 300–306. [CrossRef] [PubMed]
142. Pšenička, M.; Saito, T.; Rodina, M.; Dzyuba, B. Cryopreservation of early stage Siberian sturgeon Acipenser baerii germ cells, comparison of whole tissue and dissociated cells. *Cryobiology* **2016**, *72*, 119–122. [CrossRef] [PubMed]
143. Marinović, Z.; Lujić, J.; Kása, E.; Bernáth, G.; Urbányi, B.; Horváth, Á. Cryosurvival of isolated testicular cells and testicular tissue of tench Tinca tinca and goldfish Carassius auratus following slow-rate freezing. *Gen. Comp. Endocrinol.* **2017**, *245*, 77–83. [CrossRef]
144. Unni, S.; Kasiviswanathan, S.; D'Souza, S.; Khavale, S.; Mukherjee, S.; Patwardhan, S.; Bhartiya, D. Efficient cryopreservation of testicular tissue: Effect of age, sample state, and concentration of cryoprotectant. *Fertil. Steril.* **2012**, *97*, 200–208.e201. [CrossRef]
145. Donnelly, E.T.; McClure, N.; Lewis, S.E. Cryopreservation of human semen and prepared sperm: Effects on motility parameters and DNA integrity. *Fertil. Steril.* **2001**, *76*, 892–900. [CrossRef]
146. Perraguin-Jayot, S.; Audebert, A.; Emperaire, J.C.; Parneix, I. Ongoing pregnancies after intracytoplasmic injection using cryopreserved testicular spermatozoa. *Hum. Reprod.* **1997**, *12*, 2706–2709. [CrossRef]
147. Nikolettos, N.; Al-Hasani, S.; Demirel, C.; Küpker, W.; Bals-Pratsch, M.; Sandmann, J.; Fornara, P.; Schöpper, B.; Sturm, R.; Diedrich, K. Outcome of ICSI cycles using frozen-thawed surgically obtained spermatozoa in poor responders to ovarian stimulation: Cancellation or proceeding to ICSI? *Eur. J. Obstet. Gynecol. Reprod. Biol.* **2000**, *92*, 259–264. [CrossRef]
148. Friedler, S.; Raziel, A.; Soffer, Y.; Strassburger, D.; Komarovsky, D.; Ron-el, R. Intracytoplasmic injection of fresh and cryopreserved testicular spermatozoa in patients with nonobstructive azoospermia–a comparative study. *Fertil. Steril.* **1997**, *68*, 892–897. [CrossRef]
149. Gil-Salom, M.; Romero, J.; Rubio, C.; Ruiz, A.; Remohí, J.; Pellicer, A. Intracytoplasmic sperm injection with cryopreserved testicular spermatozoa. *Mol. Cell Endocrinol.* **2000**, *169*, 15–19. [CrossRef]
150. De Croo, I.; Van der Elst, J.; Everaert, K.; De Sutter, P.; Dhont, M. Fertilization, pregnancy and embryo implantation rates after ICSI with fresh or frozen-thawed testicular spermatozoa. *Hum. Reprod.* **1998**, *13*, 1893–1897. [CrossRef] [PubMed]
151. Spis, E.; Bushkovskaia, A.; Isachenko, E.; Todorov, P.; Sanchez, R.; Skopets, V.; Isachenko, V. Conventional freezing vs. cryoprotectant-free vitrification of epididymal (MESA) and testicular (TESE) spermatozoa: Three live births. *Cryobiology* **2019**, *90*, 100–102. [CrossRef]

152. Schiewe, M.C.; Rothman, C.; Spitz, A.; Werthman, P.E.; Zeitlin, S.I.; Anderson, R.E. Validation-verification of a highly effective, practical human testicular tissue in vitro culture-cryopreservation procedure aimed to optimize pre-freeze and post-thaw motility. *J. Assist. Reprod. Genet.* **2016**, *33*, 519–528. [CrossRef]
153. Huleihel, M.; Lunenfeld, E. Approaches and Technologies in Male Fertility Preservation. *Int. J. Mol. Sci.* **2020**, *21*, 5471. [CrossRef]
154. Aslam, I.; Fishel, S. Short-term in-vitro culture and cryopreservation of spermatogenic cells used for human in-vitro conception. *Hum. Reprod.* **1998**, *13*, 634–638. [CrossRef]
155. Sharma, R.; Kattoor, A.J.; Ghulmiyyah, J.; Agarwal, A. Effect of sperm storage and selection techniques on sperm parameters. *Syst. Biol. Reprod. Med.* **2015**, *61*, 1–12. [CrossRef]
156. Stanic, P.; Tandara, M.; Sonicki, Z.; Simunic, V.; Radakovic, B.; Suchanek, E. Comparison of protective media and freezing techniques for cryopreservation of human semen. *Eur. J. Obstet. Gynecol. Reprod. Biol.* **2000**, *91*, 65–70. [CrossRef]
157. Le, M.T.; Nguyen, T.T.T.; Nguyen, T.T.; Nguyen, V.T.; Nguyen, T.T.A.; Nguyen, V.Q.H.; Cao, N.T. Cryopreservation of human spermatozoa by vitrification versus conventional rapid freezing: Effects on motility, viability, morphology and cellular defects. *Eur. J. Obstet. Gynecol. Reprod. Biol.* **2019**, *234*, 14–20. [CrossRef]
158. Silva, A.M.D.; Pereira, A.F.; Comizzoli, P.; Silva, A.R. Cryopreservation and Culture of Testicular Tissues: An Essential Tool for Biodiversity Preservation. *Biopreserv. Biobank* **2020**, *18*, 235–243. [CrossRef] [PubMed]
159. Tao, Y.; Sanger, E.; Saewu, A.; Leveille, M.C. Human sperm vitrification: The state of the art. *Reprod. Biol. Endocrinol.* **2020**, *18*, 17. [CrossRef] [PubMed]
160. Arav, A.; Yavin, S.; Zeron, Y.; Natan, D.; Dekel, I.; Gacitua, H. New trends in gamete's cryopreservation. *Mol. Cell Endocrinol.* **2002**, *187*, 77–81. [CrossRef]
161. Liow, S.L.; Foong, L.C.; Chen, N.Q.; Yip, W.Y.; Khaw, C.L.; Kumar, J.; Vajta, G.; Ng, S.C. Live birth from vitrified-warmed human oocytes fertilized with frozen-thawed testicular spermatozoa. *Reprod. Biomed. Online* **2009**, *19*, 198–201. [CrossRef]
162. Schulz, M.; Risopatrón, J.; Uribe, P.; Isachenko, E.; Isachenko, V.; Sánchez, R. Human sperm vitrification: A scientific report. *Andrology* **2020**, *8*, 1642–1650. [CrossRef] [PubMed]
163. Berkovitz, A.; Miller, N.; Silberman, M.; Belenky, M.; Itsykson, P. A novel solution for freezing small numbers of spermatozoa using a sperm vitrification device. *Hum. Reprod.* **2018**, *33*, 1975–1983. [CrossRef] [PubMed]
164. Ohno, M.; Tanaka, A.; Nagayoshi, M.; Yamaguchi, T.; Takemoto, Y.; Tanaka, I.; Watanabe, S.; Itakura, A. Modified permeable cryoprotectant-free vitrification method for three or fewer ejaculated spermatozoa from cryptozoospermic men and 7-year follow-up study of 14 children born from this method. *Hum. Reprod.* **2020**, *35*, 1019–1028. [CrossRef] [PubMed]
165. Liu, S.; Li, F. Cryopreservation of single-sperm: Where are we today? *Reprod. Biol. Endocrinol.* **2020**, *18*, 41. [CrossRef]
166. Sá, R.; Cremades, N.; Malheiro, I.; Sousa, M. Cryopreservation of human testicular diploid germ cell suspensions. *Andrologia* **2012**, *44*, 366–372. [CrossRef]
167. Hammadeh, M.E.; Szarvasy, D.; Zeginiadou, T.; Rosenbaum, P.; Georg, T.; Schmidt, W. Evaluation of cryoinjury of spermatozoa after slow (programmed biological freezer) or rapid (liquid nitrogen vapour) freeze-thawing techniques. *J. Assist. Reprod. Genet.* **2001**, *18*, 364–370. [CrossRef]
168. Riva, N.S.; Ruhlmann, C.; Iaizzo, R.S.; Marcial López, C.A.; Martínez, A.G. Comparative analysis between slow freezing and ultra-rapid freezing for human sperm cryopreservation. *JBRA Assist. Reprod.* **2018**, *22*, 331–337. [CrossRef]
169. Kamath, M.S.; Muthukumar, K. Appendix B: Solid Surface Vitrification. *Methods Mol. Biol.* **2017**, *1568*, 297–307. [CrossRef]
170. Zhu, J.; Jin, R.T.; Wu, L.M.; Johansson, L.; Guo, T.H.; Liu, Y.S.; Tong, X.H. Cryoprotectant-free ultra-rapid freezing of human spermatozoa in cryogenic vials. *Andrologia* **2014**, *46*, 642–649. [CrossRef]
171. Di Santo, M.; Tarozzi, N.; Nadalini, M.; Borini, A. Human Sperm Cryopreservation: Update on Techniques, Effect on DNA Integrity, and Implications for ART. *Adv. Urol.* **2012**, *2012*, 854837. [CrossRef] [PubMed]
172. Ezzati, M.; Shanehbandi, D.; Hamdi, K.; Rahbar, S.; Pashaiasl, M. Influence of cryopreservation on structure and function of mammalian spermatozoa: An overview. *Cell Tissue Bank* **2020**, *21*, 1–15. [CrossRef] [PubMed]
173. Polge, C.; Smith, A.U.; Parkes, A.S. Revival of spermatozoa after vitrification and dehydration at low temperatures. *Nature* **1949**, *164*, 666. [CrossRef]
174. Hovatta, O.; Foudila, T.; Siegberg, R.; Johansson, K.; von Smitten, K.; Reima, I. Pregnancy resulting from intracytoplasmic injection of spermatozoa from a frozen-thawed testicular biopsy specimen. *Hum. Reprod.* **1996**, *11*, 2472–2473. [CrossRef]
175. Serafini, P.C.; Hauser, D.; Moyer, D.; Marrs, R.P. Cryopreservation of human spermatozoa: Correlations of ultrastructural sperm head configuration with sperm motility and ability to penetrate zona-free hamster ova. *Fertil. Steril.* **1986**, *46*, 691–695. [CrossRef]
176. Keros, V.; Rosenlund, B.; Hultenby, K.; Aghajanova, L.; Levkov, L.; Hovatta, O. Optimizing cryopreservation of human testicular tissue: Comparison of protocols with glycerol, propanediol and dimethylsulphoxide as cryoprotectants. *Hum. Reprod.* **2005**, *20*, 1676–1687. [CrossRef] [PubMed]
177. Brook, P.F.; Radford, J.A.; Shalet, S.M.; Joyce, A.D.; Gosden, R.G. Isolation of germ cells from human testicular tissue for low temperature storage and autotransplantation. *Fertil. Steril.* **2001**, *75*, 269–274. [CrossRef]
178. Zhang, B.; Wang, Y.; Wu, C.; Qiu, S.; Chen, X.; Cai, B.; Xie, H. Freeze-thawing impairs the motility, plasma membrane integrity and mitochondria function of boar spermatozoa through generating excessive ROS. *BMC Vet. Res.* **2021**, *17*, 127. [CrossRef]
179. Medrano, L.; Enciso, M.; Gomez-Torres, M.J.; Aizpurua, J. First birth of a healthy infant following intra-cytoplasmic sperm injection using a new permeable cryoprotectant-free sperm vitrification protocol. *Cryobiology* **2019**, *87*, 117–119. [CrossRef]

180. Isachenko, E.; Isachenko, V.; Katkov, I.I.; Rahimi, G.; Schöndorf, T.; Mallmann, P.; Dessole, S.; Nawroth, F. DNA integrity and motility of human spermatozoa after standard slow freezing versus cryoprotectant-free vitrification. *Hum. Reprod.* **2004**, *19*, 932–939. [CrossRef]
181. Fahy, G.M.; MacFarlane, D.R.; Angell, C.A.; Meryman, H.T. Vitrification as an approach to cryopreservation. *Cryobiology* **1984**, *21*, 407–426. [CrossRef]
182. Desai, N.N.; Blackmon, H.; Goldfarb, J. Single sperm cryopreservation on cryoloops: An alternative to hamster zona for freezing individual spermatozoa. *Reprod. Biomed. Online* **2004**, *9*, 47–53. [CrossRef]
183. Liu, F.; Zou, S.S.; Zhu, Y.; Sun, C.; Liu, Y.F.; Wang, S.S.; Shi, W.B.; Zhu, J.J.; Huang, Y.H.; Li, Z. A novel micro-straw for cryopreservation of small number of human spermatozoon. *Asian J. Androl.* **2017**, *19*, 326–329. [CrossRef]
184. Desai, N.; Goldberg, J.; Austin, C.; Sabanegh, E.; Falcone, T. Cryopreservation of individually selected sperm: Methodology and case report of a clinical pregnancy. *J. Assist. Reprod. Genet.* **2012**, *29*, 375–379. [CrossRef]
185. Diaz-Jimenez, M.; Dorado, J.; Pereira, B.; Ortiz, I.; Consuegra, C.; Bottrel, M.; Ortiz, E.; Hidalgo, M. Vitrification in straws conserves motility features better than spheres in donkey sperm. *Reprod. Domest. Anim.* **2018**, *53* (Suppl. 2), 56–58. [CrossRef]
186. Cohen, J.; Garrisi, G.J. Micromanipulation of gametes and embryos: Cryopreservation of a single human spermatozoon within an isolated zona pellucida. *Hum. Reprod. Update* **1997**, *3*, 453. [CrossRef] [PubMed]
187. Hsieh, Y.Y.; Tsai, H.D.; Chang, C.C.; Lo, H.Y. Sperm cryopreservation with empty human or mouse zona pellucidae. A comparison. *J. Reprod. Med.* **2000**, *45*, 383–386. [PubMed]
188. Walmsley, R.; Cohen, J.; Ferrara-Congedo, T.; Reing, A.; Garrisi, J. The first births and ongoing pregnancies associated with sperm cryopreservation within evacuated egg zonae. *Hum. Reprod.* **1998**, *13* (Suppl. 4), 61–70. [CrossRef]
189. Just, A.; Gruber, I.; Wöber, M.; Lahodny, J.; Obruca, A.; Strohmer, H. Novel method for the cryopreservation of testicular sperm and ejaculated spermatozoa from patients with severe oligospermia: A pilot study. *Fertil. Steril.* **2004**, *82*, 445–447. [CrossRef] [PubMed]
190. Herrler, A.; Eisner, S.; Bach, V.; Weissenborn, U.; Beier, H.M. Cryopreservation of spermatozoa in alginic acid capsules. *Fertil. Steril.* **2006**, *85*, 208–213. [CrossRef] [PubMed]
191. Araki, Y.; Yao, T.; Asayama, Y.; Matsuhisa, A. Single human sperm cryopreservation method using hollow-core agarose capsules. *Fertil. Steril.* **2015**, *104*, 1004–1009. [CrossRef] [PubMed]
192. Tomita, K.; Sakai, S.; Khanmohammadi, M.; Yamochi, T.; Hashimoto, S.; Anzai, M.; Morimoto, Y.; Taya, M.; Hosoi, Y. Cryopreservation of a small number of human sperm using enzymatically fabricated, hollow hyaluronan microcapsules handled by conventional ICSI procedures. *J. Assist. Reprod. Genet.* **2016**, *33*, 501–511. [CrossRef] [PubMed]
193. Endo, Y.; Fujii, Y.; Kurotsuchi, S.; Motoyama, H.; Funahashi, H. Successful delivery derived from vitrified-warmed spermatozoa from a patient with nonobstructive azoospermia. *Fertil. Steril.* **2012**, *98*, 1423–1427. [CrossRef] [PubMed]
194. Endo, Y.; Fujii, Y.; Shintani, K.; Seo, M.; Motoyama, H.; Funahashi, H. Simple vitrification for small numbers of human spermatozoa. *Reprod. Biomed. Online* **2012**, *24*, 301–307. [CrossRef]
195. Schuster, T.G.; Keller, L.M.; Dunn, R.L.; Ohl, D.A.; Smith, G.D. Ultra-rapid freezing of very low numbers of sperm using cryoloops. *Hum. Reprod.* **2003**, *18*, 788–795. [CrossRef]
196. Desai, N.; Culler, C.; Goldfarb, J. Cryopreservation of single sperm from epididymal and testicular samples on cryoloops: Preliminary case report. *Fertil. Steril.* **2004**, *82*, S264–S265. [CrossRef]
197. Stein, A.; Shufaro, Y.; Hadar, S.; Fisch, B.; Pinkas, H. Successful use of the Cryolock device for cryopreservation of scarce human ejaculate and testicular spermatozoa. *Andrology* **2015**, *3*, 220–224. [CrossRef]
198. Wang, X.L.; Zhang, X.; Qin, Y.Q.; Hao, D.Y.; Shi, H.R. Outcomes of day 3 embryo transfer with vitrification using Cryoleaf: A 3-year follow-up study. *J. Assist. Reprod. Genet.* **2012**, *29*, 883–889. [CrossRef]
199. Sun, J.; Chen, W.; Zhou, L.; Hu, J.; Li, Z.; Zhang, Z.; Wu, Y. Successful delivery derived from cryopreserved rare human spermatozoa with novel cryopiece. *Andrology* **2017**, *5*, 832–837. [CrossRef]
200. Mansilla, M.A.; Merino, O.; Risopatrón, J.; Isachenko, V.; Isachenko, E.; Sánchez, R. High temperature is essential for preserved human sperm function during the devitrification process. *Andrologia* **2016**, *48*, 111–113. [CrossRef]
201. Pabón, D.; Meseguer, M.; Sevillano, G.; Cobo, A.; Romero, J.L.; Remohí, J.; de Los Santos, M.J. A new system of sperm cryopreservation: Evaluation of survival, motility, DNA oxidation, and mitochondrial activity. *Andrology* **2019**, *7*, 293–301. [CrossRef]
202. Abdelnour, S.A.; Hassan, M.A.E.; Mohammed, A.K.; Alhimaidi, A.R.; Al-Gabri, N.; Al-Khaldi, K.O.; Swelum, A.A. The Effect of Adding Different Levels of Curcumin and Its Nanoparticles to Extender on Post-Thaw Quality of Cryopreserved Rabbit Sperm. *Animals* **2020**, *10*, 1508. [CrossRef]
203. Hosseini, A.; Khalili, M.A.; Talebi, A.R.; Agha-Rahimi, A.; Ghasemi-Esmailabad, S.; Woodward, B.; Yari, N. Cryopreservation of Low Number of Human Spermatozoa; Which is Better: Vapor Phase or Direct Submerging in Liquid Nitrogen? *Hum. Fertil.* **2019**, *22*, 126–132. [CrossRef]
204. Valcarce, D.G.; Cartón-García, F.; Riesco, M.F.; Herráez, M.P.; Robles, V. Analysis of DNA damage after human sperm cryopreservation in genes crucial for fertilization and early embryo development. *Andrology* **2013**, *1*, 723–730. [CrossRef]
205. Len, J.S.; Koh, W.S.D.; Tan, S.X. The roles of reactive oxygen species and antioxidants in cryopreservation. *BioSci. Rep.* **2019**, *39*. [CrossRef] [PubMed]

206. Gualtieri, R.; Kalthur, G.; Barbato, V.; Di Nardo, M.; Adiga, S.K.; Talevi, R. Mitochondrial Dysfunction and Oxidative Stress Caused by Cryopreservation in Reproductive Cells. *Antioxidants* **2021**, *10*, 337. [CrossRef] [PubMed]
207. Lusignan, M.F.; Li, X.; Herrero, B.; Delbes, G.; Chan, P.T.K. Effects of different cryopreservation methods on DNA integrity and sperm chromatin quality in men. *Andrology* **2018**, *6*, 829–835. [CrossRef] [PubMed]
208. Tongdee, P.; Sukprasert, M.; Satirapod, C.; Wongkularb, A.; Choktanasiri, W. Comparison of Cryopreserved Human Sperm between Ultra Rapid Freezing and Slow Programmable Freezing: Effect on Motility, Morphology and DNA Integrity. *J. Med. Assoc Thai* **2015**, *98* (Suppl. 4), S33–S42. [PubMed]
209. Vutyavanich, T.; Piromlertamorn, W.; Nunta, S. Rapid freezing versus slow programmable freezing of human spermatozoa. *Fertil. Steril.* **2010**, *93*, 1921–1928. [CrossRef]
210. Oraiopoulou, C.; Vorniotaki, A.; Taki, E.; Papatheodorou, A.; Christoforidis, N.; Chatziparasidou, A. The impact of fresh and frozen testicular tissue quality on embryological and clinical outcomes. *Andrologia* **2021**, *53*, e14040. [CrossRef] [PubMed]
211. Vernaeve, V.; Tournaye, H.; Osmanagaoglu, K.; Verheyen, G.; Van Steirteghem, A.; Devroey, P. Intracytoplasmic sperm injection with testicular spermatozoa is less successful in men with nonobstructive azoospermia than in men with obstructive azoospermia. *Fertil. Steril.* **2003**, *79*, 529–533. [CrossRef]
212. Martin, R.H.; Greene, C.; Rademaker, A.W.; Ko, E.; Chernos, J. Analysis of aneuploidy in spermatozoa from testicular biopsies from men with nonobstructive azoospermia. *J. Androl.* **2003**, *24*, 100–103.
213. Mulder, C.L.; Catsburg, L.A.E.; Zheng, Y.; de Winter-Korver, C.M.; van Daalen, S.K.M.; van Wely, M.; Pals, S.; Repping, S.; van Pelt, A.M.M. Long-term health in recipients of transplanted in vitro propagated spermatogonial stem cells. *Hum. Reprod.* **2018**, *33*, 81–90. [CrossRef]
214. Sharma, R.; Biedenharn, K.R.; Fedor, J.M.; Agarwal, A. Lifestyle factors and reproductive health: Taking control of your fertility. *Reprod. Biol. Endocrinol.* **2013**, *11*, 66. [CrossRef]
215. Semião-Francisco, L.; Braga, D.P.; Figueira, R.e.C.; Madaschi, C.; Pasqualotto, F.F.; Iaconelli, A.; Borges, E. Assisted reproductive technology outcomes in azoospermic men: 10 years of experience with surgical sperm retrieval. *Aging Male* **2010**, *13*, 44–50. [CrossRef] [PubMed]
216. Jellad Ammar, S.; Arfaoui, R.; Hammami, F.; Souayah, N.; Chibani, M.; Rachdi, R. Does cryopreservation of testicular sperm affect ICSI outcomes in azoospermia? *Tunis Med.* **2020**, *98*, 581–587. [PubMed]
217. Ernandez, J.; Berk, B.; Han, T.; Abou Ghayda, R.; Kathrins, M. Evaluating the quality of reported outcomes for microsurgical TESE in men with non-obstructive azoospermia: A methodological analysis. *Andrology* **2021**. [CrossRef]
218. Khan, I.M.; Cao, Z.; Liu, H.; Khan, A.; Rahman, S.U.; Khan, M.Z.; Sathanawongs, A.; Zhang, Y. Impact of Cryopreservation on Spermatozoa Freeze-Thawed Traits and Relevance OMICS to Assess Sperm Cryo-Tolerance in Farm Animals. *Front. Vet. Sci.* **2021**, *8*, 609180. [CrossRef]
219. Vermeulen, M.; Poels, J.; de Michele, F.; des Rieux, A.; Wyns, C. Restoring Fertility with Cryopreserved Prepubertal Testicular Tissue: Perspectives with Hydrogel Encapsulation, Nanotechnology, and Bioengineered Scaffolds. *Ann. Biomed. Eng.* **2017**, *45*, 1770–1781. [CrossRef] [PubMed]
220. Shahin, M.A.; Khalil, W.A.; Saadeldin, I.M.; Swelum, A.A.; El-Harairy, M.A. Comparison between the Effects of Adding Vitamins, Trace Elements, and Nanoparticles to SHOTOR Extender on the Cryopreservation of Dromedary Camel Epididymal Spermatozoa. *Animals* **2020**, *10*, 78. [CrossRef] [PubMed]
221. Del Vento, F.; Vermeulen, M.; Ucakar, B.; Poels, J.; des Rieux, A.; Wyns, C. Significant Benefits of Nanoparticles Containing a Necrosis Inhibitor on Mice Testicular Tissue Autografts Outcomes. *Int. J. Mol. Sci.* **2019**, *20*, 5833. [CrossRef]
222. Saadeldin, I.M.; Khalil, W.A.; Alharbi, M.G.; Lee, S.H. The Current Trends in Using Nanoparticles, Liposomes, and Exosomes for Semen Cryopreservation. *Animals* **2020**, *10*, 2281. [CrossRef] [PubMed]
223. Du, J.; Shen, J.; Wang, Y.; Pan, C.; Pang, W.; Diao, H.; Dong, W. Boar seminal plasma exosomes maintain sperm function by infiltrating into the sperm membrane. *Oncotarget* **2016**, *7*, 58832–58847. [CrossRef] [PubMed]
224. Mokarizadeh, A.; Rezvanfar, M.A.; Dorostkar, K.; Abdollahi, M. Mesenchymal stem cell derived microvesicles: Trophic shuttles for enhancement of sperm quality parameters. *Reprod. Toxicol.* **2013**, *42*, 78–84. [CrossRef] [PubMed]
225. Stremersch, S.; Vandenbroucke, R.E.; Van Wonterghem, E.; Hendrix, A.; De Smedt, S.C.; Raemdonck, K. Comparing exosome-like vesicles with liposomes for the functional cellular delivery of small RNAs. *J. Control. Release* **2016**, *232*, 51–61. [CrossRef] [PubMed]
226. Sullivan, R.; Saez, F. Epididymosomes, prostasomes, and liposomes: Their roles in mammalian male reproductive physiology. *Reproduction* **2013**, *146*, R21–R35. [CrossRef] [PubMed]
227. Jiang, Y.; Zhu, W.Q.; Zhu, X.C.; Cai, N.N.; Yang, R.; Cai, H.; Zhang, X.M. Cryopreservation of calf testicular tissues with knockout serum replacement. *Cryobiology* **2020**, *92*, 255–257. [CrossRef] [PubMed]
228. Bahmyari, R.; Zare, M.; Sharma, R.; Agarwal, A.; Halvaei, I. The efficacy of antioxidants in sperm parameters and production of reactive oxygen species levels during the freeze-thaw process: A systematic review and meta-analysis. *Andrologia* **2020**, *52*, e13514. [CrossRef]
229. Arkoun, B.; Galas, L.; Dumont, L.; Rives, A.; Saulnier, J.; Delessard, M.; Rondanino, C.; Rives, N. Vitamin E but Not GSH Decreases Reactive Oxygen Species Accumulation and Enhances Sperm Production during In Vitro Maturation of Frozen-Thawed Prepubertal Mouse Testicular Tissue. *Int. J. Mol. Sci.* **2019**, *20*, 5380. [CrossRef]

230. Leão, A.P.A.; Souza, A.V.; Mesquita, N.F.; Pereira, L.J.; Zangeronimo, M.G. Antioxidant enrichment of rooster semen extenders—A systematic review. *Res. Vet. Sci.* **2021**, *136*, 111–118. [CrossRef]
231. Schlegel, P.N. Nonobstructive azoospermia: A revolutionary surgical approach and results. *Semin. Reprod. Med.* **2009**, *27*, 165–170. [CrossRef]
232. Mehmood, S.; Aldaweesh, S.; Junejo, N.N.; Altaweel, W.M.; Kattan, S.A.; Alhathal, N. Microdissection testicular sperm extraction: Overall results and impact of preoperative testosterone level on sperm retrieval rate in patients with nonobstructive azoospermia. *Urol. Ann.* **2019**, *11*, 287–293. [CrossRef] [PubMed]
233. Gross, K.X.; Hanson, B.M.; Hotaling, J.M. Round Spermatid Injection. *Urol. Clin. N. Am.* **2020**, *47*, 175–183. [CrossRef] [PubMed]
234. Tanaka, A.; Suzuki, K.; Nagayoshi, M.; Takemoto, Y.; Watanabe, S.; Takeda, S.; Irahara, M.; Kuji, N.; Yamagata, Z.; Yanagimachi, R. Ninety babies born after round spermatid injection into oocytes: Survey of their development from fertilization to 2 years of age. *Fertil. Steril.* **2018**, *110*, 443–451. [CrossRef]
235. Pabuccu, R.; Sertyel, S.; Pabuccu, E.; Aydos, K.; Haliloglu, A.H.; Demirkıran, D.; Keles, G.; Tanaka, A. Live Births with a Novel ROSI Technique Using Elongating Spermatids for Non Obstructive Azoospermia Patients: A European Cohort Study. In Proceedings of the ESHRE 36th Annual Meeting, Copenhagen, Denmark, 5–8 July 2020; p. O-125.
236. Sousa, M.; Cremades, N.; Alves, C.; Silva, J.; Barros, A. Developmental potential of human spermatogenic cells co-cultured with Sertoli cells. *Hum. Reprod.* **2002**, *17*, 161–172. [CrossRef] [PubMed]
237. Sato, T.; Katagiri, K.; Gohbara, A.; Inoue, K.; Ogonuki, N.; Ogura, A.; Kubota, Y.; Ogawa, T. In vitro production of functional sperm in cultured neonatal mouse testes. *Nature* **2011**, *471*, 504–507. [CrossRef] [PubMed]
238. Yokonishi, T.; Sato, T.; Komeya, M.; Katagiri, K.; Kubota, Y.; Nakabayashi, K.; Hata, K.; Inoue, K.; Ogonuki, N.; Ogura, A.; et al. Offspring production with sperm grown in vitro from cryopreserved testis tissues. *Nat. Commun* **2014**, *5*, 4320. [CrossRef] [PubMed]
239. Perrard, M.H.; Sereni, N.; Schluth-Bolard, C.; Blondet, A.; D Estaing, S.G.; Plotton, I.; Morel-Journel, N.; Lejeune, H.; David, L.; Durand, P. Complete Human and Rat Ex Vivo Spermatogenesis from Fresh or Frozen Testicular Tissue. *Biol. Reprod.* **2016**, *95*, 89. [CrossRef]
240. de Michele, F.; Poels, J.; Vermeulen, M.; Ambroise, J.; Gruson, D.; Guiot, Y.; Wyns, C. Haploid Germ Cells Generated in Organotypic Culture of Testicular Tissue from Prepubertal Boys. *Front. Physiol* **2018**, *9*, 1413. [CrossRef]
241. Portela, J.M.D.; de Winter-Korver, C.M.; van Daalen, S.K.M.; Meißner, A.; de Melker, A.A.; Repping, S.; van Pelt, A.M.M. Assessment of fresh and cryopreserved testicular tissues from (pre)pubertal boys during organ culture as a strategy for in vitro spermatogenesis. *Hum. Reprod.* **2019**, *34*, 2443–2455. [CrossRef]
242. Medrano, J.V.; Vilanova-Pérez, T.; Fornés-Ferrer, V.; Navarro-Gomezlechon, A.; Martínez-Triguero, M.L.; García, S.; Gómez-Chacón, J.; Povo, I.; Pellicer, A.; Andrés, M.M.; et al. Influence of temperature, serum, and gonadotropin supplementation in short- and long-term organotypic culture of human immature testicular tissue. *Fertil. Steril.* **2018**, *110*, 1045–1057.e1043. [CrossRef] [PubMed]
243. Komeya, M.; Hayashi, K.; Nakamura, H.; Yamanaka, H.; Sanjo, H.; Kojima, K.; Sato, T.; Yao, M.; Kimura, H.; Fujii, T.; et al. Pumpless microfluidic system driven by hydrostatic pressure induces and maintains mouse spermatogenesis in vitro. *Sci. Rep.* **2017**, *7*, 15459. [CrossRef]
244. Ibtisham, F.; Honaramooz, A. Spermatogonial Stem Cells for In Vitro Spermatogenesis and In Vivo Restoration of Fertility. *Cells* **2020**, *9*, 745. [CrossRef]
245. Nasiri, Z.; Hosseini, S.M.; Hajian, M.; Abedi, P.; Bahadorani, M.; Baharvand, H.; Nasr-Esfahani, M.H. Effects of different feeder layers on short-term culture of prepubertal bovine testicular germ cells in-vitro. *Theriogenology* **2012**, *77*, 1519–1528. [CrossRef] [PubMed]
246. Qian, C.; Meng, Q.; Lu, J.; Zhang, L.; Li, H.; Huang, B. Human amnion mesenchymal stem cells restore spermatogenesis in mice with busulfan-induced testis toxicity by inhibiting apoptosis and oxidative stress. *Stem Cell Res. Ther.* **2020**, *11*, 290. [CrossRef]
247. Liang, J.; Wang, N.; He, J.; Du, J.; Guo, Y.; Li, L.; Wu, W.; Yao, C.; Li, Z.; Kee, K. Induction of Sertoli-like cells from human fibroblasts by NR5A1 and GATA4. *Elife* **2019**, *8*. [CrossRef]
248. Yang, S.; Ping, P.; Ma, M.; Li, P.; Tian, R.; Yang, H.; Liu, Y.; Gong, Y.; Zhang, Z.; Li, Z.; et al. Generation of haploid spermatids with fertilization and development capacity from human spermatogonial stem cells of cryptorchid patients. *Stem Cell Rep.* **2014**, *3*, 663–675. [CrossRef]
249. Marh, J.; Tres, L.L.; Yamazaki, Y.; Yanagimachi, R.; Kierszenbaum, A.L. Mouse round spermatids developed in vitro from preexisting spermatocytes can produce normal offspring by nuclear injection into in vivo-developed mature oocytes. *Biol. Reprod.* **2003**, *69*, 169–176. [CrossRef] [PubMed]
250. Lee, J.H.; Kim, H.J.; Kim, H.; Lee, S.J.; Gye, M.C. In vitro spermatogenesis by three-dimensional culture of rat testicular cells in collagen gel matrix. *Biomaterials* **2006**, *27*, 2845–2853. [CrossRef]
251. Abu Elhija, M.; Lunenfeld, E.; Schlatt, S.; Huleihel, M. Differentiation of murine male germ cells to spermatozoa in a soft agar culture system. *Asian J. Androl.* **2012**, *14*, 285–293. [CrossRef]
252. Lee, J.H.; Gye, M.C.; Choi, K.W.; Hong, J.Y.; Lee, Y.B.; Park, D.W.; Lee, S.J.; Min, C.K. In vitro differentiation of germ cells from nonobstructive azoospermic patients using three-dimensional culture in a collagen gel matrix. *Fertil. Steril.* **2007**, *87*, 824–833. [CrossRef]

253. Gholami, K.; Pourmand, G.; Koruji, M.; Sadighigilani, M.; Navid, S.; Izadyar, F.; Abbasi, M. Efficiency of colony formation and differentiation of human spermatogenic cells in two different culture systems. *Reprod. Biol.* **2018**, *18*, 397–403. [CrossRef] [PubMed]
254. Yi, H.; Xiao, S.; Zhang, Y. Stage-specific approaches promote in vitro induction for spermatogenesis in vitro. *Cell. Dev. Biol. Anim.* **2018**, *54*, 217–230. [CrossRef] [PubMed]
255. Cremades, N.; Bernabeu, R.; Barros, A.; Sousa, M. In-vitro maturation of round spermatids using co-culture on Vero cells. *Hum. Reprod.* **1999**, *14*, 1287–1293. [CrossRef]
256. Tanaka, A.; Nagayoshi, M.; Awata, S.; Mawatari, Y.; Tanaka, I.; Kusunoki, H. Completion of meiosis in human primary spermatocytes through in vitro coculture with Vero cells. *Fertil. Steril.* **2003**, *79* (Suppl. 1), 795–801. [CrossRef]
257. Movahedin, M.; Ajeen, A.; Ghorbanzadeh, N.; Tiraihi, T.; Valojerdi, M.R.; Kazemnejad, A. In vitro maturation of fresh and frozen-thawed mouse round spermatids. *Andrologia* **2004**, *36*, 269–276. [CrossRef] [PubMed]
258. Tesarik, J.; Bahceci, M.; Ozcan, C.; Greco, E.; Mendoza, C. Restoration of fertility by in-vitro spermatogenesis. *Lancet* **1999**, *353*, 555–556. [CrossRef]
259. Tesarik, J.; Greco, E.; Mendoza, C. Assisted reproduction with in-vitro-cultured testicular spermatozoa in cases of severe germ cell apoptosis: A pilot study. *Hum. Reprod.* **2001**, *16*, 2640–2645. [CrossRef]
260. Solomon, R.; AbuMadighem, A.; Kapelushnik, J.; Amano, B.C.; Lunenfeld, E.; Huleihel, M. Involvement of Cytokines and Hormones in the Development of Spermatogenesis In Vitro from Spermatogonial Cells of Cyclophosphamide-Treated Immature Mice. *Int. J. Mol. Sci.* **2021**, *22*, 1672. [CrossRef]
261. Liu, S.; Tang, Z.; Xiong, T.; Tang, W. Isolation and characterization of human spermatogonial stem cells. *Reprod. Biol. Endocrinol.* **2011**, *9*, 141. [CrossRef]
262. Mohammadzadeh, E.; Mirzapour, T.; Nowroozi, M.R.; Nazarian, H.; Piryaei, A.; Alipour, F.; Modarres Mousavi, S.M.; Ghaffari Novin, M. Differentiation of spermatogonial stem cells by soft agar three-dimensional culture system. *Artif. Cells Nanomed. Biotechnol.* **2019**, *47*, 1772–1781. [CrossRef] [PubMed]
263. Pramod, R.K.; Mitra, A. In vitro culture and characterization of spermatogonial stem cells on Sertoli cell feeder layer in goat (Capra hircus). *J. Assist. Reprod. Genet.* **2014**, *31*, 993–1001. [CrossRef] [PubMed]
264. Nowroozi, M.R.; Ahmadi, H.; Rafiian, S.; Mirzapour, T.; Movahedin, M. In vitro colonization of human spermatogonia stem cells: Effect of patient's clinical characteristics and testicular histologic findings. *Urology* **2011**, *78*, 1075–1081. [CrossRef]
265. Jabari, A.; Sadighi Gilani, M.A.; Koruji, M.; Gholami, K.; Mohsenzadeh, M.; Rastegar, T.; Khadivi, F.; Ghanami Gashti, N.; Nikmahzar, A.; Mojaverrostami, S.; et al. Three-dimensional co-culture of human spermatogonial stem cells with Sertoli cells in soft agar culture system supplemented by growth factors and Laminin. *Acta Histochem.* **2020**, *122*, 151572. [CrossRef] [PubMed]
266. Hasegawa, H.; Terada, Y.; Ugajin, T.; Yaegashi, N.; Sato, K. A novel culture system for mouse spermatid maturation which produces elongating spermatids capable of inducing calcium oscillation during fertilization and embryonic development. *J. Assist. Reprod. Genet.* **2010**, *27*, 565–570. [CrossRef] [PubMed]
267. Roulet, V.; Denis, H.; Staub, C.; Le Tortorec, A.; Delaleu, B.; Satie, A.P.; Patard, J.J.; Jégou, B.; Dejucq-Rainsford, N. Human testis in organotypic culture: Application for basic or clinical research. *Hum. Reprod.* **2006**, *21*, 1564–1575. [CrossRef] [PubMed]
268. Majumdar, S.S.; Sarda, K.; Bhattacharya, I.; Plant, T.M. Insufficient androgen and FSH signaling may be responsible for the azoospermia of the infantile primate testes despite exposure to an adult-like hormonal milieu. *Hum. Reprod.* **2012**, *27*, 2515–2525. [CrossRef]
269. Heidargholizadeh, S.; Aydos, S.E.; Yukselten, Y.; Ozkavukcu, S.; Sunguroglu, A.; Aydos, K. A differential cytokine expression profile before and after rFSH treatment in Sertoli cell cultures of men with nonobstructive azoospermia. *Andrologia* **2017**, *49*, e12647. [CrossRef]
270. Komeya, M.; Kimura, H.; Nakamura, H.; Yokonishi, T.; Sato, T.; Kojima, K.; Hayashi, K.; Katagiri, K.; Yamanaka, H.; Sanjo, H.; et al. Long-term ex vivo maintenance of testis tissues producing fertile sperm in a microfluidic device. *Sci. Rep.* **2016**, *6*, 21472. [CrossRef]
271. Sato, T.; Katagiri, K.; Kojima, K.; Komeya, M.; Yao, M.; Ogawa, T. In Vitro Spermatogenesis in Explanted Adult Mouse Testis Tissues. *PLoS ONE* **2015**, *10*, e0130171. [CrossRef]
272. Reuter, K.; Schlatt, S.; Ehmcke, J.; Wistuba, J. Fact or fiction: In vitro spermatogenesis. *Spermatogenesis* **2012**, *2*, 245–252. [CrossRef] [PubMed]
273. Galdon, G.; Atala, A.; Sadri-Ardekani, H. In Vitro Spermatogenesis: How Far from Clinical Application? *Curr. Urol. Rep.* **2016**, *17*, 49. [CrossRef] [PubMed]

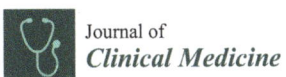

Review

Microfluidic Systems for Isolation of Spermatozoa from Testicular Specimens of Non-Obstructive Azoospermic Men: Does/Can It Improve Sperm Yield?

Gary D. Smith [1,*], Clementina Cantatore [2] and Dana A. Ohl [3]

[1] Reproductive Sciences Program, Departments of Obstetrics/Gynecology, Physiology, and Urology, University of Michigan, Ann Arbor, MI 48103, USA
[2] Reproductive and IVF Unit, Department of Maternal and Child Health, Asi Bari, 70014 Conversano (BA), Italy; clemecant@yahoo.it
[3] Department of Urology, University of Michigan, Ann Arbor, MI 48103, USA; daohl@med.umich.edu
* Correspondence: smithgd@umich.edu; Tel.: +1-734-764-4134

Abstract: Intracytoplasmic sperm injection (ICSI) has allowed reproduction options through assisted reproductive technologies (ARTs) for men with no spermatozoa within the ejaculate (azoospermia). In men with non-obstructive azoospermia (NOA), the options for spermatozoa retrieval are testicular sperm extraction (TESE), testicular sperm aspiration (TESA), or micro-surgical sperm extraction (microTESE). At the initial time of spermatozoa removal from the testis, spermatozoa are immobile. Independent of the means of spermatozoa retrieval, the subsequent steps of removing spermatozoa from seminiferous tubules, determining spermatozoa viability, identifying enough spermatozoa for oocyte injections, and isolating viable spermatozoa for injection are currently performed manually by laboratory microscopic dissection and collection. These laboratory techniques are highly labor-intensive, with yield unknown, have an unpredictable efficiency and/or success rate, and are subject to inter-laboratory personnel and intra-laboratory variability. Here, we consider the potential utility, benefits, and shortcomings of developing technologies such as motility induction/stimulants, microfluidics, dielectrophoresis, and cell sorting as andrological laboratory add-ons to reduce the technical burdens and variabilities in viable spermatozoa isolation from testicular samples in men with NOA.

Keywords: non-obstructive azoospermia; testicular spermatozoa; processing; microfluidics; new technologies

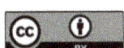

1. NOA Background

Clinical infertility is a disease of the reproductive system defined by the failure to achieve a clinical pregnancy after 12 months or more of regularly unprotected sexual intercourse [1]. The worldwide prevalence of clinical infertility is approximately 9%, with 56% of couples seeking medical interventions [2]. Male factor infertility describes couples in whom the inability to conceive is associated with compromised reproductive function in the male partner. Broadly, this can be due to (1) compromised semen parameters involving semen volume, sperm numbers, motility, morphology, or viability; (2) abnormal sperm function; or (3) normal semen/sperm parameters, yet conditions that prevent sperm deposition in the vagina during intercourse involving male reproductive tract obstructions and/or ejaculatory dysfunction [3]. Males are solely responsible for approximately 20–30% of these clinical infertility cases and contribute to approximately 50% of cases overall (male factor and female factor). The absence of sperm in an ejaculate is termed azoospermia and occurs in less than 1% of the general male population and an estimated 10% of men with infertility. Azoospemia may be caused by an obstruction of the male reproductive tract, which is termed obstructive azoospermia (OA) and makes up approximately 40% of azoospermic cases [4]. Additionally, azoospermia may be a result of inadequate spermatogenesis in the seminiferous tubules of the testis, which is termed non-obstructive azoospermia (NOA). The introduction of intracytoplasmic sperm injection (ICSI; injection of a single sperm into a single oocyte) revolutionized the treatment of male factor infertility, OA, and NOA [5–7]. NOA is considered the most severe and difficult form of azoospermia to treat with assisted reproductive technologies (ARTs) for at least three primary reasons: (1) the method of gamete retrieval; (2) the variable and unpredictable degree of compromised spermatogenesis and success of spermatozoa retrieval/isolation; (3) the initial non-motile nature of retrieved testicular sperm. In this review, we will not address the pros and cons of gamete retrieval methods (as this is specifically addressed in other manuscripts within this series). However, in men with NOA, the following questions arise: (1) Are there focal sites of spermatogenesis within the testes available for spermatozoa isolation? (2) What is the best method to access these focal sites of spermatogenesis? In early studies, testicular sperm extraction (TESE) was used, whereby a single-site testicular biopsy was performed in attempting spermatozoa isolation [8–10]. A retrospective review of first-TESE in NOA from 1994 to 2009 (714 cycles) demonstrated 41% success of spermatozoa retrieval [11]. A modified approach to TESE is testicular sperm aspiration (TESA), which involves the placement of a needle (often a butterfly needle) with negative pressure into the testis, aspiration of fluid and tissue, and movement into multiple regions of the testis without removal from the testes, to "sample" fluid and tissue from numerous focal areas [12]. Subsequent studies using TESA reported variance in spermatozoa retrieval success ranging from 59% [13] to 54% [14]. In contrast to TESE and TESA, microTESE is another form of spermatozoa isolation in NOA. This procedure involves a urologist/surgeon bisecting the testis and using surgical microscopy and 15–20× magnification to identify and isolate dilated/plump seminiferous tubules. Though this surgical procedure is considered more invasive than TESE and TESA, it is a regionally selective biopsy of visualized and isolated seminiferous tubules—resulting in less tissue removal and the ability for spermatozoa identification from isolated tubules to be confirmed by an andrologist in the surgical suite. MicroTESE-isolated seminiferous tubules are subsequently placed into 37 °C processing media and transported to the andrology laboratory, where they are manually dissected under microscope observation. Ramasamy and colleagues [15] demonstrated that the success of spermatozoa retrieval by microTESE diminished with greater operative time, yet overall was successful in 52% of cases. The success of spermatozoa isolation from microTESE-isolated seminiferous tubules was shown to be highest in cases of dilated/plump tubule selective biopsy (90%) versus non-dilated tubule removal (7%) [16].

2. Current Laboratory Techniques for Spermatozoa Isolation from NOA Testicular Samples

Independent of the process used to collect testicular tissue/seminiferous tubules (TESE, TESA, or microTESE), the first steps in the andrology laboratory are to isolate and evaluate seminiferous tubules for the presence of active spermatogenesis (dilated/plump) or lack of spermatogenesis (not dilated/skinny/transparent; Figure 1A). Compared to TESA samples, the amount of testicular somatic or connective tissue is higher in TESE samples, which can make this process of manual seminiferous tubule isolation more difficult. TESA samples tend to yield individualized seminiferous tubules that resemble "unraveled yarn" in the collection media/tube. Within the laboratory, both TESE and TESA samples can require mincing in 37 °C processing media (simple HEPES-buffered media such as human tubule fluid (HTF)-HEPES + protein (human serum albumin (HSA)) to: (1) release the seminiferous tubules from connective tissue; (2) reduce the size of individualized seminiferous tubules; (3) produce clean-cut edges to seminiferous tubules that will facilitate collection of tubule contents. Mincing can be performed on a dissecting microscope in a drop of processing media, with tissue placed on a Petri dish with tweezers and a scalpel. This manual mincing method is useful for seminiferous tubule isolation from TESE samples. One can use a similar manual method for TESA samples or use tuberculin syringe/26–27-gauge needles to cut tubules into manageable sizes. Due to the surgical and selective nature of seminiferous tubule isolation in micro-TESE, the tubules are already isolated in a truncated and pure state and usually do not require laboratory tubule isolation and mincing.

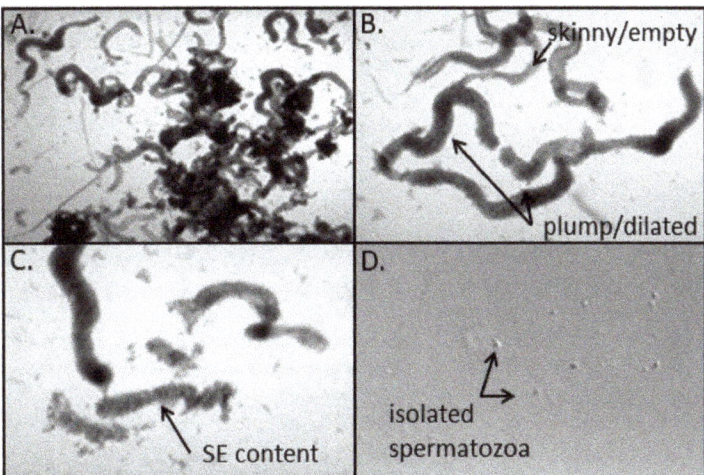

Figure 1. Composite micrographs of laboratory manual processing of testicular aspirate for spermatozoa isolation. (**A**) Minced seminiferous tubules (ST) in processing media. (**B**) Isolated truncated ST with indication of plump/dilated ST with presumed active spermatogenesis and skinny/empty ST (also transparent) with presumed absence of spermatogenesis. (**C**) Seminiferous tubules with one ST processed with tuberculin syringe and needles to squeeze out seminiferous epithelium (SE). (**D**) Following pulled glass pipet dispersion of SE into single cells, the isolation of non-motile testicular spermatozoa. Magnifications: (**A**)—100×, (**B,C**)—200×, (**D**)—400×.

Once the individualized dilated/plump tubules are isolated and truncated, they can be moved into a clean drop of 37 °C processing media (Figure 1B) for further manual processing. At this point, under microscopic observation, a pair of tuberculin syringe/26–27-gauge needles can be used to squeeze the seminiferous tubule contents out of each short dilated/plump tubule segment (Figure 1C). This results in seminiferous tubule content that can be aspirated easily into a small-bore (~15–20 μm inner diameter) flame-pulled glass pipet. This allows one to expel the seminiferous tubule contents into a separate fresh drop of 37 °C processing media as a single-cell suspension, which will contain germ cells of varying degrees of development, supportive cells, and—hopefully—mature spermatozoa (Figure 1D). These testicular-isolated spermatozoa will likely be non-motile; this is especially observed in samples from NOA men [17].

The culture time and conditions have been evaluated for both OA and NOA spermatozoa samples, demonstrating that 24–48 h culture of testicular spermatozoa in complex media (Ham's F10 + albumin) can benefit spermatozoa maturation and motility induction [18–20]. These maturation conditions can be tested on individuals having testicular spermatozoa retrieval in a diagnostic manner, prior to a therapeutic procedure coordinated with egg retrieval. These "diagnostic" testicular spermatozoa retrievals, maturation/motility initiation, and cryopreservation of isolated "rare" spermatozoa [21–23] can be quite successful and have been nicely reviewed and critiqued [24].

The above-described laboratory procedure of spermatozoa isolation from testicular samples relies primarily on manual, mechanical, microscopic processing and can be quite labor- and time-intensive. There are numerous limitations to the current mechanical method of spermatozoa isolation from testicular samples that need to be addressed. The success and efficiency of spermatozoa isolation are influenced by human experience, examiner fatigue, and the slight procedural variations used to yield single-cell suspensions and visualize individual spermatozoa. These laboratory microscopic mechanical procedures can take 2–12 h, depending on testicular sample purity and volume, number of spermatozoa, volumes of media used for procedures, and laboratory personnel experience. As time spent searching for spermatozoa increases, the success of spermatozoa isolation decreases, which can impact subsequent pregnancy rates [15]. Cases with spermatozoa isolation taking < 2 h had significantly higher pregnancy rates (89%) compared to cases taking > 4 h (37%). There have been numerous reports of using enzymatic treatment of testicular samples to aid the recovery of testicular spermatozoa [25–27]; however, its advantages are debated. These enzymatic techniques usually use collagenase type IA or IV to digest the collagen within the basement membrane and extracellular matrix within seminiferous tubules. However, these collagenases have been demonstrated to digest cell surface proteins [28] that may have influence on downstream sperm function in fertilization, pronuclear formation, and embryo development. Additionally, enzymatic methods incorporate centrifugation, which, as discussed below, can have a detrimental impact on spermatozoa DNA integrity. Before discussion of the potential future of microfluidics for spermatozoa isolation from testicular samples of men with NOA, we need to acknowledge that achieving a level of single-cell suspension (as discussed above) will still be required; thus, a significant amount of mechanical and manual processing is still required.

3. Microfluidics and Potential Use in Spermatozoa Isolation from NOA Testicular Samples

Microfluidics is defined as a multidisciplinary field of study and design whereby fluid behaviors are accurately controlled and manipulated with small-scale geometric constraints that yield dominance of surface forces over volumetric forces. While past procedures in the ART laboratory have been successful, they have been more macroscale approaches to microscale cellular biological events [29]. Integration of microfluidics into the ART laboratory has at least four foreseeable advantages: (1) allowing precisely controlled fluidic gamete/embryo manipulations; (2) providing biomimetic environments for culture; (3) facilitating microscale genetic and molecular bioassays; (4) enabling miniaturization and automation. The basic utility and advantages of individual microfluidic devices for isolation of motile spermatozoa have been studied and reported over the last two decades. These can generally be categorized as microfluidic means of motile sperm isolation by three similar but slightly discrete biophysical means.

First, motile sperm can be enriched by using a microfluidic-generated laminar flow and sperm motility-enabled crossing of the meniscus or interstream line formed by the laminar flow [30,31]. These devices allow a separation of motile spermatozoa from seminal plasma, non-motile sperm, dead cells, and debris without centrifugation or resulting potential lethal and sublethal spermatozoa damage. The technical parameters of the device were designed to optimize the isolation of motile human spermatozoa with the inflow channel (semen; 100 µm × 50 µm; width × depth), inflow channel (media; 300 µm × 50 µm), common mid-channel (laminar flow; 500 µm × 50 µm × 100 mm length). Centrifugation can negatively influence sperm motility [32], mitochondrial function [33], intact acrosomal status [33], and DNA integrity [34]. Using the microfluidic laminar flow and inertia spermatozoa isolation, it was demonstrated that isolated motile spermatozoa had significantly less DNA damage compared to processing sperm with centrifugation, density gradient and centrifugation, and swim-up of overlaid semen [35–37]. Using a microfluidic device without laminar flow but with microchannel hydrodynamic constrain to isolate motile sperm and the sperm chromatin dispersion assay, which detects primarily single-strand DNA breaks, Quinn and colleagues [38] demonstrated significantly reduced DNA fragmentation index (DFI) in microfluidic isolated motile sperm (median: 0%; intraquartile ranges (IQR): 0–2.4) compared to motile sperm isolated with density-gradient centrifugation with swim-up (median—6%; intraquartile ranges (IQR): 3–11.5).

The second microfluidic method for motile sperm isolation involves multiple narrow channels and sperm inertia [39]. These microfluidic devices incorporate a radial array of hundreds of microchannels, with motile sperm swimming from the inlet to the outlets away from dead cells, debris, and seminal plasma—resulting in a highly motile population of sperm, again with reduced DNA damage compared to other conventional centrifugation-based semen-processing methods. Recently, these investigators have demonstrated the potential practical use of this design for human sperm isolation for clinical intracytoplasmic sperm injection [40].

Third, Wu and coworkers [41] have developed a microfluidic device that is able to generate an impeding flow field for isolating human motile sperm in a high-throughput manner. While a highly motile population of sperm is isolated in this device, the influence on sperm DNA integrity is unknown; yet, in theory, one would expect reduced processing-induced DNA fragmentation as demonstrated by the other microfluidic methods mentioned above. It is important to appreciate that these microfluidic devices do not directly improve sperm DNA integrity, but they do allow isolation of motile sperm—whereas raw samples have both motile (live) and non-motile (many times dead and DNA fragmented)—without processing-induced DNA damage. Finally, it is important to recognize that all of the above microfluidic devices and methods rely on spermatozoa motility for isolation. As mentioned earlier, testicular spermatozoa at the initial time of retrieval are predominantly non-motile; thus, other creative microfluidic methods or combinations of methods need to be considered in non-motile spermatozoa isolation from NOA testicular samples.

As mentioned above, microfluidics can circumvent centrifugation and deleterious influence on spermatozoa form and function experienced in conventional sperm processing. If one is using enzymatic processing of testicular samples to yield spermatozoa, then centrifugation can be part of the process. However, manual/mechanical processing does not necessarily entail centrifugation. An advantage of microfluidics isolation of spermatozoa from NOA testicular samples compared to other developing methods (magnetic-activated cell sorting (MACS) and fluorescence-activated cell sorting (FACS)—reviewed in Mangum et al., 2020 [42]) is the ability to isolate testicular spermatozoa without biochemical fluorescent or bead labeling of cells [43], which presents safety issues that are yet to be fully evaluated in gametes, fertilization, and offspring health [44]. Magnum and colleagues very nicely have provided a summary table of the advantages and disadvantages of these developing technologies. There are additional microfluidic approaches with potential for isolating non-motile testicular spermatozoa that have been proposed or proof-of-concept tested in animal models, such as combined microfluidics and dielectrophoresis cell sorting [45] and pinched flow fractionation [46,47]. Whether these microfluidic approaches and add-ons will be useful and/or beneficial in isolation of non-motile spermatozoa from human testicular samples of NOA men remains to be demonstrated.

4. Spiral Microfluidics, Inertial Separation, and Cell Size

As testicular resident spermatozoa are largely non-motile, the use of microfluidic laminar flow for isolation is not useful. Son and colleagues [48] demonstrated an ingenious and novel application of spiral microfluidics to effectively and efficiently separate non-motile spermatozoa (or beads of similar size) from non-motile cells of differing size. This spiral inertial microfluidic device yields separation of particles or cells based on size and shape. Spiral microchannel dimensions were calculated with specific consideration in relation to the cellular constituents of a single-cell suspension of a human testicular sample (spermatozoa, white blood cells (WBCs), and germ cells of a more immature state). This prototype spiral microfluidic device had a single inlet and multiple outlets to separate particles/cells at their equilibrium positions as they exit the device. Calculations were performed considering the differing cell sizes, various flow rates, and best conditions for cell focusing (microchannel height—50 µm, microchannel width—150 µm, space between microchannels—310 µm, initial radius—700 µm, and final radius—899 µm). The authors were able to demonstrate separation and isolation of spermatozoa from WBCs. More recently, Vasilescu and coworkers [49] used a similar spiral microchannel device produced by 3D printing to demonstrate rapid spermatozoa recovery from heterogeneous cell suspension of spermatozoa, WBCs, red blood cells, epithelial cells, and leukemic cancer cells. This study demonstrated rapid (5 min) separation of spermatozoa from other cell types and, very importantly, that this spiral microfluidic processing had no detrimental influence on spermatozoa viability, morphology, or DNA integrity. Collectively, these are exciting findings in the quest for future means of isolating immobile spermatozoa from testicular samples, yet there are some issues that remain uninvestigated and require testing. First, does spermatozoa shape/size asymmetry impact isolation efficiency? Second, while most testicular spermatozoa are non-motile, some testicular sperm can exhibit a form of motility termed "twitching"—how that might impact spiral microfluidic separation and focus isolation remains to be determined. This gives rise to a secondary issue of the need for determining the viability of spiral microfluidic testicular non-motile sperm post-isolation prior to use in ICSI. However, future combinations of spiral inertial microfluidic testicular spermatozoa isolation with a short culture period to induce maturation/some motility [20] or a non-terminal viability test, such as the hypo-osmotic swelling test of spermatozoa membrane integrity [50], may aid in addressing this issue.

5. Practical and Future Considerations of Using Microfluidics in Spermatozoa Isolation from NOA Testicular Samples

When initially considering the use of microfluidic applications with existing methods of gamete isolation, in vitro fertilization, embryo culture, gamete/embryo analysis, and/or cryopreservation, we need to first examine the practical shortcomings of the existing techniques, the potential benefits of incorporating microfluidics, and the potential hurdles that this incorporation of microfluidics may have in individual ART procedures. This leads to the practical question of why one might use microfluidics for non-motile spermatozoa isolation from retrieved NOA testicular samples. At a basic level, use of microfluidics would be justified if it does: (1) something we cannot do today; (2) something we do today, but is more efficient or provides a better sample; (3) something we do today, but is less expensive or requires less work, supplies, or personnel effort; (4) something we do today, as well as reduces intra-laboratory personnel and/or inter-laboratory variability; or (5) something we do today, but facilitates future automation and associated benefits [51]. While current methodologies of spermatozoa isolation from NOA testicular samples are manually burdensome and tedious, they do work on most occasions. Whether microfluidics will reduce the cases of "no spermatozoa found for ICSI", increase efficiency, and/or produce a better sample in relation to fertilization rates, embryo development, and live-birth rates remains to be demonstrated. Use of microfluidics to isolate sperm from testicular samples will not become less expensive unless the personnel workload is significantly reduced. This could be the case in the future; however, it is important to recognize that most of the burdensome and tedious manual work in processing testicular samples is in producing a single-cell suspension, which is still needed for current microfluidic application to non-motile spermatozoa isolation from testicular samples. This brings up the potential hurdle of microfluidic application to non-motile spermatozoa isolation—specifically, the lack of microchannel functionality and/or clogging that can and will occur if input samples are not in a single-cell suspension. Notwithstanding the above discussion, the potential use of microfluidics in isolating non-motile spermatozoa from NOA testicular samples should continue to be investigated in rigorous and practical ways. Integration of multiple technologies—existing and of the future—will likely facilitate the use of microfluidics for improving success, reducing technical signatures and variation, and providing bridges over current limitations. Potential examples include combined spiral microfluidics [48,49] with subsequent short-term culture to assess viability/motility [20] and Raman spectroscopy to non-invasively interrogate sperm DNA integrity [52,53].

Author Contributions: Conceptualization, G.D.S., C.C., D.A.O.; Resources, G.D.S.; writing—original, G.D.S.; writing—review, C.C. and D.A.O. All authors have read and agreed to the published version of the manuscript.

Funding: Work in our laboratories on microfluidics for gamete/embryo biology have been supported by National Research Initiative Competitive Grant from the USDA National Institutes of Food and Agriculture (2005-35203-16148), the Coulter Foundation, and the University of Michigan Reproductive Science Program Collaborative Pilot Grant Program. The APC was funded by the University of Michigan Reproductive Sciences Program Collaborative Pilot Grant to GDS.

Acknowledgments: We would like to thank Sarah Block for her editorial comments. We would also like to acknowledge the scientific contributions of many in microfluidics and andrology that unfortunately have not been referenced in this review due to content and size constraints.

Conflicts of Interest: The authors declare no conflict of interest.

References

1. Zegers-Hochschild, F.; Adamson, G.D.; de Mouzon, J.; Ishihara, O.; Mansour, R.; Nygren, K.; Sullivan, E.; Vanderpoel, S.; International Committee for Monitoring Assisted Reproductive Technology; World Health Organization. International Committee for Monitoring Assisted Reproductive Technology (ICMART) and the World Health Organization (WHO) revised glossary of ART terminology, 2009. *Fertil. Steril.* **2009**, *92*, 1520–1524. [CrossRef] [PubMed]
2. Boivin, J.; Bunting, L.; Collins, J.A.; Nygren, K.G. International estimates of infertility prevalence and treatment-seeking: Potential need and demand for infertility medical care. *Hum. Reprod.* **2007**, *22*, 1506–1512. [CrossRef] [PubMed]
3. Schlegel, P.N.; Girardi, S.K. Clinical review 87: In vitro fertilization for male factor infertility. *J. Clin. Endocrinol. Metab.* **1997**, *82*, 709–716. [CrossRef]
4. Jarow, J.P.; Espeland, M.A.; Lipshultz, L.I. Evaluation of the azoospermic patient. *J. Urol.* **1989**, *142*, 62–65. [CrossRef]
5. Palermo, G.; Joris, H.; Devroey, P.; Van Steirteghem, A.C. Pregnancies after intracytoplasmic injection of single spermatozoon into an oocyte. *Lancet* **1992**, *340*, 17–18. [CrossRef]
6. Schoysman, R.; Vanderzwalmen, P.; Nijs, M.; Segal, L.; Segal-Bertin, G.; Geerts, L.; van Roosendaal, E.; Schoysman, D. Pregnancy after fertilisation with human testicular spermatozoa. *Lancet* **1993**, *342*, 1237. [CrossRef]
7. Devroey, P.; Liu, J.; Nagy, Z.; Goossens, A.; Tournaye, H.; Camus, M.; Van Steirteghem, A.; Silber, S. Pregnancies after testicular sperm extraction and intracytoplasmic sperm injection in non-obstructive azoospermia. *Hum. Reprod.* **1995**, *10*, 1457–1460. [CrossRef]
8. Devroey, P.; Liu, J.; Nagy, Z.; Tournaye, H.; Silber, S.J.; Van Steirteghem, A.C. Normal fertilization of human oocytes after testicular sperm extraction and intracytoplasmic sperm injection. *Fertil. Steril.* **1994**, *62*, 639–641. [CrossRef]
9. Silber, S.J.; van Steirteghem, A.; Nagy, Z.; Liu, J.; Tournaye, H.; Devroey, P. Normal pregnancies resulting from testicular sperm extraction and intracytoplasmic sperm injection for azoospermia due to maturation arrest. *Fertil. Steril.* **1996**, *66*, 110–117. [CrossRef]
10. Tournaye, H.; Camus, M.; Vandervorst, M.; Nagy, Z.; Joris, H.; Van Steirteghem, A.; Devroey, P. Surgical sperm retrieval for intracytoplasmic sperm injection. *Int. J. Androl.* **1997**, *20* (Suppl. 3), 69–73.
11. Vloeberghs, V.; Verheyen, G.; Haentjens, P.; Goossens, A.; Polyzos, N.P.; Tournaye, H. How successful is TESE-ICSI in couples with non-obstructive azoospermia? *Hum. Reprod.* **2015**, *30*, 1790–1796. [CrossRef]
12. Lewin, A.; Weiss, D.B.; Friedler, S.; Ben-Shachar, I.; Porat-Katz, A.; Meirow, D.; Schenker, J.G.; Safran, A. Delivery following intracytoplasmic injection of mature sperm cells recovered by testicular fine needle aspiration in a case of hypergonadotropic azoospermia due to maturation arrest. *Hum. Reprod.* **1996**, *11*, 769–771. [CrossRef] [PubMed]
13. Lewin, A.; Reubinoff, B.; Porat-Katz, A.; Weiss, D.; Eisenberg, V.; Arbel, R.; Bar-el, H.; Safran, A. Testicular fine needle aspiration: The alternative method for sperm retrieval in non-obstructive azoospermia. *Hum. Reprod.* **1999**, *14*, 1785–1790. [CrossRef]
14. Khadra, A.A.; Abdulhadi, I.; Ghunain, S.; Kilani, Z. Efficiency of percutaneous testicular sperm aspiration as a mode of sperm collection for intracytoplasmic sperm injection in nonobstructive azoospermia. *J. Urol.* **2003**, *169*, 603–605. [CrossRef]
15. Ramasamy, R.; Fisher, E.S.; Ricci, J.A.; Leung, R.A.; Schlegel, P.N. Duration of microdissection testicular sperm extraction procedures: Relationship to sperm retrieval success. *J. Urol.* **2011**, *185*, 1394–1397. [CrossRef] [PubMed]
16. Caroppo, E.; Colpi, E.M.; Gazzano, G.; Vaccalluzzo, L.; Piatti, E.; D'Amato, G.; Colpi, G.M. The seminiferous tubule caliber pattern as evaluated at high magnification during microdissection testicular sperm extraction predicts sperm retrieval in patients with non-obstructive azoospermia. *Andrology* **2019**, *7*, 8–14. [CrossRef] [PubMed]
17. Tabbara, S.O.; Covell, J.L.; Abbitt, P.L. Diagnosis of endometriosis by fine-needle aspiration cytology. *Diagn. Cytopathol.* **1991**, *7*, 606–610. [CrossRef] [PubMed]
18. Zhu, J.; Meniru, G.I.; Craft, I. In vitro maturation of human testicular sperm in patients with azoospermia. *J. Assist. Reprod. Genet.* **1997**, *14*, 361–363. [CrossRef]
19. Wu, B.; Wong, D.; Lu, S.; Dickstein, S.; Silva, M.; Gelety, T.J. Optimal use of fresh and frozen-thawed testicular sperm for intracytoplasmic sperm injection in azoospermic patients. *J. Assist. Reprod. Genet.* **2005**, *22*, 389–394. [CrossRef]
20. Morris, D.S.; Dunn, R.L.; Schuster, T.G.; Ohl, D.A.; Smith, G.D. Ideal culture time for improvement in sperm motility from testicular sperm aspirates of men with azoospermia. *J. Urol.* **2007**, *178*, 2087–2091; discussion 2091. [CrossRef]
21. Schuster, T.G.; Keller, L.M.; Dunn, R.L.; Ohl, D.A.; Smith, G.D. Ultra-rapid freezing of very low numbers of sperm using cryoloops. *Hum. Reprod.* **2003**, *18*, 788–795. [CrossRef]

22. Desai, N.; Goldberg, J.; Austin, C.; Sabanegh, E.; Falcone, T. Cryopreservation of individually selected sperm: Methodology and case report of a clinical pregnancy. *J. Assist. Reprod. Genet.* **2012**, *29*, 375–379. [CrossRef]
23. Kathrins, M.; Abhyankar, N.; Shoshany, O.; Liebermann, J.; Uhler, M.; Prins, G.; Niederberger, C. Post-thaw recovery of rare or very low concentrations of cryopreserved human sperm. *Fertil. Steril.* **2017**, *107*, 1300–1304. [CrossRef] [PubMed]
24. Verheyen, G.; Vernaeve, V.; Van Landuyt, L.; Tournaye, H.; Devroey, P.; Van Steirteghem, A. Should diagnostic testicular sperm retrieval followed by cryopreservation for later ICSI be the procedure of choice for all patients with non-obstructive azoospermia? *Hum. Reprod.* **2004**, *19*, 2822–2830. [CrossRef] [PubMed]
25. Crabbe, E.; Verheyen, G.; Silber, S.; Tournaye, H.; Van de Velde, H.; Goossens, A.; Van Steirteghem, A. Enzymatic digestion of testicular tissue may rescue the intracytoplasmic sperm injection cycle in some patients with non-obstructive azoospermia. *Hum. Reprod.* **1998**, *13*, 2791–2796. [CrossRef] [PubMed]
26. Baukloh, V.; German Society for Human Reproductive, B. Retrospective multicentre study on mechanical and enzymatic preparation of fresh and cryopreserved testicular biopsies. *Hum. Reprod.* **2002**, *17*, 1788–1794. [CrossRef]
27. Ramasamy, R.; Reifsnyder, J.E.; Bryson, C.; Zaninovic, N.; Liotta, D.; Cook, C.A.; Hariprashad, J.; Weiss, D.; Neri, Q.; Palermo, G.D.; et al. Role of tissue digestion and extensive sperm search after microdissection testicular sperm extraction. *Fertil. Steril.* **2011**, *96*, 299–302. [CrossRef]
28. Taghizadeh, R.R.; Cetrulo, K.J.; Cetrulo, C.L. Collagenase Impacts the Quantity and Quality of Native Mesenchymal Stem/Stromal Cells Derived during Processing of Umbilical Cord Tissue. *Cell Transplant.* **2018**, *27*, 181–193. [CrossRef]
29. Smith, G.D.; Takayama, S. Application of microfluidic technologies to human assisted reproduction. *Mol. Hum. Reprod.* **2017**, *23*, 257–268. [CrossRef]
30. Cho, B.S.; Schuster, T.G.; Zhu, X.; Chang, D.; Smith, G.D.; Takayama, S. Passively driven integrated microfluidic system for separation of motile sperm. *Anal. Chem.* **2003**, *75*, 1671–1675. [CrossRef] [PubMed]
31. Schuster, T.G.; Cho, B.; Keller, L.M.; Takayama, S.; Smith, G.D. Isolation of motile spermatozoa from semen samples using microfluidics. *Reprod. Biomed. Online* **2003**, *7*, 75–81. [CrossRef]
32. Matas, C.; Decuadro, G.; Martinez-Miro, S.; Gadea, J. Evaluation of a cushioned method for centrifugation and processing for freezing boar semen. *Theriogenology* **2007**, *67*, 1087–1091. [CrossRef]
33. Raad, G.; Bakos, H.W.; Bazzi, M.; Mourad, Y.; Fakih, F.; Shayya, S.; McHantaf, L.; Fakih, C. Differential impact of four sperm preparation techniques on sperm motility, morphology, DNA fragmentation, acrosome status, oxidative stress, and mitochondrial activity: A prospective study. *Andrology* **2021**. [CrossRef]
34. Zini, A.; Finelli, A.; Phang, D.; Jarvi, K. Influence of semen processing technique on human sperm DNA integrity. *Urology* **2000**, *56*, 1081–1084. [CrossRef]
35. Schulte, R.T.; Chung, Y.K.; Ohl, D.A.; Takayama, S.; Smith, G.D. Microfluidic sperm sorting device provides a novel method for selecting motile sperm with higher DNA integrity. *Fertil. Steril.* **2007**, *88*, S76. [CrossRef]
36. Shirota, K.; Yotsumoto, F.; Itoh, H.; Obama, H.; Hidaka, N.; Nakajima, K.; Miyamoto, S. Separation efficiency of a microfluidic sperm sorter to minimize sperm DNA damage. *Fertil. Steril.* **2016**, *105*, 315–321.e1. [CrossRef]
37. Nagata, M.P.B.; Endo, K.; Ogata, K.; Yamanaka, K.; Egashira, J.; Katafuchi, N.; Yamanouchi, T.; Matsuda, H.; Goto, Y.; Sakatani, M.; et al. Live births from artificial insemination of microfluidic-sorted bovine spermatozoa characterized by trajectories correlated with fertility. *Proc. Natl. Acad. Sci. USA* **2018**, *115*, E3087–E3096. [CrossRef]
38. Quinn, M.M.; Jalalian, L.; Ribeiro, S.; Ona, K.; Demirci, U.; Cedars, M.I.; Rosen, M.P. Microfluidic sorting selects sperm for clinical use with reduced DNA damage compared to density gradient centrifugation with swim-up in split semen samples. *Hum. Reprod.* **2018**, *33*, 1388–1393. [CrossRef] [PubMed]
39. Nosrati, R.; Vollmer, M.; Eamer, L.; San Gabriel, M.C.; Zeidan, K.; Zini, A.; Sinton, D. Rapid selection of sperm with high DNA integrity. *Lab Chip* **2014**, *14*, 1142–1150. [CrossRef] [PubMed]
40. Xiao, S.; Riordon, J.; Simchi, M.; Lagunov, A.; Hannam, T.; Jarvi, K.; Nosrati, R.; Sinton, D. FertDish: Microfluidic sperm selection-in-a-dish for intracytoplasmic sperm injection. *Lab Chip* **2021**, *21*, 775–783. [CrossRef] [PubMed]
41. Wu, J.K.; Chen, P.C.; Lin, Y.N.; Wang, C.W.; Pan, L.C.; Tseng, F.G. High-throughput flowing upstream sperm sorting in a retarding flow field for human semen analysis. *Analyst* **2017**, *142*, 938–944. [CrossRef]
42. Mangum, C.L.; Patel, D.P.; Jafek, A.R.; Samuel, R.; Jenkins, T.G.; Aston, K.I.; Gale, B.K.; Hotaling, J.M. Towards a better testicular sperm extraction: Novel sperm sorting technologies for non-motile sperm extracted by microdissection TESE. *Transl. Androl. Urol.* **2020**, *9*, S206–S214. [CrossRef]
43. Gossett, D.R.; Weaver, W.M.; Mach, A.J.; Hur, S.C.; Tse, H.T.; Lee, W.; Amini, H.; Di Carlo, D. Label-free cell separation and sorting in microfluidic systems. *Anal. Bioanal. Chem.* **2010**, *397*, 3249–3267. [CrossRef]
44. Said, T.M.; Land, J.A. Effects of advanced selection methods on sperm quality and ART outcome: A systematic review. *Hum. Reprod. Update* **2011**, *17*, 719–733. [CrossRef]
45. de Wagenaar, B.; Dekker, S.; de Boer, H.L.; Bomer, J.G.; Olthuis, W.; van den Berg, A.; Segerink, L.I. Towards microfluidic sperm refinement: Impedance-based analysis and sorting of sperm cells. *Lab Chip* **2016**, *16*, 1514–1522. [CrossRef] [PubMed]
46. Horsman, K.M.; Barker, S.L.; Ferrance, J.P.; Forrest, K.A.; Koen, K.A.; Landers, J.P. Separation of sperm and epithelial cells in a microfabricated device: Potential application to forensic analysis of sexual assault evidence. *Anal. Chem.* **2005**, *77*, 742–749. [CrossRef] [PubMed]

47. Liu, W.; Chen, W.; Liu, R.; Ou, Y.; Liu, H.; Xie, L.; Lu, Y.; Li, C.; Li, B.; Cheng, J. Separation of sperm and epithelial cells based on the hydrodynamic effect for forensic analysis. *Biomicrofluidics* **2015**, *9*, 044127. [CrossRef]
48. Son, J.; Samuel, R.; Gale, B.K.; Carrell, D.T.; Hotaling, J.M. Separation of sperm cells from samples containing high concentrations of white blood cells using a spiral channel. *Biomicrofluidics* **2017**, *11*, 054106. [CrossRef] [PubMed]
49. Vasilescu, S.A.; Khorsandi, S.; Ding, L.; Bazaz, S.R.; Nosrati, R.; Gook, D.; Warkiani, M.E. A microfluidic approach to rapid sperm recovery from heterogeneous cell suspensions. *Sci. Rep.* **2021**, *11*, 7917. [CrossRef] [PubMed]
50. Casper, R.F.; Meriano, J.S.; Jarvi, K.A.; Cowan, L.; Lucato, M.L. The hypo-osmotic swelling test for selection of viable sperm for intracytoplasmic sperm injection in men with complete asthenozoospermia. *Fertil. Steril.* **1996**, *65*, 972–976. [CrossRef]
51. Holland, I.; Davies, J.A. Automation in the Life Science Research Laboratory. *Front. Bioeng. Biotechnol.* **2020**, *8*, 571777. [CrossRef] [PubMed]
52. Mallidis, C.; Wistuba, J.; Bleisteiner, B.; Damm, O.S.; Gross, P.; Wubbeling, F.; Fallnich, C.; Burger, M.; Schlatt, S. In situ visualization of damaged DNA in human sperm by Raman microspectroscopy. *Hum. Reprod.* **2011**, *26*, 1641–1649. [CrossRef] [PubMed]
53. Da Costa, R.; Amaral, S.; Redmann, K.; Kliesch, S.; Schlatt, S. Spectral features of nuclear DNA in human sperm assessed by Raman Microspectroscopy: Effects of UV-irradiation and hydration. *PLoS ONE* **2018**, *13*, e0207786. [CrossRef] [PubMed]

Review

Endocrine Follow-Up of Men with Non-Obstructive Azoospermia Following Testicular Sperm Extraction

Evangelia Billa [1,*,†], George A. Kanakis [2,*,†] and Dimitrios G. Goulis [1]

[1] Unit of Reproductive Endocrinology, 1st Department of Obstetrics and Gynecology, Medical School, Aristotle University of Thessaloniki, 56403 Thessaloniki, Greece; dgg@auth.gr
[2] IVF Unit, Department of Endocrinology, Athens Naval and Veteran Affairs Hospital, 11521 Athens, Greece
* Correspondence: evbilla@gmail.com (E.B.); fyleas52@gmail.com (G.A.K.)
† Equal contribution.

Abstract: Testicular sperm extraction (TESE) is a surgical procedure which, combined with intracytoplasmic sperm injection, constitutes the main treatment for achieving biological parenthood for patients with infertility due to non-obstructive azoospermia (NOA). Although it is effective, TESE procedures might cause structural testicular damage leading to Leydig cell dysfunction and, consequently, temporary or even permanent hypogonadism with long-term health consequences. To a lesser extent, the same complications have been reported for microdissection TESE, which is considered less invasive. The resulting hypogonadism is more profound and of longer duration in patients with Klinefelter syndrome compared with other NOA causes. Most studies on serum follicle-stimulating hormone and luteinizing hormone concentrations negatively correlate with total testosterone concentrations, which depends on the underlying histology. As hypogonadism is usually temporary, and a watchful waiting approach for about 12 months postoperative is suggested. In cases where replacement therapy with testosterone is indicated, temporary discontinuation of treatment may promote the expected recovery of testosterone secretion and revise the decision for long-term treatment.

Keywords: hypogonadism; intracytoplasmic sperm injection; Sertoli cell-only syndrome

1. Introduction

Testicular sperm extraction (TESE) is a surgical procedure which, in combination with intracytoplasmic sperm injection (ICSI), is currently used to enable men with non-obstructive azoospermia (NOA) to produce their biological children. Several TESE techniques have been reported including simple or multi-biopsy conventional TESE (cTESE), microdissection TESE (micro-TESE, mTESE), and testicular sperm aspiration (TESA) [1]. Their development was imposed by the need for focused, less invasive, and more effective techniques for sperm retrieval, as spermatogenesis is focal in many patients with NOA [2].

The cTESE procedure involves random single or multiple testicular incisions in different testicular regions with a resection of a variable volume of tissue until sperm are identified and extracted [3]. In mTESE, a larger longitudinal or equatorial incision is made through the tunica albuginea under the observation of an operating microscope. The exposed seminiferous tubules are then studied. The larger, more opaque, whitish ones are selectively removed since they are more likely to contain sperm [4]. There is a lack of strong evidence concerning the superiority of one technique over the other in terms of sperm retrieval, pregnancy rates, and live birth rates. The results depend on NOA causes and testicular histology, the latter being a heterogeneous entity with distinct pathological patterns, ranging from hypospermatogenesis to Sertoli cell-only syndrome (SCOS) [5–8]. However, a recent meta-analysis indicates that mTESE has a 1.5 times higher sperm retrieval rate (SRR) compared with cTESE and 2 times higher rate compared with TESA. Therefore, mTESE should be preferred in men with NOA according to AUA/ASRM guidelines [9,10].

Concerning the postoperative complications, TESE procedures might cause structural testicular damage leading to Leydig cell dysfunction and, consequently, hypogonadism with long-term health consequences [7,11–13]. This review aims to discuss the hormonal disturbances after TESE procedures and to suggest an appropriate endocrine follow-up for men with NOA. It will be restricted mainly to hypogonadism due to the lack of evidence for other endocrinological complications.

2. Methods

The relevant literature was reviewed through the PubMed, Scopus, and CENTRAL electronic databases to identify the best available evidence concerning endocrine consequences after TESE procedures. All studies and review articles reporting hormonal evaluations and symptoms compatible with hypogonadism before and after TESE were reviewed.

3. Complications

Structural and hormonal postoperative complications have been described following TESE procedures [12–14]. These complications could be explained by the peculiarities of testicular vascularization and the detrimental effects that the TESE techniques may impose. Testicular blood supply is provided by the testicular artery (a branch of the internal spermatic artery) which enters the testis posteriorly at the level of the mid-pole beneath the epididymis, continues inferiorly to the lower pole, and then ascends along the anterior surface. By this point, it forms sub-capsular arteries, which give rise to centripetal branches that supply the adjacent testicular lobules [15]. Multiple incisions of the tunica albuginea, performed during conventional TESE, may injure sub-capsular vessels and their branches, compromising the blood supply to the corresponding parenchyma or resulting in sub-capsular hematomas. The latter may disrupt testicular function by increasing intratesticular pressure. Impaired blood flow, devascularization, hematomas, and inflammation have been reported one to three months after TESE, leading to testicular scars and calcifications [12,14]. An increase in peritubular scar tissue has also been suggested to affect Leydig cells and germ cells number [16].

mTESE, on the other hand, was initially considered less invasive compared with conventional TESE since the magnified vision minimizes the amount of tissue excised and the risk of inadvertent intra-operative vascular injury [17]. Nevertheless, the same complications have been reported, although to a lesser extent [12,18,19].

These structural disturbances have raised safety issues regarding testicular function. Several men with infertility already have impaired Leydig cell function and, therefore, lower serum testosterone (T), higher luteinizing hormone (LH) and estradiol concentrations compared with fertile men. In addition, many of them have small testicular volumes, which may get further compromised after the extraction of a considerable amount of testicular tissue for sperm retrieval during the TESE procedure [20]. Therefore, they are at high risk of developing androgen deficiency and further disturbance of spermatogenesis and Sertoli cells' function after TESE [16,21,22].

Despite the limited evidence in this field, there has been a consistent finding of a decline in total testosterone (TT) secretion of variable severity and duration after TESE procedures [8,12]. This decrease of TT concentrations is typically temporary, although two cases of testicular atrophy have been documented [14,23]. The risk of permanent hypogonadism is lesser when smaller testicular samples are taken, as serum TT concentrations return to baseline in 50–90% of patients one year after mTESE [8,11,12,17,24]. The recovery period of hypogonadism that may develop after mTESE is 12–18 months [23,25]. The range in the recovery rates is mostly due to the heterogeneous populations of men with NOA in the various studies. Factors such as the size of the removed testicular tissue, the extension of the tunic incisions, or the experience of the surgeon may also contribute to the recovery rates [8,26].

In a cohort study of highly selected eugonadal men, presenting a low risk of hypogonadism before undergoing bilateral mTESE, the mean postoperative serum TT was

88 ng/dL lower compared with the corresponding preoperative concentrations 19 months after the procedure. Of these men, 30% became biochemically hypogonadal [TT < 300 ng/dL (10.4 nmol/L)] after mTESE [8]. In another study of 435 men with non-obstructive azoospermia who underwent cTESE or mTESE, TT concentrations showed a 20% decline from baseline within three to six months following TESE. In the cTESE group, serum TT concentrations declined from 316 ng/dL to 251 ng/dL while in mTESE group they declined from 303 ng/dL to 248 ng/dL. This decline was more evident in men who underwent more than two attempts of sperm retrieval, while it was not related to the patients' age, initial TT concentrations, serum FSH concentrations, or the outcome of sperm retrieval (success vs. non-success) [17]. In addition, a study assessing the long-term effects of mTESE in 45 men with NOA (average follow-up: 2.4 years) demonstrated that postoperative T concentrations declined by 10% and that 16% of patients developed a de novo androgen deficiency during follow-up, independently of their age or testicular volume [11]. Furthermore, another study evaluating endocrinological data before and 3, 6, and 12 months after surgery in 69 NOA patients with or without Klinefelter syndrome (KS) showed a significant decrease in TT concentrations to 1.3 ± 0.2 ng/mL (46.4% of the preoperative concentrations) at 6 months after mTESE procedure in men with NOA and 46, XY karyotype. This decline was followed a different pattern according to testicular histology and was greater in patients with 47, XXY karyotype. In patients with hypospermatogenesis, preoperative serum TT concentrations were relatively high (5.2 ± 0.7 ng/mL) and decreased slightly without reaching hypogonadal concentrations. In patients with maturation arrest and SCOS preoperative serum TT concentrations were 2.9 ± 0.2 mg/mL and 3.1 ± 0.3 ng/mL, respectively, and reduced slightly at six months postoperatively to hypogonadal levels (<3.0 ng/mL) [27].

In line with the above data, a recent meta-analysis of 12 non-randomized, retrospective, uncontrolled studies showed a decrease in TT concentrations at 3, 6, 9 and 12 months following TESE procedures compared with baseline results, even reaching hypogonadal levels in some cases [7]. This decrease was more profound in men with KS [7]. In both men with NOA and a 46, XY karyotype and men with KS, the highest decrease in TT concentrations were observed six months after TESE, with a mean decrease of 78 and 118 ng/dL (2.7 and 4.1 nmol/L), respectively, which recovered to baseline at 18 and 26 months, respectively [7]. Limitations of this study include the heterogeneity of the procedures performed, including both obstructive azoospermia (OA) and NOA patients who carry a different risk for hypogonadism and flaws in patient follow-up.

Concerning hormonal disturbances in patients with KS undergoing TESE, the evidence is scarce. According to the above study, preoperative TT concentrations were relatively low (2.8 ± 1.6 ng/mL) and decreased by 30% to 35% at 1 to 12 months postoperatively [24]. In another study, preoperative TT concentrations were 2.8 ± 0.4 ng/mL and decreased significantly after mTESE [27]. A recent meta-analysis also showed decreased TT, with the strongest one being at 6 months after TESE with a mean decrease of 4.13 nmol/L [7].

The severity and duration of the decrease in the serum TT concentrations have been associated with the underlying histology of the seminiferous epithelium. Accordingly, the recovery rates 12 months after the mTESE procedure were complete in patients with hypospermatogenesis (surpassing 100% of the preoperative concentrations) and almost complete in patients with maturation arrest or SCOS (93.1% and 80.6% of the preoperative concentrations, respectively) [27]. This is not the case concerning patients with KS, in whom T concentrations were recovered in only 50% of subjects, 12 months postoperatively. This difference may be attributed to the low testicular volume of patients with KS and the severe histological disorder, which, apart from the seminiferous tubules, affects Leydig cells [24].

Evidence indicates that the prevalence of hypogonadism in men with NOA is up to 45–47% [7,14,22,28]. Men with hypospermatogenesis have normal TT concentrations, while men with maturation arrest and SCOS have lower and sometimes borderline or even low TT concentrations. The latter subgroups are presented with a greater risk of hypogonadism due to further reduction of T after TESE procedures. The reduction of

Leydig cells' number due to tissue removal has been proposed as a possible mechanism of T decrease [7]. The greater the removed tissue and the smaller the preoperative testicle volume, the larger the decline of TT concentrations is expected to reach hypogonadal levels in the subgroup with the lower preoperative levels. The reduction of T concentrations induces LH secretion through the negative feedback mechanism on the hypothalamic-pituitary-testicular axis to stimulate the remaining Leydig cells. The patients that develop post-TESE hypogonadism may have an intrinsic resistance of the cells to the stimulatory effect of LH, since some patients with NOA show an impaired response of Leydig cells in the stimulatory effect of human chorionic gonadotropin (hCG) [7,11,22]. Moreover, a decreased responsiveness of the hypothalamus and pituitary to low T may be another reason for postsurgical hypogonadism [11,27]. Additionally, the recovery of hypogonadism may be related to the Leydig cells' renewal coming from stem Leydig cells. The time and the degree of renewal may differ in NOA patients due to an underlying pathology of stem cells. Finally, as mentioned above, the inflammation and vascular damage of the testicular parenchyma may lead to Leydig cells dysfunction and/or impair the release of intratesticular T to the circulation. Especially, patients with KS have small testis with solid brown Leydig cell nodules, which may already have a degree of dysfunction responsible for their low T concentrations [29]. These abnormal Leydig cells are more vulnerable to further disruption after a TESE procedure, leading to more profound, prolonged, and even permanent hypogonadism in some cases. Furthermore, it has been implied that it may have a less responsive hypothalamic-pituitary-testicular axis [7,27,30].

Current evidence is inconsistent concerning the TESE consequences on serum follicle-stimulating hormone (FSH) and LH concentrations. Some investigators have reported an increase in the mean serum FSH and LH concentrations in patients with maturation arrest and SCOS after mTESE, while no change was found in patients with hypospermatogenesis [27]. Other studies have documented an increase in serum LH and FSH concentrations in patients with NOA and 46, XY karyotype but not in those with KS [24]. They also suggested that the change in FSH concentrations has resulted from the scar tissue with germ cell loss near the scar after the procedure [24]. In the study mentioned above, the pre-and postoperative FSH and LH concentrations remained low in patients with hypospermatogenesis and high in patients with KS. In patients with maturation arrest, both gonadotropins increased continuously after mTESE, while in patients with SCOS, they increased up to six months after surgery and decreased after that [27].

In a meta-analysis mentioned above, LH concentrations were negatively associated with TT in most studies. A role of LH in the recovery rate has also been implied since men with low TT concentrations had an adequate response, with increased TT concentrations three and four days after hCG injection. In line with this observation, in cases where LH was upregulated immediately following TESE, a faster recovery (18 months) was expected. In one study with KS patients, there was no increase in LH concentrations [24].

Symptoms associated with hypogonadism due to TESE procedures have been described, especially when T concentrations are <12 nmol/L, mainly erectile dysfunction (ED) and decrease of testicular volume [7]. In one study including 66 patients, 13 new-onset erectile dysfunction (ED) cases have been described after mTESE, which significant decreased TT concentrations from 27.1 to 9.7 nmol/L [31]. Some researchers have been reported a reduction of testicular volume of at least 2 mL in 25% of men undergoing cTESE and 2.5% of men undergoing mTESE at six months after the procedure [19]. In addition, another study reported a 0.3 and 0.6 mL decrease in mean testicular volume 3 and 12 months after mTESE [32].

4. Endocrine Follow-Up and Treatment

As there is convincing evidence for an increased risk for low TT concentrations following TESE, long-term endocrinological follow-up should be advised in these patients [7,11]. It is important to emphasize that the applied techniques should prevent testicular damage by balancing between tissue sparing and maximization of sperm retrieval rates to avoid repeated procedures [8]. In line with this approach, some researchers suggest a stepwise strategy. A single TESE sample is initially extracted, followed by an mTESE using the same testicular incision, followed by a multi-biopsy cTESE approach on the opposite testis if needed [33]. Others advocate performing a Fine Needle Aspiration (FNA) mapping before TESE. This technique relies on obtaining 18 testicular aspiration samples to represent the entire testicular surface and depth. According to its supporters, it allows the ensuing TESE to be more focused and less traumatic by avoiding areas with unfavorable cytology [8].

According to the available data, serum TT levels decline in hypogonadal levels (<300 ng/mL) in men with KS and in a proportion of NOA men without KS with the major reduction seeing at six months postoperatively. This reduction is accompanied by a corresponding increase in LH concentrations, implying the possibility and time of recovery. On this ground, evaluation of serum TT and LH concentrations at 3, 6, 12, 18 and, in some cases, 24 months is advisable. As NOA patients are at increased risk of developing hypogonadism, in general, annual estimation of TT concentrations could be, also, considered.

Since T deficiency following TESE is usually temporary, it seems prudent to wait for about 12 months postoperatively until some degree of spontaneous recovery is observed [23]. Nevertheless, some patients with T deficiency may experience symptoms such as erectile dysfunction [7]. In such a case, T replacement therapy (TRT) should be initiated based on a combination of biochemical diagnosis with symptoms of hypogonadism by the current guidelines. Temporary discontinuation of treatment may reveal the expected recovery of T secretion and revise the decision for TRT [26,34]. hCG or selective estrogen receptors modulators (SERMs) administration could be considered in highly selected, hypogonadal patients who have not completed their fertility attempts to increase intratesticular T concentration and manage the hypogonadal symptoms.

5. Conclusions

In conclusion, the current evidence suggests a considerable risk of temporary and even permanent hypogonadism following TESE procedures. It is yet unclear whether the increased hypogonadism risk is related to the number or size of testicular tissue samples excised, the number and size of the testicular tunica albuginea incisions, or the surgical experience [8]. Most probably, it is related to the NOA etiology and testicular volume as it is more profound and of longer duration in patients with KS compared with other NOA causes.

Author Contributions: E.B. and G.A.K. authors had equal contribution in conceptualization and writing of the review. D.G.G. contributed in the conceptualization, supervision, and editing. All authors have read and agreed to the published version of the manuscript.

Funding: Next Fertility Procrea Lugano, Switzerland, funded the Article Processing Charges.

Data Availability Statement: No new data were created or analyzed in this study.

Acknowledgments: The authors would like to thank the Procrea–NextClinics Institution, Milan, Italy, for the full cover of the Article Processing Charges.

Conflicts of Interest: The authors declare no conflict of interest.

References

1. Devroey, P.; Liu, J.; Nagy, Z.; Goossens, A.; Tournaye, H.; Camus, M.; Van Steirteghem, A.; Silber, S. Pregnancies after testicular sperm extraction and intracytoplasmic sperm injectioninnon-obstructiveazoospermia. *Hum. Reprod.* **1995**, *10*, 1457–1460. [CrossRef]
2. Turek, P.J.; Ljung, B.M.; Cha, I.; Conaghan, J. Diagnostic findings from testis fine needle aspiration mapping in obstructed and nonobstructed azoospermic men. *J. Urol.* **2000**, *163*, 1709–1716. [CrossRef]
3. Tournaye, H.; Verheyen, G.; Nagy, P.; Ubaldi, F.; Goossens, A.; Silber, S.; Van Steirteghem, A.C.; Devroey, P. Are there any predictive factors for successful testicular sperm recovery in azoospermic patients? *Hum. Reprod.* **1997**, *12*, 80–86. [CrossRef]
4. Schlegel, P.N. Testicular sperm extraction: Microdissection improves sperm yield with minimal tissue excision. *Hum. Reprod.* **1999**, *14*, 131–135. [CrossRef] [PubMed]

5. Caroppo, E.; Colpi, G.M. Hormonal Treatment of Men with Nonobstructive Azoospermia: What Does the Evidence Suggest? *J. Clin. Med.* **2021**, *10*, 387. [CrossRef] [PubMed]
6. Deruyver, Y.; Vanderschueren, D.; Vander Aa, F. Outcome of microdissection TESE compared with conventional TESE in non-obstructive azoospermia: A systematic review. *Andrology* **2014**, *2*, 20–24. [CrossRef]
7. Eliveld, J.; van Wely, M.; Meißner, A.; Repping, S.; van der Veen, F.; van Pelt, A.M.M. The risk of TESE-induced hypogonadism: A systematic review and meta-analysis. *Hum. Reprod. Update* **2018**, *24*, 442–454. [CrossRef] [PubMed]
8. Godart, E.S.; Turek, P.J. The evolution of testicular sperm extraction and preservation techniques. *Fac. Rev.* **2020**, *9*, 2. [CrossRef] [PubMed]
9. Bernie, A.M.; Mata, D.A.; Ramasamy, R.; Schlegel, P.N. Comparison of microdissection testicular sperm extraction, conventional testicular sperm extraction, and testicular sperm aspiration for nonobstructive azoospermia: A systematic review and meta-analysis. *Fertil. Steril.* **2015**, *104*, 1099–1103. [CrossRef] [PubMed]
10. Schlegel, P.N.; Sigman, M.; Collura, B.; De Jonge, C.J.; Eisenberg, M.L.; Lamb, D.J.; Mulhall, J.P.; Niederberger, C.; Sandlow, J.I.; Sokol, R.Z.; et al. Diagnosis and Treatment of Infertility in Men: AUA/ASRM Guideline Part I. *J. Urol.* **2021**, *205*, 36–43. [CrossRef] [PubMed]
11. Everaert, K.; DeCroo, I.; Kerckhaert, W.; Dekuyper, P.; Dhont, M.; Van der Elst, J.; De Sutter, P.; Comhaire, F.; Mahmoud, A.; Lumen, N. Long term effects of micro-surgical testicular sperm extraction on androgen status in patients with nonobstructive azoospermia. *BMC Urol.* **2006**, *6*, 9. [CrossRef] [PubMed]
12. Donoso, P.; Tournaye, H.; Devroey, P. Which is the best sperm retrieval technique for non-obstructive azoospermia? A systematic review. *Hum. Reprod. Update* **2007**, *13*, 539–549. [CrossRef] [PubMed]
13. Shin, D.H.; Turek, P.J. Sperm retrieval techniques. *Nat. Rev. Urol.* **2013**, *10*, 723–730. [CrossRef]
14. Schlegel, P.N.; Su, L.M. Physiological consequences of testicular sperm extraction. *Hum. Reprod.* **1997**, *12*, 1688–1692. [CrossRef]
15. Jarow, J.P. Clinical Significance of Intratesticular Arterial Anatomy. *J. Urol.* **1991**, *145*, 777–779. [CrossRef]
16. Tash, J.; Schlegel, P.N. The histologic effects of TESE on the testicle in men with non-obstructive azoospermia. *Urology* **2001**, *57*, 334–337. [CrossRef]
17. Ramasamy, R.; Yagan, N.; Schlegel, P.N. Structural and functional changes to the testis after conventional versus microdissection testicular sperm extraction. *Urology* **2005**, *65*, 1190–1194. [CrossRef] [PubMed]
18. Amer, M.; Atiyah, A.; Hany, R.; Zohdy, W. Prospective comparative study between microsurgical and conventional testicular sperm extraction in non-obstructive azoospermia: Follow-up by serial ultrasound examinations. *Hum. Reprod.* **2000**, *15*, 653–656. [CrossRef] [PubMed]
19. Okada, H.; Dobashi, M.; Yamazaki, T.; Hara, I.; Fujisawa, M.; Arakawa, S.; Kamino, S. Conventional versus microdissection testicular sperm extraction for non-obstructive azoospermia. *J. Urol.* **2002**, *168*, 1063–1067. [CrossRef]
20. Andersson, A.M.; Jorgensen, N.; Frydelund Larsen, L.; Rajpert-DeMeyts, E.; Skakkebaek, N.E. Impaired Leydig cell function in infertile men: A study of 357 idiopathic infertile men and 318 proven fertile controls. *J. Clin. Endocrinol. Metab.* **2004**, *89*, 3161–3167. [CrossRef] [PubMed]
21. Bouloux, P.; Warne, D.W.; Lourmaye, E.; FSH Study Group in Men's Infertility. Efficacy and safety of recombinant human follicle-stimulating hormone in men with isolated hypogonadotropic hypogonadism. *Fertil. Steril.* **2002**, *77*, 270–273. [CrossRef]
22. Schill, T.; Bals-Pratsch, M.; Kuoker, W.; Sandmann, J.; Johannisson, R.; Diedrich, K. Clinical and endocrine follow-up of patients after testicular sperm extraction. *Fertil. Steril.* **2003**, *79*, 281–286. [CrossRef]
23. Manning, M.; Junemann, K.P.; Alken, P. Decrease in testosterone blood concentrations after testicular sperm extraction for intracytoplasmic sperm injection azoospermic men. *Lancet* **1998**, *352*, 37. [CrossRef]
24. Ishikawa, T.; Yamaguchi, K.; Chiba, K.; Takenaka, A.; Fujisawa, M. Serum Hormones in patients with non-obstructive azoospermia after microdissection testicular sperm extraction. *J. Urol.* **2009**, *182*, 1495–1499. [CrossRef] [PubMed]
25. Bensalem, S.; Alhajeri, D.; Madbouly, K. Microdissection testicular sperm extraction in men with non-obstructive azoospermia: Experience of King Saud University Medical City, Riyadh, Saudi Arabia. *Urol. Ann.* **2017**, *9*, 136–140.
26. Bhasin, S.; Cunningham, G.R.; Hayes, F.J.; Matsumoto, A.M.; Snyder, P.J.; Swerdloff, R.S.; Montori, V.M.; Task Force, E.S. Testosterone therapy in men with androgen deficiency syndromes: An Endocrine Society clinical practice guideline. *J. Clin. Endocrinol. Metab.* **2010**, *95*, 2536–2559. [CrossRef]
27. Takada, S.; Tsujimura, A.; Ueda, T.; Matsuoka, Y.; Takao, T.; Miyagawa, Y.; Koga, M.; Takeyama, M.; Okamoto, Y.; Matsumiya, K.; et al. Androgen decline in patients with non-obstructive azoospermia after microdissection testicular sperm extraction. *Urology* **2008**, *72*, 114–118. [CrossRef]
28. Sussman, E.M.; Chudnovsky, A.; Niederberger, C.S. Hormonal evaluation of the infertile male: Has it evolved? *Urol. Clin. N. Am.* **2008**, *35*, 147–155. [CrossRef]
29. Koga, M.; Tsujimura, A.; Takeyama, M.; Kiuchi, H.; Takao, T.; Miyagawa, Y.; Takada, S.; Matsumiya, K.; Fujioka, H.; Okamoto, Y.; et al. Clinical comparison of successful and failed microdissection testicular sperm extraction in patients with nonmosaic Klinefelter syndrome. *Urology* **2007**, *70*, 341–345. [CrossRef]
30. Sertkaya, Z.; Tokuç, E.; Özkaya, F.; Ertaş, K.; Kutluhan, M.A.; Çulha, M.G. Acute effect of microdissection testicular sperm extraction on blood total testosterone and luteinizing hormone levels. *Andrologia* **2020**, *52*, e13655. [CrossRef]
31. Akbal, C.; Mangir, N.; Tavukçu, H.H.; Özgür, Ö.; Şimşek, F. Effect of testicular sperm extraction outcome on sexual function in patients with male factor infertility. *Urology* **2010**, *75*, 598–601. [CrossRef] [PubMed]

32. Ozturk, U.; Ozdemir, E.; Dede, O.; Sagnak, L.; Goktug, H.N.G.; Gurbuz, O.A.; Cagatay, M.; Imamoglu, M.A. Assessment of anti-sperm antibodies in couples after testicular sperm extraction. *Clin. Investig. Med.* **2011**, *34*, 179–184. [CrossRef] [PubMed]
33. Franco, G.; Scarselli, F.; Casciani, V.; DeNunzio, C.; Dente, D.; Leonardo, C.; Greco, P.F.; Greco, A.; Minasi, M.G.; Greco, E. A novel stepwise micro-TESE approach in nonobstructive azoospermia. *BMC Urol.* **2016**, *16*, 20. [CrossRef] [PubMed]
34. Corona, G.; Goulis, D.G.; Huhtaniemi, I.; Zitzmann, M.; Toppari, J.; Forti, G.; Vanderschueren, D.; Wu, F.C. European Academy of Andrology (EAA) guidelines on investigation, treatment and monitoring of functional hypogonadism in males: Endorsing organization: European Society of Endocrinology. *Andrology* **2020**, *8*, 970–987. [CrossRef] [PubMed]

MDPI
St. Alban-Anlage 66
4052 Basel
Switzerland
Tel. +41 61 683 77 34
Fax +41 61 302 89 18
www.mdpi.com

Journal of Clinical Medicine Editorial Office
E-mail: jcm@mdpi.com
www.mdpi.com/journal/jcm

www.ingramcontent.com/pod-product-compliance
Lightning Source LLC
LaVergne TN
LVHW070634100526
838202LV00012B/799